Michael St.Pierre

Gesine Hofinger

Cornelius Buerschaper

Crisis Management in Acute Care Settings

Michael St.Pierre

Gesine Hofinger

Cornelius Buerschaper

Crisis Management in Acute Care Settings

Human Factors and Team Psychology in a High Stakes Environment

With 47 Figures and 12 Tables

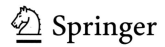

C. Buerschaper
Woehlerstrasse 12
10115 Berlin
Germany
E-mail: cornelius.buerschaper@t-online.de

G. Hofinger
Hohenheimerstrasse 104
71686 Remseck
Germany
E-mail: gesine.hofinger@t-online.de

M. St.Pierre
Department of Anesthesiology
University of Erlangen
Krankenhausstrasse 12
91054 Erlangen
Germany
E-mail: michael.st.pierre@kfa.imed.uni-erlangen.de

Library of Congress Control Number: 2007931732

ISBN 978-3-540-71061-5 Springer Berlin Heidelberg New York

Springer is a part of Springer Science+Business Media
springer.com

Editor: Dr. Ute Heilmann, Heidelberg, Germany
Desk Editor: Meike Stoeck, Heidelberg, Germany
Reproduction, typesetting and production: LE-TEX Jelonek, Schmidt & Vöckler GbR, Leipzig, Germany
Cover design: Frido Steinen-Broo, EStudio, Calamar, Spain
SPIN 11957423

Printed on acid-free paper 21/3180/YL 5 4 3 2 1 0

Preface

All of life is problem-solving
(Sir K.R. Popper)

Providing safe patient care in an acute care setting has always been, and still is, one of the greatest challenges of healthcare. On a regular basis healthcare professionals are faced with problems that are sudden, unexpected, and pose a threat to a patient's life. Worse still, these problems do not leave much time for in-depth reflection but instead demand thoughtful action despite the need for swift decisions. This, as most of us know only too well, is far easier said than done: Time pressure, uncertainty, stress, high stakes, erratic team processes, and organizational shortcomings all intermingle in a task environment which makes good decisions and successful management a critical endeavor.

The capability to master these challenges, however, requires more than profound medical knowledge and clinical expertise: A set of skills are needed that will enable healthcare professionals to reliably translate knowledge into safe patient care despite varying and often hindering circumstances. These skills are the subject of this book. Thus, you will not encounter any information concerning the clinical management of critical situations throughout the entire book: no guidelines; no algorithms; and no recommendations. Many excellent textbooks have been written on the medical aspect of crisis management in acute medical care settings; therefore, another book of that kind is not yet warranted. Instead, the present book focuses on people, on the healthcare providers from a vast array of specialties and professions who are expected to manage the unexpected: nurses; physicians; paramedics; and technicians. All of them have their defined set of technical and nontechnical skills which enables them to manage critical situations. All of them can also improve their performance by thoughtful application of basic theories on human decision-making and action.

At the same time, though, all healthcare providers suffer from inescapable cognitive limitations that contribute to errors and hinder successful crisis management. In order to help healthcare providers to better understand their strengths and weaknesses as human decision makers, this book attempts to provide an outline of the way the human mind operates. Humans think and act the way they do because the underlying psychological mechanisms provide an efficient approach to cope with environmental demands. In contrast to widespread belief, errors are not the product of an irrational or deficient psychological mechanism but instead originate from useful processes as well. Some of them, such as communication patterns, can be changed, whereas others cannot: Our perception, attention, motivations, feelings, and thoughts are not entirely subject to our will.

But not only individual performance obeys certain rules; the same is true for teamwork. As acute medical care is never a one-man show, but rather the result of many professionals on different levels of a healthcare organization cooperating for a patient's well-being, the knowledge of successful strategies to improve team performance can create an ever safer clinical environment.

Finally, errors in healthcare are not random events. They are rooted in systemic causes which are deeply embedded in the architecture of healthcare organizations and are amenable to change. The totality of these individual, team-related, and organizational factors that influence our decisions and actions are called "the human factors." The human factors are decisive for the outcome of complex socio-technical systems, such as healthcare.

There are basically two approaches you can take to this book: You can follow the text according to its inner logic, or you may prefer to read selected chapters. Both approaches are valid. The book has a modular character in which every chapter stands alone and can be read without knowledge of previous chapters. In order to avoid excessive redundancy, basic concepts are explained only once and then are cross-referenced.

Every chapter follows the same internal logic: A case study from an acute care specialty illustrates central aspects of the subject matter and is then taken as the reference point for further exposition of the topic. Every chapter provides answers to the same questions: "What is the relevance of the matter? Which problems can be explained by this particular human factor? What can we transfer into our clinical task environment and how can we apply the knowledge to improve patient safety?" To enhance practicability the chapters on individual and team factors (Chaps. 5–13) offer "tips for daily practice" which comprise many helpful clinical suggestions. Every chapter ends with a short paragraph which summarizes the essentials of the chapter.

The first section of the book addresses basic principles of errors, complexity, and human behavior. Chapter 1 sets the stage by providing a survey of published data on the incidence of human error and accidents in acute medical care. A body of research underscores the significance of the human factors in both, the development as well as the prevention and management of errors in a medical high-stakes environment. Chapter 2 describes the characteristics of acute medical care as a complex-task domain where errors are bound to occur. Chapter 3 contrasts two current perspectives on error and provides workable definitions on error. In Chap. 4 we paint a basic picture of the "psychologic" of human behavior, which will enable the reader to understand how humans arrive at decisions.

The structure of the second section follows the structure of human action as a problem-solving process. It focuses on the limitations that the basic cognitive architecture and thinking patterns of the human brain impose on decision-making and action. The individual chapters outline human perception (Chap. 5), information processing (Chap. 6), goals and plans (Chap. 7), attention (Chap. 8), and the impact of stress (Chap. 9). The final chapter of the section, Chap. 10, focuses on how healthcare providers can arrive at good decisions, the ultimate goal of the problem-solving process.

Section III broadens the perspective by shifting the focus from the individual healthcare provider to the team and the relevant human factors involved in the team process. The characteristics and pitfalls of teamwork (Chap. 11) are followed by an outline of communication (Chap. 12) and leadership (Chap. 13), the two main factors of successful teamwork.

Section IV focuses on the influence that healthcare organizations have on the performance of their providers. Basic organizational theories as well as systemic models that enhance patient safety are presented (Chap. 14). The final chapter (Chap. 15) develops an outline for a comprehensive concept of organizational development which could help healthcare institutions to avoid and better manage clinical errors.

The clinical relevance and the practicability of this book has been our major concern; therefore, we tried to formulate the text in an easy-to-read and common language, devoid of psychological jargon. As we tried to build every chapter around a case study from different acute medical care environments, we hope to have brought even more sophisticated psychological theories "down to earth." In writing this book we had in mind physicians, nurses, technicians, and paramedics as target groups. Hopefully, they will all be able to benefit from the book.

For us, creating this book was teamwork experience at its best. The writing process was very challenging yet certainly fruitful. We are grateful to have learned a great deal from the different perspectives clinicians and psychologists have on the same problem, and from the divergent approaches to problem-solving. We hope that the reader will benefit from this process as well.

Finally, because all of us contributed to every chapter, all of us take responsibility for the inevitable errors as well. We are grateful for any remarks concerning the content of this book as well as for clues to misperceptions and/or errors in the text.

Acknowledgements

Our ideas have been shaped by many colleagues, among whom we must single out Dietrich Dörner, head of the Department of Psychology at the University of Bamberg (Germany). He has been a great teacher and we are grateful for the many years of collaboration. His book "Logic of Failure" has been a great inspiration to us, exemplifying how even the most sophisticated matters of psychology can be made accessible and readable. In addition, we thank our colleagues of the Department of Psychology at the University of Bamberg for their friendship, support, and ideas. Prof. Schüttler, chair of the Department of Anesthesiology, University of Erlangen (Germany), has been, and still is, one of Germany's leading proponents of simulation-based training in acute medical care. His personal support has encouraged us to pursue our goal of providing a comprehensive handbook on human factors for healthcare providers. Many healthcare professionals, both physicians and nurses, contributed to the final version of this book. Their critical review of the manuscript and their helpful corrections added much to the clarity and understandability of our thoughts; however, the translated and revised edition of the German original would not have taken its current shape without the encouragement and support of our valued friend Robert Simon, Center for Medical Education, Boston, and the very practical assistance of Alina Lazar and Jonathan Bernardini, both anesthesia residents at Harvard Medical School, who edited all of the case studies.

Last but not least, our families have contributed considerably to the success of our work: thank you to Ulrike St. Pierre and Michael Brenner, and to seven very patient children.

Finally, one of the authors would like to dedicate this book to his father, Roland St. Pierre, for whom a dream has come true.

July 2007
Michael St.Pierre
Erlangen

Gesine Hofinger
Remseck

Cornelius Buerschaper
Berlin

Contents

IV   The Organization

I Basic Principles: Error, Complexity, and Human Behavior

The first section of the book addresses the relevance of human error as a contributory factor to incidents and accidents in acute medical care. Basic principles of human error, complexity, and human action are outlined.

Chapter 1 focuses on "the human factors" which provide both, the potential to trigger critical situations as well as the skills to master them. An overview of published data on the incidence of human error and accidents in acute medical care underscores the fact that human behavior dominates the risk to modern socio-technical systems such as healthcare. Nevertheless, the human factors should never be equated with "risk factors," because they also include "nontechnical skills" which enable healthcare providers to cope with critical situations.

Healthcare in a high-stakes environment has a number of properties that make it considerably more challenging than decision-making in an every day context. Chapter 2 describes these characteristics which psychologists call the "complexity of a working environment." The response of healthcare professionals corresponds with the levels of familiarity with a task or an environment. These varying levels at which behavior is controlled are described.

Chapter 3 provides workable definitions on error and contrasts two current perspectives (consequential and causal classification) which give rise to two different approaches to deal with human fallibility (person-based and system-based approach). Emphasis is placed on the fact that accidents occur as a result of latent conditions which combine with other factors and local triggering events to breach the defensive barriers of the system.

Chapter 4 attempts to provide understanding about how humans arrive at decisions. The "psycho-logic" of human action regulation is presented which conceptualizes that human behavior does not strictly follow the consistency of logical arguments but instead is always influenced by motivation and emotions. The combination of all three factors gives rise to decisions and, hence, action.

1 The Human Factors: Errors and Skills

1.1   Case Study

During an afternoon shift two hemodynamically unstable patients were admitted to the cardiac ICU (CCU), one immediately after the other. The physician's attempt to stabilize both patients at the same time completely overwhelmed him. Because of this, he was unable to give adequate attention to a patient being anticoagulated with warfarin who had several episodes of coffee-ground emesis during the previous 2 h. After finally stabilizing the two new admissions, the resident prepared for an upper endoscopy, but the patient suddenly became hemodynamically unstable. The patient had a recent hemoglobin value of 6.9 g/dl. With the working diagnosis of acute upper gastrointestinal (GI) bleeding, the patient received several peripheral IV lines. Crystalloid infusions were started. Six units of cross-matched packed red blood cells (PRBCs) were ordered from the blood bank, which was short of personnel and unusually burdened by many orders for blood products. The 6 units of PRBCs were sent together with 2 units of PRBCs for another patient in the CCU. The blood products arrived in the CCU while one of the recently admitted patients was being stabilized. After a quick glance at the bag containing the PRBCs, the resident asked the nurse to start the blood transfusion. Within minutes of starting the first infusion of blood, the patient complained of dizziness and shortness of breath and began to deteriorate rapidly. The resident then focused his complete attention on the treatment of this patient. Severe and generalized erythema and edema, together with hemodynamic instability and respiratory distress, indicated a severe anaphylactic reaction. Following a comment by the nurse concerning the transfusion, the physician suspected a transfusion error and stopped the infusion immediately. The patient was then anesthetized and intubated. Controlled ventilation was difficult due to severe bronchospasm. Under high-dose continuous infusion of catecholamines, aggressive volume resuscitation, and administration of corticosteroids and histamine receptor antagonists, the resident managed to stabilize the hemodynamic situation and improve the bronchospasm. In the course of the following hours the patient developed severe disseminated intravascular coagulation (DIC) which led to uncontrollable upper GI bleeding. Despite massive transfusion with coagulation factors and blood products, the patient died several hours later as a result of his uncontrolled bleeding.

An intensive care patient suffers harm from a medical error. Despite maximum therapeutic efforts, the patient died several hours later as a consequence of a massive transfusion reaction. At first sight, the cardiology resident could be readily identified as the responsible agent. He was the person in direct contact with the patient, he gave orders for the transfusion, and he did not adhere to standard treatment protocols, thus displaying negligence in the transfusion process. A closer look, however, reveales additional factors which contributed to the adverse event: a share of workload which overwhelmed the resident; staff shortage in the blood bank; the simultaneous arrival of PRBCs for two different patients; and the acceptance of final responsibility for the transfusion on behalf of the nurse. None of these factors alone would have been able to compromise patient safety. Taken together, however, all these factors combined and managed to breach the defensive barriers of the system. The unlikely combination of several contributing factors on different levels within an organization created a condition where a single moment of inattention on behalf of the resident sufficed to trigger a deadly outcome. "Human error" was one link only in a longer chain of human factors.

Faulty actions, however, represent only one aspect of human factors in a medical high-stakes environment. It is often overlooked that the ability to rapidly detect, diagnose, and treat a medical emergency is rooted in human factors as well. Healthcare providers can only perform successfully in critical situations because the "human factors" enable them to do so. More often than not, healthcare professionals can provide safe and efficient patient care even under the most unfortunate circumstances.

1.2   Human Factors in Healthcare: the Problem

Almost a decade ago the Quality of Healthcare in America Committee of the Institute of Medicine (IOM) issued their report "To Err Is Human: Building a Safer Healthcare System" (Kohn et al. 1999), which examined the quality of the U.S. healthcare delivery system. The numbers presented were alarming and stirred up healthcare systems all around the globe: Year for year a staggering figure of 44,000 people, and perhaps as many as 98,000 people, died in U.S. hospitals as a result of preventable medical error. Even when using the lower estimate, the number of deaths attributable to preventable medical errors exceeded the mortality rate of severe trauma, breast cancer, and HIV.

The IOM report spurred patient safety initiatives all around the globe and triggered an unparalleled endeavor within the healthcare community to identify medical errors and to design interventions to prevent and mitigate their effect. One of the report's main conclusions was in diametrical opposition to hitherto existing assumptions within the healthcare community: that the majority of medical errors did not result from individual recklessness, but instead were caused by faulty systems, processes, and conditions that led people to make mistakes or failed to prevent them. Although new to many within healthcare, the idea of a "systemic approach" to safety was no novelty: A sizable body of knowledge and successful experiences from other high-risk industries had proven all along that mistakes can best be prevented by systematically designing safety into processes thereby breaking down a culture of blame. Healthcare, despite the considerable efforts within the past years, is still in its infancy when compared with efforts of other high-risk industries to ensure basic safety.

For over three decades interdisciplinary research groups from the field of cognitive and social psychology, anthropology, sociology, and reliability engineering have been investigating human and organizational factors that shape the behavior of human beings in high-risk socio-technical systems. The analysis of catastrophic breakdowns of high-hazard enterprises (e.g., Three Mile Island, Bhopal, Cernobyl, Challenger) betrayed a recurrent pattern: Independently from the task environment 70–80% of the accidents were not caused by technological problems but by inadequacies in problem-solving, faulty decision-making, and substandard or non-existent team work: The so-called human error. Despite the results from industrial accident investigations, the medical community was reluctant for a long time to participate in discussions of human error. For the obvious reason of exposure to litigation, the medical community avoided public scrutiny of medical errors. Only in the past two decades has the medical community become open to taking a close look at medical error. As a result of the increasing openness, the 70–80% contribution of human error as trigger for incidents and accidents has been confirmed for the medical high-stakes environment (e.g., Cooper et al. 1978; Hollnagel 1993; Reason 1997; Williamson et al. 1993; Wright et al. 1991).

1.3 Levels of Human Factors

Human behavior clearly dominates the risk to modern socio-technical systems. Figures around 80–90% are not surprising considering that people design, build, operate, maintain, organize, and manage these systems. Human error, however, in contrast to prevailing assumptions, cannot be equated with negligence, sloppiness, incompetence, or lack of motivation on the part of the healthcare provider. On the contrary, serious errors are often committed by highly motivated and experienced people (Amalberti and Mosneron-Dupin 1997). Most of the time human error is the result of an unlikely confluence and interaction of several causal streams originating not in the corruption of human nature but rather in the interaction with normal cognitive processes and "upstream" systemic factors. This assessment is also true for the dynamics of accident causation in the presented case study: A multitude of organizational factors (e.g., human resource allocation, lack of supervision, staff qualification; ▶ Chaps. 14, 15) were hidden as latent failures within the system for considerable time until they combined with other factors and local triggering events (▶ Chap. 3). The unforeseen combination of factors opened a limited window of accident opportunity. All it needed to trigger the accident was a moment of inattention by a healthcare professional.

In order to fully understand human error with all its implications, an understanding of the basic principles of human cognition and action regulation of both, the individual and the team, is indispensable. The same principles apply to management and organizational levels, and on an even larger scale, to the political and legal framework of the healthcare system (▢ Fig. 1.1).

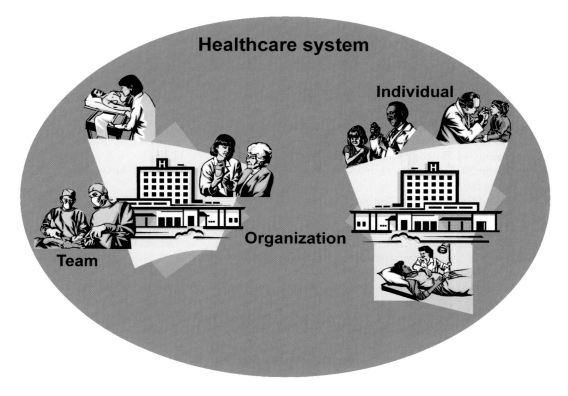

■ **Fig. 1.1** The different levels of patient care which human-factors research addresses

1.3.1 The Individual

Although human error can manifest in various ways, there are nevertheless only a few cognitive principles which contribute to these failures. These principles can be identified on the level of perception, information management, and decision-making. Some examples that are explained in Chaps. 4–10 are as follows:

- Behavior always follows the "psycho-logic" of action regulation (▶ Chap. 4). There is no such thing as a "purely rational" action.
- Humans do not perceive reality but rather "construct" their worldview on a level as early as visual perception.
- Humans tend to "adjust" information to their preferred mental model instead of challenging their current point of view. Data is selected and distorted to fit present assumptions.
- Humans try to defend the feeling of competence at any cost. More important than the solution of

a problem, as vital as it may be, will be the necessity of the feeling that the situation, or at least some relevant aspect of it, is under control.
- Problem-solving and decision-making are impaired by many factors.

In the case study, the physician's perceptual error – he did not notice the wrong name on the blood packs – is obvious. Errors in information processing are not as easily observable; here we rely on theories from cognitive psychology (▶ Chap. 4).

1.3.2 The Team

Compared with an individual, teams represent increased cognitive resources which can contribute a substantial amount of information, situational models, and proposed courses of action. In addition, workload can be shouldered by all team members. The physician in the case study lacked this kind of support. The presence of others, however, can degrade the performance of an individual team member. If basic principles of a successful team process are neglected, or if teams get under stress, internal team dynamics may develop which will lead to a lower performance (▶ Chaps. 11–13). In such a case the following occurs:

— Team members tend to conform their opinion to the majority in the team. Legitimate concerns are not articulated, and criticism is withheld.
— Misunderstanding may result from the use of ambiguous and nontechnical terminology as well as from relational problems.
— Groups tend to centralize information flow and decision-making when external pressure arises.

1.3.3   The Organization

Healthcare delivery has become one of the largest and most complex systems in western culture. This system is composed of many organizations as subsystems (e.g., prehospital emergency medical service, hospitals, outpatient clinics, manufacturers) with each having a distinct culture and differing financial, technical, and personal resources. Healthcare organizations try to achieve explicit goals which often are mutually exclusive: The delivery of safe patient care and medical excellence vs economy and cost reduction.

In the case study, examples for organizational factors influencing the transfusion error would be the staffing of ICU and blood bank as well as the hierarchical culture that prevented the nurse from challenging unsafe decisions.

Organizations can influence the quantity and quality of healthcare by influencing the following variables (▶ Chaps. 14–15):

— Structure and processes
— Equipment and technologies
— Human resource management
— Teamwork and leadership
— Communication
— Organizational culture

1.3.4   The Health Care System

Healthcare organizations have to operate within a political and legal framework that limits the scope for organizing patient care. The influence of these factors is more difficult to trace in concrete cases than individual or organizational factors, but the data presented in the following section shows their importance on a larger scale. Some of the factors beyond influence of individual healthcare organizations are as follows:

— The increasing economic pressure on cost explosion within healthcare
— The funding of healthcare systems (e.g., general taxation, social health insurance, voluntary or private health insurance)
— Working time directives
— Regulations enacted by federal governments
— Professional development

1.3.5   Errors in Acute Patient Care

In the mid-1980s several interdisciplinary research groups started to investigate the issue of human error in medical high-stakes environments. Because anesthetists understood that their task characteristics have much in common with those of more widely studied groups in industrial high-risk settings (e.g., pilots, process control), they were the first to initiate collaborations with human factors specialists (e.g., Cooper et al. 1978; Currie 1989). Because the characteristics of the high-stakes medical work environment can challenge human problem-solving, decision-making, and teamwork considerably (▶ Chap. 2), it would be quite natural to expect that the likelihood for active failures in acute patient care is higher than the error rate in routine task environments (e.g., on ward).

The past decade has witnessed an increased awareness of the contribution of human error to suboptimal patient care and adverse events. Despite a large body of scientific work, the attempt to present an overview on errors in acute patient care is highly problematic. On one hand, too many issues surrounding the identification of errors and adverse events in a medical high-stakes environment are still unresolved: Which form of data collection is the most appropriate? Retrospective chart reviews, mandatory reportings, solicited voluntary reportings, surveillance systems, or a direct observation approach (Handler et al. 2000)? On the other hand, the data available provides a very heterogeneous picture, as study design, local structure of the respective hospital, and the healthcare systems studied vary greatly. Given the differing methodological approaches, it is almost impossible to draw sound conclusions about the "real" magnitude of the problem. It is only with these limitations that we present the following data; neither do they claim completeness nor do they provide an adequate picture of the problem. All they can do is to give the reader an idea of the nature and scale of errors in acute care medicine.

1.3.5.1   Errors in the Prehospital Emergency Medical Service

Reports on errors in the Emergency Medical Service (EMS) focus on two aspects of emergency medical care: the *appropriateness of on-scene performance* and the *reliability of the primary diagnosis* as compared with the discharge diagnosis. Incorrect therapeutic measures included drug-related errors (e.g., unfamiliarity with drugs due to infrequent use of the medication, dosage calculation errors, incorrect dosage given), nonadherence to guidelines or standardized treatment protocols, and choice of an unsuitable means of transportation (Arntz et al. 1996; Rittenberger et al. 2005).

Severe errors of assessment included unrecognized life-threatening conditions, underestimation of the severity of injury, and an on-site diagnosis different to the discharge diagnosis. The majority of data seem to confirm the reliability of prehospital diagnoses for adult patients independently of national prehospital medical care strategies (e.g., physician based: Arntz et al. 1996; EMS/paramedic system: Buduhan and McRitchie 2000; Enderson et al. 1990; Esposito et al. 1999). For the treatment of the pediatric population, however, there seems to be still some need for further improvement and training of healthcare providers (e.g., Esposito et al. 1999; Peery et al. 1999).

Despite a growing body of scientific knowledge about clinical errors in healthcare, there is still scarce information concerning the performance and error rate of healthcare professionals in the prehospital emergency care setting. The question of whether or not emergency medical care on-site (characterized by constantly changing environments, uncertainty and time pressure, performance as ad-hoc teams) carries an inherently higher risk for committing an error as compared with the provision of patient care in familiar working situations

☐ **Table 1.1** Incidence of diagnostic and therapeutic errors in prehospital emergency care

Incidence of error	References
8–24% of all injuries in adult trauma patients are missed	Buduhan and McRitchie (2000) Linn et al. (1997)
Severe errors of assessment by the emergency physician in 3% of cases	Arntz et al. (1996)
9% preventable trauma deaths and 16% inappropriate care for pediatric trauma patients	Esposito et al. (1999)
EMS on-scene evaluation misdiagnosed 28% of stroke/TIA patients	Kothari et al. (1995)
Self-reported incidence of medication administration errors in 9.1%	Vilke et al. (2007)
Medical team's scene diagnostic accuracy of spinal injury was 31%	Flabouris (2001)
The incidence of missed injuries in pediatric trauma to be 20%	Peery et al. (1999)

(i.e., in-hospital) has still to be answered. An overview of errors in the EMS is given in ▪ Table 1.1.

1.3.5.2 Errors in the Emergency Department

Many of the sickest patients enter the Emergency Department (ED) and are at increased risk of adverse events because of the serious nature of their presentation and time constraint on diagnosis. Adverse events involving emergency medicine providers are attributed to task complexity (▶ Chap. 2) and time constraints: Errors in care delivery are facilitated by the necessity of multitasking, constant interruptions (Chisholm et al. 2000), a quick turnaround of patients with insufficient time to be thorough, and inadequate supervision (Hendrie et al. 2007). In addition, the large number of differential diagnoses contributes to the element of diagnostic uncertainty and may be responsible for the high rate of negligence attributed to diagnostic errors (Thomas et al. 2000). Because many EDs around the world are not subspecialized, emergency healthcare providers are confronted with nearly any type of injury or disease.

This puts especially the pediatric population at risk: Staff without specialized pediatric training and with little experience is expected to provide adequate patient care in infants and children, often without the supplies necessary for handling pediatric emergencies (IOM 2006). As EDs in many large cities are overcrowded and operate at or near full capacity, even a multiple-car highway crash can create havoc in an ED. A major disaster with many casualties would be something that many hospitals have no adequate capacity to handle.

Because of the nature of task performance and the many obstacles, teamwork plays an important role in detecting and preventing adverse events. Active failures in trauma patient care include problems arising from the interaction of the trauma team with the patient or other team members (Schaefer et al. 1994). ▪ Table 1.2 shows some of the typical teamwork-associated problems and errors frequently encountered in the ED. As with prehospital patient care, the question of whether or not acute patient care in an emergency is more error-prone than routine patient care remains unanswered.

▪ Table 1.2 Incidence of diagnostic and therapeutic errors in the Emergency Department (ED)

Incidence of errors	References
27% of patients with acute myocardial infarction were missed in the ED due to absence of chest pain or lack of ST elevation in the ECG	Chan et al. (1998)
3% of all adverse events occur in the ED; a high rate is associated with negligence in diagnostics	Kohn et al. (1999)
5.9% of all trauma patient deaths were considered preventable. The most common single error was failure to appropriately evaluate the abdomen	Davis et al. (1992)
In 9% of patients injuries are missed during the initial work-up	Enderson et al. (1990)
3.5 errors per patients with spinal/cerebral injury are committed; errors contribute to neurological disability	McDermott et al. (2004)
2–3% of patients with acute myocardial infarction or unstable angina are not hospitalized after presenting at the ED	Pope et al. (2000) McCarthy et al. (1993)
23% of all airway management cases show performance deficiencies	Mackenzie et al. (1996)
Per case an average of 8.8 teamwork failures occur	Risser et al. (1999)

1.3.5.3 Errors in the Intensive Care Unit

Critically ill patients require high-intensity care and may be at especially high risk of iatrogenic injury because of their underlying severe illness. Many reports confirm the notion that adverse events and serious errors involving critically ill patients are common and often potentially life-threatening (e.g., Rothschild et al. 2005). Root causes for errors in the ICU are found in the serious nature of the underlying disease as well as in structural, technical, and organizational deficiencies. Many studies ascribe adverse events to the chaotic arrangement of tubes and lines, the limited access to the patient, lighting, ambient noise, frequent interruptions, insufficiently labeled drugs, and to problems with medical devices (e.g., Donchin and Seagull 2002; Sanghera et al. 2007). In addition, poor communication between physicians and nurses has been made responsible for a multitude of adverse drug events and treatment errors: The case report is only one of countless examples that confirm this fundamental flaw of intensive patient care. Recently a review of critical incident studies in the ICU was able to identify a series of contributory factors that were associated with the lack of specific nontechnical skills (Reader et al. 2006). At present, the available data do not allow for any conclusion as to whether

⬛ **Table 1.3** Incidence of diagnostic and therapeutic errors in the intensive care unit

Incidence of errors	References
31% of all ICU patients suffer iatrogenic complications during their stay in the ICU	Donchin et al. (1995)
Medication errors and adverse drug events occur in 3.6.%; 81% are clinically important	Buckley et al. (2007)
One error for every five doses of medication administered (20%)	Kopp et al. (2006)
20.2% of critically ill patients suffer from adverse events	Rothschild et al. (2005)
15% of patients suffer consequences from an error; 92% are judged as avoidable	Graf et al. (2005)
63–83% of all critical incidents can be attributed to human error	Wright et al. (1991); Giraud et al. (1993); Beckmann et al. (1996); Buckley et al. (1997)
13–51% of all critical incidents pose a major threat for patient safety	Donchin et al. (1995); Beckmann et al. (2003)
One of 10 new patients in ICU is transferred to ICU because of a previous treatment error	Darchy et al. (1999)
For the ICU as a whole about 1.7 errors per patient per day occur. Twice a day a severe or potentially detrimental error is committed	Donchin et al. (1995)
Adverse event rates on neonatal ICUs are high: 0.75 adverse events occur per infant; 56% would have been preventable	Sharek et al. (2006)
The majority of adverse events were errors in medication (15–60%)	Giraud et al. (1993); Donchin et al. (1995)
The rate of preventable adverse drug events in ICUs is nearly twice that rate of non-ICUs	Cullen et al. (1997)
One of three errors in ICU is caused by communication problems	Giraud et al. (1993)

the frequency of errors increases when healthcare providers have to manage critical situation as compared with routine procedures. ◘ Table 1.3 illustrates the magnitude of the problem of treatment errors in the ICU.

1.3.5.4 Errors in Anesthesia and Postoperative Patient Care

The induction and maintenance of anesthesia has always been a potentially harmful undertaking without having any therapeutic benefit in itself. The use of highly potent drugs with the associated loss of consciousness and vital functions bears the risk that patients may be harmed by adverse events. As early as in the mid-1950s of the past century anesthetists were the first group of healthcare providers who systematically addressed the issue of incidence and nature of peri-operative adverse events (Beecher and Todd 1954). The increased insight into the contribution of anesthesia to

peri-operative morbidity and mortality has led to a considerable improvement in the safety and quality of anesthetic patient care. As a consequence of its leading role in the prevention and detection of medial error and in pioneering a patient safety movement, the IOM report referred to anesthesiology as the model for addressing patient safety (Kohn et al. 1999). Adverse drug events, circulatory events, problems with airway management, and pulmonary complications are among the most frequent critical situations. As a result of major improvements in technology, equipment failure has become a rare event. Patients in the postanesthesia care unit (PACU) can experience an adverse event from a residual sedative or anesthetic effect, persistent muscle-relaxant effect, inappropriate fluid management, allergic reaction, and upper airway obstruction. Human error plays a significant role in the development of these critical situations and accidents (◘ Table 1.4). Human error in anesthesia occurs on the individual level (e.g., judgment) as well as on the interpersonal level (e.g., communi-

◘ **Table 1.4** Incidence of diagnostic and therapeutic errors in anesthesia and postoperative patient care

Incidence of errors	References
31–82% of all incidents are caused by human error, 9–21% by technical failure	Cooper et al. (1978); Kumar et al. (1988); Currie (1989); Chopra et al. (1992); Webb et al. (1993); Buckley et al. (1997); Arbous et al. (2001); Bracco et al. (2001)
Critical incidents occur in 2.5 % of all pediatric anesthesia cases	Marcus (2006)
0.2% of all patients in the PACU need emergency reintubation; 70% are directly related to anesthesia management	Mathew et al. (1990)
A drug administration error occurs at a rate of 1 in 133 anesthetics. Incorrect doses (20%) and substitutions (20%) with i.v. boluses of other drugs are the most common errors	Webster et al. (2001)
4% of all incidents are caused by the patient's unpredictable reactions; 69–82% of all critical incidents could have been avoided	Arbous et al. (2001)
The most common presenting problems are related to respiratory/airway issues (43%), cardiovascular problems (24%), and drug errors (11%). Contributing factors included error of judgment (18%), communication failure (14%), and inadequate preoperative preparation (7%)	Kluger and Bullock (2002)
29% of all critical incidents lead to a major physiological disturbance and require management in intensive care unit	Kluger and Bullock (2002)

cation failure) and the organizational level (e.g., standards for preoperative management).

1.3.6 The Human Factors: Nontechnical Skills for Acute Patient Care

Poor outcomes do occur, but what is perhaps surprising given the complex circumstances of critical situations is that good outcomes happen as often as they do. Despite the manifold ways in which human factors contribute to faulty systems, processes, and conditions as well as to active failures of healthcare providers, it should not be overlooked that human factors, the way people think and feel, and interact with each other and with their environment, are the essential resource for safe patient care: Like Janus, the two-faced god of Roman mythology looking in opposite directions, human factors, too, provide both the potential to trigger as well as the skills to master a critical situation (□ Fig. 1.2). As a result, human factors should never be equated with "risk factors." Each time mindful healthcare professionals detect, diagnose, and correct a critical situation or an error before it has an opportunity to unfold, the human factors prevent patient harm (□ Fig. 1.3). Correct performance and systemic

errors are two sides of the same coin, or, perhaps more aptly, they are two sides of the same cognitive balance sheet (Reason 1990).

The past years have witnessed a growing interest in these skills, which are crucial for delivering safe and high-quality medical care but which are not directly related to technical expertise: the "nontechnical skills." Nontechnical skills include *interpersonal skills*, such as communication, teamwork, and leadership, and *cognitive skills*, such as situation awareness, planning, decision-making, and task management. The aviation industry was among the first to recognize that technical proficiency in pilots was not enough to guarantee safe flight operations and to identify the most relevant nontechnical skills (Wiener et al. 1993). Training programs were introduced which taught and reinforced nontechnical skills as a set of countermeasures against error. Because the workload profile of anesthetists shows similarities with pilots (i.e., high intensity at task initiation and completion, monitoring, and rapid response to critical events), these nontechnical skills were adopted for medical care in a high-stakes environment (e.g., Gaba et al. 1994). Because there is increasing evidence that these skills may not extrapolate directly from aviation to the medical high-stakes environment, several research groups have begun to identify and validate the specific nontechnical skills important for safety in different high-stakes medical domains (Aggarwal et al. 2004; Flin and Maran 2004; Fletcher et al. 2003; Reader et al. 2006; Yule et al. 2006).

The resident from the case report, too, experienced both sides of the human factors: After hav-

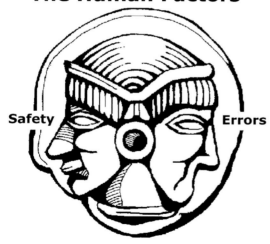

The Human Factors

Safety   Errors

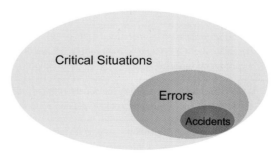

Critical Situations

Errors

Accidents

□ **Fig. 1.2** The human factors and the two faces of Janus. Similar to the god of Roman mythology, the human factors have two opposite aspects: they combine to trigger critical situations and at the same time provide the skills to master them

□ **Fig. 1.3** Human factors prevent adverse events. Because healthcare professionals detect critical situations and errors before these can cause accidents, the human factors provide a vital resource for patient safety

ing triggered the transfusion reaction, the management of the critical situation was up to him as well. As the critical situation unfolded he had to manage the emergency under utilization of all resources and team members available. He suddenly needed a broad variety of these "nontechnical" skills. He had to do the following:

- Rapidly detect and diagnose the nature of the emergency situation
- Resist the emotional strain caused by the awareness that he himself had triggered the adverse event
- Call for help
- Make good decisions under time pressure
- Know his environment and resources available
- Set priorities
- Lead a team
- Reassess the situation and make changes in his plan

The case study teaches another important lesson as well: despite maximum effort, the patient suffered irretrievable harm from the adverse event. Nontechnical skills are no magic bullet, nor are new technologies or drugs. Healthcare professionals can provide the best emergency care possible and still fail to save the patient's life.

One way to understand the relationship between technical and nontechnical skill is that of a conversation: Technical skills provide the context-specific vocabulary; nontechnical skills are the grammar which enables a meaningful interaction. The following chapters should be regarded as a kind of "grammar" which helps healthcare providers of every profession and specialty to engage in a constructive conversation with each other and with the critical situation. The most frequent "grammar errors" will demonstrate possible pitfalls of this conversation and will hopefully sharpen the providers' focus. The conversation, however, is made difficult by certain characteristics that distinguish emergency situations from any other situation in healthcare. We explore these characteristics in this book.

1.4   "The Human Factors": in a Nutshell

- The mortality rate of preventable medical error exceeds the number of deaths attributable to severe trauma, breast cancer, and HIV.

- Human behavior dominates the risk to modern socio-technical systems: 80–90% of all errors are due to "human factors."
- Available data on error in acute care medicine provides a heterogeneous picture: study design, local structure of the healthcare organization, and healthcare systems vary greatly.
- The human factors should never be equated with "risk factor." Human factors provide both, the potential to trigger for critical situations as well as the skills to master them.
- The skills necessary to manage critical situations are called "nontechnical skills." This term includes interpersonal skills (e.g., communication, teamwork, leadership) and cognitive skills (e.g., situation awareness, planning, decision-making, task management).

References

Aggarwal R, Undre S, Moorthy K, Vincent C, Darzi A (2004) The simulated operating theatre: comprehensive training for surgical teams. Qual Saf Healthcare 13 (Suppl 1):i27–i32

Amalberti R, Mosneron-Dupin F (1997) Facteurs humains et fiabilité: quelles démarches pratiques? Octares, Touluse

Arbous MS, Grobbee DE, van Kleef JW, de Lange JJ, Spoormans HH, Touw P, Werner FM, Meursing AE (2001) Mortality associated with anaesthesia: a qualitative analysis to identify risk factors. Anaesthesia 56:1141–1153

Arntz HR, Klatt S, Stern R, Willich SN, Bernecker J (1996) Are emergency physicians' diagnoses accurate? Anesthesist 45:163–70 [German]

Beckmann U, Baldwin I, Hart GK, Runciman WB (1996) The Australian Incident Monitoring Study in Intensive Care: AIMS-ICU. An analysis of the first year of reporting. Anaesth Intensive Care 24:320–329

Beckmann U, Bohringer C, Carless R, Gillies DM, Runciman WB, Wu AW, Pronovost P (2003) Evaluation of two methods for quality improvement in intensive care: facilitated incident monitoring and retrospective medical chart review. Crit Care Med 31:1006–1011

Beecher HK, Todd DP (1954) A study of the deaths associated with anesthesia and surgery. Ann Surg 140:2–34

Bracco D, Favre JB, Bissonnette B, Wasserfallen JB, Revelly JP, Ravussin P, Chiolero R (2001) Human errors in a multidisciplinary intensive care unit: a 1-year prospective study. Intensive Care Med 27:137–145

Buckley TA, Short TG, Rowbottom YM, Oh TE (1997) Critical incident reporting in the intensive care unit. Anaesthesia 52:403–409

Buckley MS, Erstad BL, Kopp BJ, Theodorou AA, Priestley G (2007) Direct observation approach for detecting medication errors and adverse drug events in a pediatric intensive care unit. Pediatr Crit Care Med 31 [Epub ahead of print]

Buduhan G, McRitchie DI (2000) Missed injuries in patients with multiple trauma. J Trauma 49: 600–605

Chan WK, Leung KF, Lee YF, Hung CS, Kung NS, Lau FL (1998) Undiagnosed acute myocardial infarction in the accident and emergency department: reasons and implications. Eur J Emerg Med 5:219–224

Chisholm CD, Collison, EK, Nelson DR, Cordell WH (2000) Emergency department workplace interruptions: Are emergency physicians "interrupt-driven" and "multitasking"? Acad Emerg Med 7:1239–1243

Chopra V, Bovill JG, Spierdijk J, Koornneef F (1992) Reported significant observations during anaesthesia: A prospective analysis over an 18-month period. Br J Anaesth 68:13–18

Cooper JB, Newbower RS, Long CD, McPeek B (1978) Preventable anesthesia mishaps: a study of human factors. Anesthesiology 49:399–406

Cullen DJ, Sweitzer BJ, Bates DW, Burdick E, Edmondson A, Leape LL (1997) Preventable adverse drug events in hospitalised patients. A comparative study of intensive care and general care units. Crit Care Med 25:1289–1297

Currie M (1989) A prospective survey of anaesthetic critical events in a teaching hospital. Anaesth Intensive Care 17:403–411

Darchy B, Le Miere E, Figueredo B (1999) Iatrogenic diseases as a reason for admission to the intensive care unit: incidence, causes and consequences. Arch Intern Med 159:71–78

Davis JW, Hoyt DB, McArdle MS, Mackersie RC, Eastman AB, Virgilio RW, Cooper G, Hammill F, Lynch FP (1992) An analysis of errors causing morbidity and mortality in a trauma system: a guide for quality improvement. J Trauma 32:660–665

Donchin Y, Seagull FJ (2002) The hostile environment of the intensive care unit. Curr Opin Crit Care 8:316–320

Donchin Y, Gopher D, Olin M, Badihi Y, Biesky M, Sprung CL, Pizov R, Cotev S (1995) A look into the nature and causes of human errors in the intensive care unit. Crit Care Med 23:294–300

Enderson BL, Reath DB, Meadors J, Dallas W, DeBoo JM, Maull KI (1990) The tertiary trauma survey: a prospective study of missed injury. J Trauma 30:666–669

Esposito TJ, Sanddal ND, Dean JM, Hansen JD, Reynolds SA, Battan K (1999) Analysis of preventable pediatric trauma deaths and inappropriate trauma care in Montana. J Trauma 47:243–251

Flabouris A (2001) Clinical features, patterns of referral and out of hospital transport events for patients with suspected isolated spinal injury. Injury 32:569–575

Fletcher G, Flin R, McGeorge P, Glavin R, Maran N, Patey R (2003) Anaesthetists' Non-Technical Skills (ANTS): evaluation of a behavioural marker system. Br J Anaesth 90:580–588

Flin R, Maran N (2004) Identifying and training non-technical skills for teams in acute medicine. Qual Saf Healthcare 13 (Suppl 1):i80–i84

Gaba DM, Fish KJ, Howard SK (1994) Crisis management in anesthesia. Churchill Livingstone, New York

Giraud T, Dhainaut J, Vaxelaire J (1993) Iatrogenic complications in adult intensive care units: a prospective two-center study. Crit Care Med 21:40–51

Graf J, Driesch A von den, Koch KC, Janssens U (2005) Identification and characterization of errors and incidents in a medical intensive care unit. Acta Anaesthesiol Scand 49:930–939

Handler JA, Gillam M, Sanders AB, Klasco R (2000) Defining, identifying, and measuring error in emergency medicine. Acad Emerg Med 7:1183–1188

Hendrie J, Sammartino L, Silvapulle M, Braitberg G (2007) Experience in adverse events detection in an emergency department: nature of events. Emerg Med Austral 19:9–15

Hollnagel E (1993) Reliability of cognition: foundations of human reliability analysis. Academic Press, London

IOM (2006) Emergency care for children. Growing pains. Committee on the future of Emergency Care in the United States Health System Board on Healthcare Services. Academic Press, Washington

Kluger MT, Bullock MF (2002) Recovery room incidents: a review of 419 reports from the Anaesthetic Incident Monitoring Study (AIMS). Anaesthesia 57:1060–1066

Kohn L, Corrigan J, Donaldson M (1999) To err is human: building a safer health system. Committee on Quality of Healthcare in America, Institute of Medicine (IOM). National Academy Press, Washington

Kopp BJ, Erstad BL, Allen ME, Theodorou AA, Priestley G (2006) Medication errors and adverse drug events in an intensive care unit: direct observation approach for detection. Crit Care Med 34:415–425

Kothari R, Barsan W, Brott T, Broderick J, Ashbrock S (1995) Frequency and accuracy of prehospital diagnosis of acute stroke. Stroke 26:937–941

Kumar V, Barcellos WA, Mehta MP, Carter JG (1988) An analysis of critical incidents in a teaching department for quality assurance: a survey of mishaps during anaesthesia. Anaesthesia 43:879–883

Linn S, Knoller N, Giligan CG, Dreifus U (1997) The sky is a limit: errors in prehospital diagnosis by flight physicians. Am J Emerg Med 15:316–320

Mackenzie CF, Jefferies NJ, Hunter WA, Bernhard WN, Xiao Y (1996) Comparison of self-reporting of deficiencies in airway management with video analyses of actual performance. LOTAS Group. Level One Trauma Anesthesia Simulation. Hum Factors 38:623–635

Marcus R (2006) Human factors in pediatric anesthesia incidents. Paediatr Anaesth 16:242–250

Mathew JP, Rosenbaum SH, O'Connor T, Barash PG (1990) Emergency tracheal intubation in the postanesthesia care unit: physician error or patient disease? Anesth Analg 71:691–697

McCarthy BD, Beshansky JR, D'Agostino RB, Selker HP (1993) Missed diagnoses of myocardial infarction in the emergency department: results from a multicenter study. Ann Emerg Med 22:579–582

McDermott FT, Rosenfeld JV, Laidlaw JD, Cordner SM, Tremayne AB (2004) Evaluation of management of road trauma survivors with brain injury and neurologic disability in Victoria. J Trauma 56:137–149

Peery CL, Chendrasekhar A, Paradise NF, Moorman DW, Timberlake GA (1999) Missed injuries in pediatric trauma. Am Surg 65:1067–1069

Pope JH, Aufderheide TP, Ruthazer R, Woolard RH, Feldman JA, Beshansky JR, Griffith JL, Selker HP (2000) Missed diagnoses of acute cardiac ischemia in the emergency department. N Engl J Med 342:1163–1170

Reader T, Flin R, Lauche K, Cuthbertson B (2006) Non-technical skills in the intensive care unit. Br J Anaesth 96:551–559

Reason J (1990) Human error. Cambridge University Press, Cambridge

Reason J (1997) Managing the risks of organizational accidents. Ashgate, Aldershot

Risser DT, Rice MM, Salisbury ML, Simon R, Jay GD, Berns SD (1999) The potential for improved teamwork to reduce medical errors in the emergency department. The MedTeams Research Consortium. Ann Emerg Med 34:373–383

Rittenberger JC, Beck PW, Paris PM (2005) Errors of omission in the treatment of prehospital chest pain patients. Prehosp Emerg Care 9:2–7

Rothschild JM, Landrigan CP, Cronin JW, Kaushal R, Lockley SW, Burdick E, Stone PH, Lilly CM, Katz JT, Czeisler CA, Bates DW (2005) The Critical Care Safety Study: the incidence and nature of adverse events and serious medical errors in intensive care. Crit Care Med 33:1694–1700

Sanghera IS, Franklin BD, Dhillon S (2007) The attitudes and beliefs of healthcare professionals on the causes and reporting of medication errors in a UK intensive care unit. Anaesthesia 62:53–61

Schaefer HG, Helmreich RL, Scheidegger D (1994) Human factors and safety in emergency medicine. Resuscitation 28:221–225

Sharek PJ, Horbar JD, Mason W, Bisarya H, Thurm CW, Suresh G, Gray JE, Edwards WH, Goldmann D, Classen D (2006) Adverse events in the neonatal intensive care unit: development, testing, and findings of an NICU-focused trigger tool to identify harm in North American NICUs. Pediatrics 118:1332–1340

Thomas EJ, Studdert DM, Burstin HR et al. (2000) Incidence and types of adverse events and negligent patient care in Utah and Colorado. Med Care 38:261–271

Vilke GM, Tornabene SV, Stepanski B, Shipp HE, Ray LU, Metz MA, Vroman D, Anderson M, Murrin PA Davis DP, Harley J (2007) Paramedic self-reported medication errors. Prehosp Emerg Care 11:80–84

Webb RK, Currie M, Morgan CA, Williamson JA, Mackay P, Russell WJ, Runciman WB (1993) The Australian Incident Monitoring Study: an analysis of 2000 incident reports. Anaesth Intensive Care 21:520–528

Webster CS, Merry AF, Larsson L, McGrath KA, Weller J (2001) The frequency and nature of drug administration error during anaesthesia. Anaesth Intensive Care 29:494–500

Wiener E, Kanki B, Helmreich R (1993) Cockpit resource management. Academic Press, San Diego

Williamson JA, Webb RK, Sellen A, Runciman WB (1993) Human failure: an analysis of 2000 incident reports. Anaesth Intensive Care 21:678–683

Wright D, Mackenzie SJ, Buchan I, Cairns CS, Price LE (1991) Critical incidents in the intensive therapy unit. Lancet 338:676–678

Yule S, Flin R, Paterson-Brown S, Maran N (2006) Non-technical skills for surgeons in the operating room: a review of the literature. Surgery 139:140–149

2 The Challenge of Acute Healthcare

2.1   Case Study

A 32-year-old trauma patient was admitted to the emergency department with severe head trauma, maxillofacial injuries, blunt thoracic trauma, an open fracture of the femur, and the suspicion of a contained subcapsular hematoma of the spleen. Following the initial work-up, the patient was transferred to the OR and was simultaneously operated on by trauma surgeons and maxillofacial surgeons. Twenty minutes after the incision, the patient developed increasingly high peak inspiratory pressures, the tidal volumes began to decrease, and the saturation dropped. The flow-volume curve on the monitor showed an incomplete expiratory phase; however, lung auscultation was normal. Suspecting bronchospasm, the anesthesiologist initiated broncholytic therapy which failed to improve the ventilatory parameters. At the anesthesiologist's request, the surgeons explored the oral cavity and noticed that the endotracheal tube was kinked. After unkinking the tube, the peak pressure, tidal volumes, and saturation normalized. Twenty minutes later, the peak pressure increased, the tidal volumes decreased and the saturation dropped again; however, this time the flow-volume curve did not indicate an obstructive pattern. Instead, lung auscultation revealed diminished right-sided breath sounds. In addition, the invasive arterial line tracing showed a significant decrease in the blood pressure. The anesthesiologist attributed these changes to a possible tension pneumothorax which could have occurred at the time of insertion of the central line in the right subclavian vein. She communicated her findings to the trauma surgeons, who inserted a chest tube. Subsequently, the ventilation, oxygenation, and vital signs returned to normal values. Forty-five minutes later, the patient became unstable again. The peak pressure gradually increased and the tidal volumes decreased to 150 ml. The saturation also dropped, although at a slower pace than the first two times. The lungs were ventilated with increasing difficulty and rales were identified on auscultation. Despite increasing the inspiratory pressure, adding PEEP and ventilating with 100% oxygen, the saturation continued to drop to the 80s. The anesthesiologist contacted the ICU and requested an intensive care ventilator. The new ventilator improved the oxygenation and ventilation, and the patient was rendered stable enough to be transferred to the ICU. The ventilatory parameters were: tidal volume of 400 ml; respiratory rate of 14; peak pressure of 32 mbar; PEEP of 15 mbar; and the F_1O_2 was 100%. Bilateral densities on the chest X-ray confirmed early-stage acute respiratory distress syndrome (ARDS).

A multiple-injured trauma patient undergoes an emergency operation. After an initial uneventful period the patient develops a series of ventilatory problems. Each time the problems lead to a rapid deterioration of the patient's oxygenation status, which puts the anesthetist under time pressure. She has to find the cause of the clinical deterioration and has to take therapeutic measures before the patient is seriously harmed. The circumstances of this series of ventilation problems, however, are very challenging for the anesthetist: Every time the pathophysiological disturbances present with an almost identical set of symptoms and monitor parameters, but the underlying cause is always a different one. Furthermore, the physician has difficulty diagnosing the problem because the apparent changes of one organ systems are caused by concealed alterations of another system: The significant decrease in the blood pressure is caused by a pulmonary problem (i.e., tension pneumothorax) and a decrease in arterial saturation is due to performance limitations of an anesthesia machine (when ventilating a patient with ARDS).

2.2   Medical Emergencies and Critical Situations

Emergencies are among the most challenging situations in medicine. The need for immediate life-saving treatment, the necessity of swift decisions, and actions in the absence of complete information, time pressure, the sudden rush of anxiety, the awareness that a human life is at stake, the interaction with team members from different specialties – all this creates a potent mix of stressful demands for the healthcare provider. Because emergency situations often appear very dramatic and sometimes are characterized by chaos and disorganization, they seem to be incomparable to situations in daily life. From a cognitive psychologist's perspective, however, an emergency situation represents only a specific type of decisional situation with a specific situational context: a situation in which human decision-making and task performance have an immediate impact on the current state and further development of the situation. Because the future course of events hangs in the balance for good or bad, we call these situations *critical* (Badke-Schaub 2002).

For the healthcare provider it is basically irrelevant whether the *critical situation* was triggered by an *external* (e.g., trauma, equipment malfunction) or *internal* event (e.g., cardiac dysrhythmia, myocardial infarction, pulmonary embolis, stroke) or by an *error* committed by a healthcare provider (e.g., transfusion error). The requirements and difficulties for successful problem-solving and quality patient care are similar. As in the case report, a medical emergency may be composed of multiple critical situations. Each of those critical situations can be analyzed and treated as a separate entity: An unforeseen event interrupts routine patient care and calls forth a decision. Once the critical situation has passed, task performance can return to routine (Badke-Schaub 2002; ◘ Fig. 2.1).

In the literature on acute medical care critical situations are either termed "emergencies," "complications" (Atlee 2007; Gravenstein and Kirby 1995; Taylor and Major 1987), or "crisis" (Gaba et al. 1994). The major emphasis of this perspective lies on the clinical picture of an emergency and on the knowledge and skills necessary to manage it. In this book we use the term "critical situation," as our focus is on the *cognitive and behavioral aspects* of these situations, and on the factors that influence human decision-making, task performance, and teamwork. With the focus on decision-making,

"critical situation" includes emergencies but also minor incidents or minimal events that require decisions to avoid harm to the patient.

2.3 Complexity and Human Behavior

Despite sharing several characteristics with everyday decisional situations, the provision of healthcare in a high-stakes environment has a number of properties that make it significantly different from and considerably more challenging than the provision of patient care in other medical domains. Whereas healthcare providers traditionally have been taught technical proficiency and clinical decision-making, the cognitive process of detecting and correcting critical situations in a high-stakes environment necessitates a broader set of capabilities. The reasons lie in several characteristics which apply to critical situations in a high-stakes environment.

The case study illustrates several of these characteristics which cognitive psychologists subsume under the term "complexity of a working environment." Complexity has found widespread interest among all fields concerned with human problem-solving (e.g., cognitive science, human factors approach, reliability engineering), because complexity places many specific demands on decision makers and affects the kinds and quality of cognitive processes carried out by people. Most of the scientific

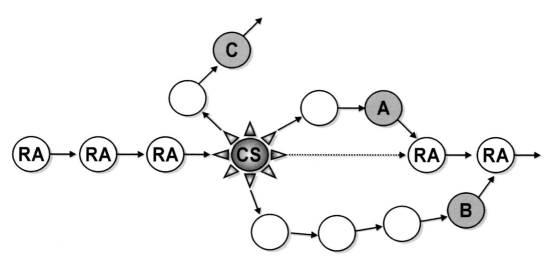

◘ **Fig. 2.1** Critical situations. Routine actions (RA) are interrupted by a critical situation (CS). If this situation is successfully managed, actions will return sooner (A) or later (B) to routine; however, some decisions result in a deviating treatment pathway for the patient (C). (Modified from Badke-Schaub 2002)

evidence comes from industrial or military high-risk environments where human behavior in complex man-made systems was studied.

Systems theorists and psychologists have advanced several different conceptual frameworks of what exactly the characteristics of complexity are. Despite the diversity in definition, there is nevertheless a general acceptance about basic features of complexity (e.g., Cook and Woods 2001; Dörner 1996; Dörner and Schaub 1994; Frensch and Funke 1995; Perrow 1999; Rasmussen and Lind 1981; Reason 1997; Sterman 1984; Woods 1988). On a most basic level complexity has a dual nature (◘ Fig. 2.2). It is (a) a characteristic of the task environment, and (b) an obstacle for the problem solver.

2.3.1   Complexity: a Characteristic of the Task Environment

Several dimensions have been identified which influence the way humans perceive their environment. In general, when we describe a task or a situation as "simple" this usually refers to the fact that the below-stated characteristics are only weekly expressed; however, if an environment is described as "complex," this means that the situational characteristics are strongly represented. The dimensions of a complex task environment are (Dörner and Schaub 1994; Frensch and Funke 1995):

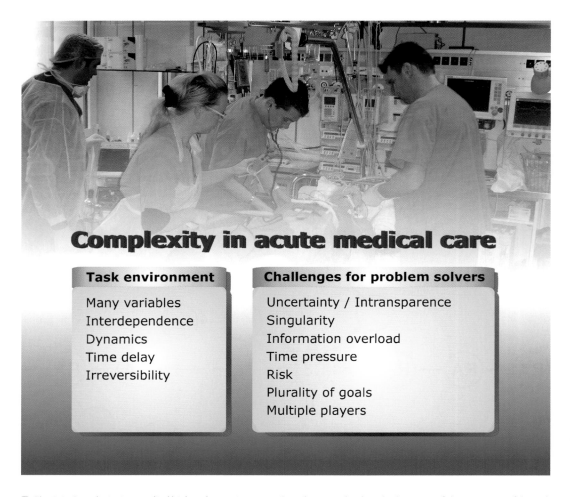

Complexity in acute medical care

Task environment	Challenges for problem solvers
Many variables	Uncertainty / Intransparence
Interdependence	Singularity
Dynamics	Information overload
Time delay	Time pressure
Irreversibility	Risk
	Plurality of goals
	Multiple players

◘ **Fig. 2.2** Complexity in a medical high-stakes environment. Complexity can be described in terms of characteristics of the task environment as well as the characteristics of the problem-solving approach

2.3.1.1 Many Variables

Depending on the nature of a critical situation (e.g., multiple trauma, the patient's pathophysiology, previous medical history, invasiveness of procedures) many variables and their interrelation have to be handled. As human conscious thinking is neither very fast nor capable of processing very much information per time unit, people will have great difficulty in taking all variables into account. As a result, the large number of variables will make it easy for decision makers to overlook them and to make false assumptions about the state of the system.

2.3.1.2 Interdependence/Interrelatedness

Because humans can easily get an incorrect or incomplete understanding of the system they operate in, they often tend to overlook the interdependence ("coupling"; ► Chap. 14) between the variables as well. If variables constitute a network of interdependencies, an action that affects one part of the system will also affect other parts of it. Interdependence leads to side effects and long-term repercussions, even of actions aimed at only one variable. The decrease in arterial blood pressure caused by the tension pneumothorax and the desaturation due to performance limits of the anesthesia machine exemplify interdependence. The more links exist between the variables, the more difficulty decision makers will experience in predicting the consequences of their actions. Not regarding side effects of actions would be a typical error in complex systems. In addition, one action can have multiple immediate consequences. Most importantly, interdependence of variables defines the task environment as *a system*, not as an accumulation of disconnected items. Failure to approach a critical situation from a system perspective is one major obstacle to successful decision-making under complexity. If a problem solver tries to manipulate variables in isolation, he or she most certainly will fail to predict a system's developmental trends realistically.

2.3.1.3 Dynamics

Complex situations can be slower or faster. If they are event driven with rapid time constants, such as the above-described critical incident, they are highly dynamic. An emergency situation does not, like in a game of chess, simply wait for a player to make moves. The pace of decision is determined by external events, and these events will progress, with or without participation of the actors (Dörner 1996). While the healthcare provider is still busy searching for a solution, the problem changes. This creates the necessity to maintain an up-to-date "mental model" (► Chap. 6) of what is often a rapidly changing situation. These dynamics narrow down the freedom of action: If we wait too long before we act, we will lose opportunities. A therapeutic measure which could help the patient now may already have become obsolete in near future; thus, healthcare professionals must often do with tentative solutions because time pressure forces them to act before they have gathered complete information or have outlined a comprehensive plan. Time pressure, however, is not only forced upon the healthcare professional from outside events, it can be an unavoidable consequence of necessary therapeutic actions as well: Once anesthesia has been induced, the patient's ventilation has to be secured, no matter how.

2.3.1.4 Time Delay

Side effects and long-term repercussions are not necessarily obvious right away; instead, they can appear with considerable time delay thus making it difficult for the healthcare professional to correlate symptoms with the triggering event: The shaldoncatheter was inserted into the right subclavian vein during the initial work-up in the emergency room. The tension pneumothorax, however, did not manifest until several hours later in the operating room. As with interdependence, time delay can obscure the result of therapeutic measures. Whether or not a certain strategy was successful may take quite a while to become apparent and be overlaid by the effects of other measures.

2.3.1.5 Irreversibility

Pathophysiological changes in a patient often take a one-way direction. As a consequence, there can be a "too late" for organ systems to recover and a narrow therapeutic window to prevent irretrievable harm. Actions, too, can have irretrievable consequences. When faced with a critical situation, healthcare providers often have one chance only to choose the correct action. Behavior following the principle of trial and error is far too risky.

2.3.2   Complexity: an Obstacle for the Problem Solver

Complexity is in part defined by the situational characteristics described above. Described from the perspective of an actor, complexity is defined by requirements for successful action. Healthcare providers who have to cope with a complex situation will experience characteristics of complexity as obstacles to gathering information, integrating findings, and designing effective actions (e.g., Dörner 1996; Frensch and Funke 1995; Sterman 1994).

2.3.2.1   Uncertainty and Intransparence

Many problems in a medical high-stakes environment are ambiguous and underspecified (e.g., dropping saturation, low arterial blood pressure). What the healthcare provider really wants to know about the patient is not visible and critical information might not be available. Because man, in contrast to man-made systems, does not provide detailed information on (patho)physiological processes, healthcare professionals are often faced with very unspecific symptoms. In contrast to decision makers in the industrial or aviation setting, problem solvers in acute medical care have no direct access to information about the situation they must address, so they must make decisions affecting a system whose momentary features they can only see partially, unclearly, in blurred and shadowy outline. Monitoring provides access to the patient's underlying condition only via weak external signals and cannot give more than hints as to what the problem exactly might be (Gaba 1992). There is no monitor that could tell the physician "the sats drop because your patient starts to develop an ARDS" or "the peak airway pressure is high because the endotracheal tube is kinked." It is only from ambiguous patterns of different variables that healthcare professionals can draw conclusions concerning the medical problem. Intransparence thus injects another element of uncertainty into planning and decision-making. In a medical high-stakes environment the main problem in problem-solving is not "What should I do?" Rather, the main task is to lift the veil and to answer the question: "What exactly is the problem" (Klein 1992)?

2.3.2.2   Singularity of the Situation

Once the problem has been defined (by giving a diagnosis) there is another danger waiting for the decision maker: He or she might miss subtle situational clues which would indicate that this critical situation differs slightly, but in important features, from previously experienced ones. If unobtrusive but important details are missed – or are not even looked for – the resulting behavior will take the form "strong-but-wrong" (Reason 1990): The planning process is skipped, established patterns of actions are activated, and the action will be more in keeping with past practice than with the current situational demands. Rather than choosing an action because it has worked many times before ("*methodism*" Dörner 1996; "*cognitive conservatism*" Reason 1990; ► Chap. 7) healthcare providers should be flexible in their approach to decision-making; thus, *flexibility* is a key characteristic of successful problem-solving in critical situations.

2.3.2.3   Information Overload and Lack of Information

In critical situations, much of the information needed at the time of a decision is not (yet) available. On the other hand, multiple sources of concurrent information may overwhelm the healthcare provider. Data have to be assessed for relevance and reliability and either integrated into a situational model or discarded. The healthcare provider has to constantly decide how much information is enough and when to stop information gathering. Will rough-cut information do because the evidence points overwhelmingly to a diagnosis, or do new lines of inquiry have to be pursued because greater detail is needed? In order to successfully balance these contradicting requirements, healthcare professionals have to pursue problem-oriented *information management*. The aim of information management is to arrive at a cohesive picture of the situation which is supported by the data available (► Chap. 6). The integration of all team members available in this process of generating and evaluating information is an important step towards a more consistent mental model of the situation (Salas et al. 1992).

2.3.2.4 Time Pressure

Time pressure limits the possibilities for data collection, problem analysis, goal formulation, and action. Once the saturation starts to drop, there is not much time left to find out why. Even if you are told differently after a critical situation, there is no way a healthcare provider could act under time pressure and at the same time gather complete information. In complex situations, information management will never be comprehensive. Instead, as the need for a rapid decision increases, *transfer of previous knowledge* will replace problem-oriented information management. Mental models of past experience with similar situations will define current assumptions and preestablished patterns of actions will govern behavior.

Emotions and "intuition," which are both forms of implicit knowledge, will replace explicit efforts of situation assessment, but as own emotions in a risky situation will interfere with "felt knowledge," it is dangerous to rely on emotions only; thus, decision-making under time pressure is error-prone.

2.3.2.5 Risk

Decisions under complexity are always risky: The odds are high that our model of reality could be wrong and that the actions we take will not solve, but rather aggravate, the problem; therefore, the question for healthcare providers can never be *if* they actually are willing to take risks, but rather under which circumstances they will do so and for which reason. Unfortunately, judgment of risks can only be based on perceived risk and not on objective facts. Risk assessment is therefore a highly subjective undertaking and prone to error. Acute medical care is a high-stakes environment because of the ever-present danger of actually harming the patient with therapeutic measures. The possibility of causing irreversible patient harm, or even death, by triggering a critical situation and then being unable to manage it suspends like the sword of Damocles over the head of the healthcare provider. One moment of inattention can develop into

a personal, human and economic disaster for the healthcare professional. The awareness of this potential to harm can become the major stressor in critical situations (▶ Chap. 9); thus, what healthcare professionals need is the competency to decide under risk.

2.3.2.6 Plurality of Goals

Goals should tell the healthcare professional where to go. They should be "beacons for human action." Goals should help the healthcare provider to regain control over a critical situation and to satisfy as many concurrent needs as possible without creating new problems. The reality of acute medical care, however, is different: Healthcare professionals frequently have to cope with shifting, ill-defined, or competing goals; thus, in a high-stakes medical environment the formulation of an adequate goal can turn out to be the central cognitive task (Dörner 1996; ▶ Chap. 7). Goals can be clear, unclear, explicit, implicit, general, or specific. In addition, sometimes goal criteria are linked inversely: If one is satisfied, another will necessary fail, e.g., to focus on oxygenation by increasing ventilation in the presence of a tension pneumothorax would worsen the hemodynamic situation of a patient; therefore, complexity makes it necessary that decision makers pursue multiple goals at the same time. This implies that we have to attend to many factors and satisfy several criteria at once. One of the main task requirements when faced with a plurality of goals is the ability to prioritize and to compromise.

2.3.2.7 Multiple Players

Teamwork is a characteristic feature of acute medical care; however, as every medical specialty or professional group may have a specific approach to an emergency situation, standards of performance and expectations may differ. Different mental models can result in conflicts if team members fail to communicate appropriately (e.g., speed of technical rescue vs stabilization of a patient's vital parameters). The major prerequisite for successful teamwork with an inter-disciplinary or inter-professional team is the development of a shared mental model among all healthcare professionals involved (▶ Chap. 11).

2.3.3 Complexity and Expertise

Having listed the dual characteristics of complexity, it is important to stress that complexity is not a static or objective characteristic of a task, but instead a subjective one: "Complexity is not a thing per se, complexity is a situation to be investigated" (Rasmussen 1979). Complexity and intransparency must be understood in terms of the specific individual and his or her experience with the situation. For the beginner almost any clinical task will be a complex business that demands full attention. The more experienced he or she becomes, the more the conglomerate of individual variables will turn into meaningful patterns thereby reducing the need for conscious thinking. The experienced clinician finally will respond to the situation as a "Gestalt" (► Chap. 5), a meaningful whole which has reduced the multitude of features into one. From this point of view complexity can be described as "mental construction" of the clinician: depending on his or her familiarity with the environment or task a different "level" of cognitive activity will be necessary. Experience even provides several meaningful patterns for a set of symptoms and monitor parameters; thus, the anesthetist was able to choose from among several "Gestalten" (► Chap. 6.) to explain the pathophysiological disturbances.

2.4 The Skills, Rules, Knowledge (SRK) Framework

This fundamental correspondence of levels of familiarity with a task or an environment with levels at which behavior is controlled has been conceptualized by the Rasmussen distinction of "skills, rules, and knowledge" (Rasmussen 1983, 1987; ◘ Fig. 2.3). The Skills, Rules, Knowledge (SRK) taxonomy divides cognitive operations intro three levels of abstraction and defines three ways in which information is processed and actions are executed. This distinction has been particularly helpful in characterizing the cognitive mechanisms behind different categories of errors (► Chap. 3). When faced with a situation people generally try to delegate control of behavior to the most routine level (i.e., skills). This provides an economical use of the limited resources of attention and conscious thinking (► Chap. 6); however, if the routine level is not effective, a change is made to one of the other levels (i.e., rules, knowledge).

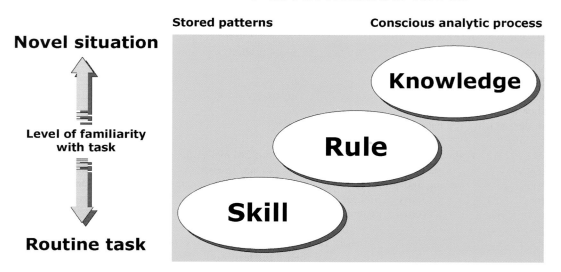

◘ **Fig. 2.3** Rasmussen's "Skills–Rules–Knowledge" (SRK) framework of cognitive behavioral control. The model distinguishes three levels of cognitive control which are related to a decreasing familiarity with the task at hand. (From Rasmussen 1983)

When the novice or an experienced clinician is faced with a critical situation, they will differ in the cognitive control mechanisms they need in order to perform adequately; thus, both parties will differ from each other in the following areas:

— Automaticity of response (i.e., highly integrated patterns of behavior)
— Level of abstraction on which problems are represented
— Amount of clinical rules available
— Knowledge available
— Problem-solving strategies

2.4.1 Skill-Based Behavior

A skill-based behavior represents a type of action that requires very little or no conscious control to perform once an intention is formed. This kind of behavior, also known as *sensorimotor behavior*, is smooth and consists of highly integrated patterns of performance. Much of this behavior is not available to conscious thought or verbalization, it is "automated." *Automaticity* (i.e., the ability to perform tasks without allocating attention) allows humans to free up cognitive resources which can then be used for higher cognitive functions such as problem-solving. As there are a multitude of routine tasks in critical situations which demand skill-based behavior (e.g., intubation, placement of peripheral and central IV lines, thoracocentesis, CPR), it is predictable when and under which circumstances certain skills are required. Skill-based behavior becomes an issue in critical situations if the healthcare professional does not possess these skills, if he or she applies them wrongly, or if the behavior cannot be applied for whatever reason. If skills are available, the requirement lies in the accurate execution and continuous check for deviation.

2.4.2 Rule-Based Behavior

Rule-based behavior is a conscious activity and is characterized by the use of rules and procedures to select a course of action in a familiar work situation (Rasmussen 1983). The rules can be acquired by experience or instructions given by supervisors and clinical teachers. Rules-based behavior is needed in situations that are rarer than skill-based tasks so that the expected actions are not automated. If rules are known, there is no need for finding a solution, and the healthcare professional is provided with a set of correct responses. Rule-based behavior follows an "if-then" logic: "If this is A, then do B." If the healthcare professional correctly recognizes a situation or condition, then he or she can apply a stored rule to steer towards a known goal. As the case report clearly demonstrates, the *diagnosis* of the problem rather than the adequate response will be the main challenge for the healthcare professional (Klein 1992). As in acute patient care in a high-stakes environment, time for thinking is scarce, and wrong actions can cause patients harm; thus, healthcare providers must adhere to as many rules as possible to avoid potential problems.

2.4.3 Knowledge-Based Behavior and Problem-solving

Knowledge-based tasks are those that are new, unfamiliar, or unique to the healthcare professional. The unfamiliarity can have many causes: lack of experience; inadequate clinical training; or simply forgetfulness. Most of the time, however, complexity and coupling create an unexpected and rare combination of events, thereby giving the healthcare professional an unpleasant surprise. Because they are caused by random factors, critical situations like these cannot be anticipated, no learned rule can be applied. Instead, a more advanced level of reasoning, problem-solving, is needed to successfully manage the task. Healthcare providers need to build a comprehensive model of the situation, have to form explicit goals based on their current analysis of the system, have to make a plan, and finally have to execute the plan. The cognitive workload for finding higher-level analogies or analyzing more abstract relations between structure and function is much greater than when using skill- or rule-based behaviors. Successful use of knowledge or problem-solving depends heavily upon the performer's fundamental knowledge, diagnosis, and analysis skills. Because many critical situations unfold without warning the surprise effect is significant. Errors in managing the critical situation derive from a complex interplay of imperfect rationality, faulty mental models of the situation, and a strong emotional component (Tversky and Kahneman 1974; Kahneman et al. 1982). Because these critical situations demand a quick response, on the one hand, but cannot be addressed by precompiled responses, on the other hand, they can rapidly develop into a vital threat to patient safety. Fortunately, problem-solving can be practiced, for example, by confronting learners with different types of emergencies. By regularly training skill- and rule-based behaviors for critical situations, more cognitive resources may be released to knowledge-based behavior when faced with an unanticipated event.

2.5 "The Challenge of Acute Medical Care": in a Nutshell

In conclusion, the challenge of acute medical care is as follows:
- Healthcare in a high-stakes environment has a number of properties that make it considerably more challenging than decision-making in an everyday context. Cognitive psychologists call these characteristics "complexity of a working environment."
- Complexity has a dual nature: It is a characteristic of the task environment as well as set of demands imposed on the problem solver.
- The characteristics of a complex task environment are: many features; interdependence; dynamics; time delay; and irreversibility.
- Problem-solving in complex environments is rendered difficult by uncertainty, intransparency, singularity of the situation, information overload or lack of information, time pressure, risk, plurality of goals, and the presence of many players.
- Complexity is not a static or objective characteristic of a task domain but instead a subjective one. It is a "mental construction" and depends on the experience of an individual with a specific situation or certain task demands.
- The correspondence of levels of familiarity with a task or an environment with levels at which behavior is controlled has been conceptualized by Rasmussen's tripartite distinction of "skills, rules, and knowledge."
- Automaticity allows humans to free up cognitive resources, which can then be used for higher cognitive functions such as problem-solving.

References

Atlee JL (2007) Complications in anesthesia. Saunders, Philadelpha

Badke-Schaub P (2002) Kritische Situationen als Analyseeinheit komplexer Handlungen [Critical situations as unit for analyzing complex actions]. In: Trimpop R, Zimolong B, Kalveram A (eds) Psychologie der Arbeitssicherheit und Gesundheit, Neue Welten – alte Welten [Psychology of work safety and health]. Asanger, Heidelberg, pp 137–142

Cook R, Woods D (2001) Operating at the sharp end: the complexity of human error. In: Salas E, Bowers C, Edens E (eds) Improving teamwork in organizations: applications of resource management training. Erlbaum, Mahwah, New Jersey, pp 255–310

Dörner D (1996) The Logic of failure. Recognizing and avoiding error in complex situations. Metropolitan Books, New York

Dörner D, Schaub H (1994) Errors in planning and decision-making and the nature of human information processing. Appl Psychol Int Rev 43:433–453

Frensch A, Funke J (eds) (1995) Complex problem-solving: the European Perspective. Erlbaum, Hillsdale, New Jersey

Gaba D (1992) Dynamic decision-making in anesthesiology: cognitive models and training approaches. In: Evans DA, Patel VL (eds) Advanced models of cognition for medical training and practice. Springer, Berlin Heidelberg New York, pp 123–148

Gaba DM, Fish KJ, Howard SK (1994) Crisis management in anesthesia. Churchill Livingstone, New York

Gravenstein N, Kirby RR (1995) Complications in anaesthesiology. Lippincott-Raven, Philadelphia

Kahneman D, Slovic P, Tversky A (1982) Judgment under uncertainty: heuristics and biases. Cambridge University Press, Cambridge

Klein G (1992) A recognition-primed decision (RPD) model of rapid decision-making. In: Klein G, Orasanu J, Calderwood R, Zsamboka E (eds) Decision-making in action: models and methods. Ablex, New Jersey, pp 138–47

Perrow C (1999) Normal accidents. Living with high-risk technologies. Princeton University Press, Princeton, New Jersey

Rasmussen J (1979) On the structure of knowledge: a morphology of mental models in a man–machine systems context. Technical Report Riso-M-2192. Riso National Laboratory, Roskilde, Denmark

Rasmussen J (1983) Skills, rules, knowledge: signals, signs and symbols and other distinctions in human performance models. IEEE Trans Systems, Man and Cybernetics, vol SMC-13, no. 3, pp 257–267

Rasmussen J (1987) Cognitive control and human error mechanisms. In: Rasmussen J, Duncan K, Leplat J (eds) New technology and human error. Wiley, Chichester, pp 53–61

Rasmussen J, Lind M (1981) Coping with complexity. Technical Report Riso-M-2293. Riso National Laboratory, Roskilde, Denmark

Reason J (1990) Human error. Cambridge University Press, Cambridge UK

Reason J (1997) Managing the risks of organizational accidents. Ashgate, Aldershot

Salas E, Dickinson TL, Converse SA, Tannenbaum SI (1992) Toward an understanding of team performance and training. In: Swezey RW, Salas E (eds) Teams: their training and performance. Ablex, Norwood, New Jersey, pp 3–30

Sterman JD (1994) Learning in and about complex systems. Syst Dyn Rev 10:291–330

Taylor TH, Major E (1987) Hazards and complications in anaesthesia. Churchill Livingstone, Edinburgh UK

Tversky A, Kahneman D (1974) Judgment under uncertainty: heuristics and biases. Science 185:1124–1131

Woods D (1988) Coping with complexity: the psychology of human behaviour in complex systems. In: Goodstein L, Andersen H, Olsen S (eds) Tasks, errors and mental models. Taylor Francis, London, pp 128–147

3 The Nature of Error

3.1   Case Study

An anesthesia resident physician in his second year of training anesthetized a 76-year-old patient scheduled for a laryngectomy and bilateral neck dissection. The medical history revealed coronary artery disease and liver cirrhosis. As a result of the associated coagulopathy, the surgeon had difficulty achieving adequate hemostasis and therefore repeatedly applied epinephrine-soaked swabs to the surgical site. The undiluted epinephrine was rapidly absorbed into circulation and caused sinus tachycardia and polymorphic premature ventricular contractions. Unaware of the surgeon's use of undiluted epinephrine, the resident did not attribute the PVCs to the hemostatic treatment and hence did not urge the surgeon to stop the application. Instead, he decided to treat the arrhythmia with an ampule of lidocaine. Distracted by the ECG, he did not pay close attention and mistakenly used an ampule of metoprolol instead of lidocaine 2%. This drug error was facilitated by the fact that both ampules, adjacent to each other in the anesthesia cart, had similar labels. The bolus of the β-blocker led to cardiac arrest. Immediate CPR was started. After calling the attending anesthesiologist to the operating room, the patient was successfully resuscitated. The patient was discharged from ICU the following day without any neurological deficits.

3.2   What is an "Erorr"?

Without question the heading contains an error. But what exactly is the error in "erorr"? Is it the false orthography in the typed word? Or is it the fact that someone, while typing the word, swapped the letters, perhaps due to distraction? What at first may seem to be splitting hairs – in fact, both points of view seem to agree that the intention to correctly write the word "error" failed – turns out to be an everyday example of two distinct perspectives on error (◘ Fig. 3.1). One way to look at errors is to classify them by their consequences. *Consequential classifications* are the most widely used in medicine. Consequential classifications emphasize strongly the result of an action (e.g., a wrong drug was given to the patient). The point of interest here is what happened to the patient. Why and under which circumstances the error occurred is of little interest.

Causal classifications, on the other hand, make assumptions about mechanisms implicated in generating the error. The point of interest is why a planned activity did not result in its intended outcome. In this conceptual framework the focus is shifted toward possible psychological precursors and systemic interactions which led to the wrong action.

As already mentioned, people do not seem to distinguish between those two perspectives in everyday practice: "A drug error occurred in the OR" seems to be the same as "The resident injected the wrong drug." If only one person seems to be involved in the medication error, a clear cause-and-effect attribution seems justified: His or her wrong actions led to the undesired result. If even in such simple cases such an assessment is doubtful, it becomes difficult when accidents occur in a dynamic setting with multiple healthcare providers involved. In the first perspective on error it is easy

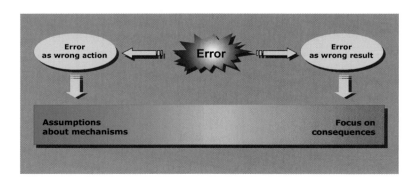

◘ **Fig. 3.1** Different perspectives on error

to find the wrong result, to identify the error. If in looking for causes we try to find *the* wrong action, and the (one) person who did it, we speak of the "person-based approach" to errors.

3.2.1 Person-Based Approach

The "person approach" remains the dominant tradition in healthcare for the response to human error. The longstanding and widespread tradition of the person approach focuses on the unsafe acts of people with direct patient contact.

According to the person approach it is the healthcare provider's fault if something goes wrong: He or she either did not have the necessary knowledge, did not pay attention, or was not willing to do their best. Errors are attributed to missing knowledge, or to aberrant mental processes such as forgetfulness, not paying attention, poor motivation, and negligence. As a consequence, assuming that bad things happen because "bad" (i.e., lazy, stupid, or reckless) people did them, errors become moral issues as well. The result is a culture of "naming, blaming, and shaming."

When viewed from this perspective, solutions to errors lie in improving knowledge (training, education), and in improving motivation by exhortations ("be more careful the next time"), disciplinary measures, or threat of litigation. Especially motivation seems to be the key to error-free performance: "If you concentrate, you will not swap ampules."

From an organizational perspective this approach is attractive: Instead of looking for institutional responsibility, it is easier to target individuals. In addition, in most countries this approach is legally more convenient, even if not expected. The person approach, however, misses the point by isolating unsafe acts from their system context. Far from being random, mishaps tend to fall into recurrent patterns. The same set of circumstances can provoke similar errors, regardless of the healthcare provider involved. This explains why error is not the monopoly of an unfortunate few: Accident analyses from technological high-stakes environments (e.g., civil aviation) demonstrate that it is often the best people who make the worst mistakes. Over and above not being appropriate and helpful, the person approach may even impede the pursuit of greater safety by focusing on individuals rather than seeking out and removing the error-provoking properties within the system at large.

3.2.2 System-Based Approach

If people advocate a "systemic approach" to the study and prevention of safety-critical errors, the focus will shift from the person at the sharp end to organizational processes and the system as a whole. Instead of looking for the one defining action (and hence the one responsible person) which caused the accident, all levels of the organization are scrutinized for contributing factors. The basic premise in the system approach is that humans are fallible and errors are to be expected, even in the best organizations. Whenever errors are studied this should not be done as a separate, pathological category of behavior fragments; the object of study should instead be the cognitive control of behavior in complex environments (Rasmussen 1990). In this conceptual framework accidents are seen as the result of an unlikely confluence and interaction of several causal streams originating not in the perversity of human nature but rather in the interaction with normal cognitive processes and "upstream" systemic factors. Systemic dimensions greatly influence a system's susceptibility to accidents: As soon as socio-technological systems have become sufficiently complex, accidents will be inevitable or "normal" (▶ Chap. 14; Perrow 1999). In this view the people are the inheritors, rather than the instigators, of an accident sequence. The concept of an "organizational accident" replaces the notion of "human error" (Reason 1995). Within the systemic framework countermeasures are based on the assumption that although the human condition cannot be changed, the conditions under which humans work *can* be. The vulnerability of a system can be reduced by strengthening system defenses.

Finally, when an adverse event does occur and patients are harmed the important issue will not be: "Who blundered?", but rather "Why and how did the defenses fail? What were the upstream systemic factors?" To focus on the system and its weakness will provide valuable information for further improvement. Thus, the question "Whose fault is it?" should be abandoned and replaced by the following:

— *What* exactly went wrong? What different types of failures occurred? Is a temporal reconstruction of key events possible?
— *Why* did things go wrong? Which psychological mechanisms may have contributed to the development of the accident?
— *In which ways* did the various organizational and human factors *combine* to create the accident?

3.3   How Can Errors Be Classified?

Since Sigmund Freud's "Psychopathology of Everyday Life" (Freud 1901), which searched for the roots of error in the subconscious, the unconscious, and the psycho-sexual state of the individual, many different taxonomies on error have been proposed (for an overview: Reason 1990; Senders and Moray 1991; Dekker 2002, 2005; Strauch 2002). There is still no one conceptual framework, however, which gives us a comprehensive picture of human error. This is not surprising, because different classifications serve different needs; however, there is widespread agreement that speaking of an "error" implies that there was (a) an intentional action, (b) aiming at a goal, and (c) at least one alternative so that it could have been done differently.

Also, all classifications agree on the distinction between whether something was done wrongly (execution failure) or whether something wrong was done (planning failure).

Within the healthcare community the most influential classification was introduced by the cognitive psychologist James Reason (1990) who proposed three important distinctions (◘ Fig. 3.2):
1. At what level of action control was the error committed? (Execution failure vs planning failure)

2. Was an action executed in the way intended? (Error vs violation)
3. How long before the accident and at which level of the organization was the error committed? (Active vs latent error)

In addition to the psychological and systemic perspective on errors, another type of error plays an important role in the high-stakes medical environment: errors in teamwork.

Faulty communication, insufficient leadership, and inadequate allocation of resources are responsible for incidents and accidents in acute patient care.

3.3.1   Execution Failure vs Planning Failure

The term "error" applies to intentional actions only: An error is a planned sequence of mental or physical activities that fails to achieve its intended outcome (Reason 1990). The reason can be twofold (Norman 1981):
— *Execution failure:* A planned action fails to achieve the desired outcome because the actions did not go as planned.

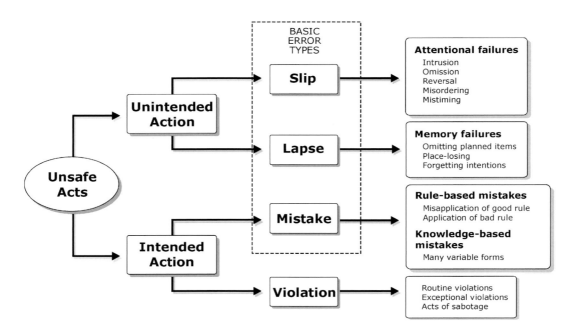

◘ **Fig. 3.2** Taxonomy of error according to Reason. (Adapted from Reason 1990)

— *Planning failure*: A planned action fails to achieve the desired outcome because the plan was inadequate.

3.3.1.1 Execution Failure

The planned action is adequate to achieve its objective but the action deviates from the intended course. This distinction gives rise to two other working definitions:

— *Slips* result from failure in the execution of an action sequence *(attentional failure)*. Slips, which are potentially observable as externalized "actions-not-as-planned" occur predominantly with familiar tasks.
— *Lapses* are a more covert form of execution failure and result from failure of memory. Steps within the sequence of action are omitted because they have been forgotten.

Because the resident's attention was bound for a brief moment by the pathological ECG, he did not pay sufficient attention to the drug he drew from the anesthesia cart. A slip was the triggering event of the cardiac arrest in the ENT patient.

3.3.1.2 Planning Failure

Whereas slips and lapses hinder an adequate plan going as intended, the problem of planning failure lies in the adequacy of the plan itself.

Mistakes are defined as deficiencies or failures in the cognitive processes with which a problem was addressed. Mistakes are independent of whether or not the action sequence executed resulted in the desired outcome.

Mistakes can happen when problem-solving has to be applied (knowledge-based mistake) or when rules are used (rule-based mistake). In the latter case mistakes can manifest as:

— The application of a bad rule, because it remained uncorrected in the repertoire of problem solutions.
— The misapplication of a "good" rule, because countersigns (i.e., inputs such as contraindications that indicate that the more general rule is inapplicable) are not taken into account.
— The nonapplication of a "good" rule, because the healthcare provider was unfamiliar with the rule or unable to remember it in time.

The resident's decision to inject lidocaine for the treatment of PVCs would be an example for the misapplication of a "good" rule for antiarrhythmic therapy, because he missed the specifics of the situation: Not the patient's cardiac status, but rather the excessive (but short-lived) plasma level of epinephrine was responsible for the electrophysiological alterations.

3.3.2 Errors in Problem-solving

Every time a healthcare professional encounters a novel situation that lies outside the range of his or her precompiled responses, problem-solving becomes necessary. Instead of applying rules to a problem the healthcare provider has to utilize knowledge to address the situation. Conscious thinking, however, the very "tool" we need for problem-solving, is highly error-prone for several reasons:

— Conscious thought works slowly. It has limited capacity and prompts us to use our scarce resources as efficiently as possible. We therefore avoid conscious thinking whenever possible and instead take shortcuts or resort to rule-based behavior (▶ Chap. 6).
— Any plan has to be based on a mental model of the current situation. Unfortunately, mental models are often incomplete or even incorrect. Resulting actions will therefore be faulty right from the start.
— Complexity, uncertainty, and high risk create the uneasy feeling of incompetence. As human beings prefer to maintain a simple and stable mental model that guards their own feeling of competence, models of the world that support it are selected while contradictory evidence is discarded (Kahneman et al. 1982; Dörner 1996).

A closer look at the process of problem-solving reveals that it can be further subdivided into several steps (◘ Table 3.1; ▶ Chap. 10).

Errors in problem-solving can occur at every single step. Research on human problem-solving capabilities has identified several "cardinal errors" (◘ Table 3.2; Dörner 1996).

Errors in problem-solving are much more difficult to detect than execution failures, because slips and laps s can become apparent while a person is still ..ng. Mistakes, however, can pass unnoticed

◻ **Table 3.1** Five Steps in the organization of complex action

1. Preparedness
2. Analysis of the situation
– Gathering of information
– Building of mental models
3. Planning of actions
– Formulation of goals
– Risk assessment
– Planning of action sequences
– Decision-making
4. Execution of action
5. Review of effects
– Review of actions
– Revision of strategy
– Self-reflection

◻ **Table 3.2** "Cardinal errors" in problem-solving

Nobody suspects or anticipates any problems ("planning optimism")
Only information supporting initial assumptions are selected ("confirmation bias")
People skip the process of planning and defining goals and immediately start to act. This results in "repair-service behavior" or blind activism
Unawareness of conflicting goals
Side effects, long-term repercussions, and risks are not taken into account
The effects of actions are not re-evaluated on a regular basis

for lengthy periods and become apparent only after actions failed to achieve the intended outcome. Even if the issue of faulty planning is raised, the pros and cons of a plan can still be debated. Chapters 6 and 7 deal with errors on different levels of the outward and visible order of action in more detail.

3.3.3   Errors vs Violations

Up to now deviating behavior has been addressed from the perspective of individual cognitive processes. Most healthcare providers, however, do not act in isolation but within a regulated social context (i.e., organization, department). In this perspective, deviations from safe operating procedures, standards, or rules provided by the social context are called violations. Such deviations can be deliberate or erroneous. In contrast to error, *violations* intend the particular action executed, though not the possible bad consequences. While errors arise primarily from cognitive problems, violations are a motivational and goal issue. Violations do not originate from irrational or deficient psychological mechanisms but are caused by a regular psychological process (►Chap. 4): the choice between competing intentions. The intention to provide safe patient care is outweighed by stronger intentions: to save time, to prove competence, to go to bed as early as possible, etc. Also, it is possible that the rule is seen as unnecessary for "someone as experienced as I am" – this is no goal conflict but a matter of risk assessment. Violations are facilitated by a general learning principle: If safety regulations are equipped with a lot of "buffer" and violations are not immediately sanctioned, people learn via positive feedback that such regulations can be broken without consequence. If rules are broken and corners are cut whenever the opportunity arises, violations can become a personal habit (routine violations) and part of a working culture (Vaughan 1997). Violations are only seen as problematic if the behavior leads to patient harm. Whereas errors can be addressed by strategies of information management, violations require motivational as well as organizational remedies (e.g., by addressing issues of low work morale, poor supervisory example, failure to sanction noncompliance, etc.).

3.3.4 Active Errors vs Latent Conditions

For the understanding of how people contribute to critical situations and accidents a third distinction is important (Reason 1990, 1997): Errors threatening a patient's safety can be committed by the person treating the patient at the moment or they can be the result of decisions far away from the actual patient encounter (e.g., management, equipment manufacturer). These failures lie dormant within the system and can take considerable time until they contribute to an unwanted event. In summary, active errors and latent conditions differ in two points: (a) the place/level in an organization where they occur; and (b) the length of time that passes before human they show an adverse impact on safety.

3.3.4.1 Active Errors

Active errors are committed by people in close proximity to the human–system interface (e.g., when operating with medical equipment) or healthcare provider–patient interface. These interfaces are the so-called "sharp end" of an organization. Active errors are visible and trigger incidents or accidents directly, thus leading to immediate consequences. Because active errors are easily identified, they are the object of public scrutiny and often lead to sanctions of the "responsible" individual. Swapping drug ampules and injecting the wrong drug are clearly active errors on the anesthetist's side.

3.3.4.2 Latent Conditions

Safety critical decisions can be made at great distance to the patient from people who are neither in time nor space involved in patient care, who work at the "blunt end" of the organization. If these decisions threaten the safety of a system, they are called "latent conditions." These decisions are made at all levels of the organization: Top-level decisions as well as administrative regulations create conditions that facilitate accidents in the work place. Latent conditions can be hidden in structures (e.g., architecture of acute care facilities, medical equipment, and software) as well as in processes (e.g., operational procedures, staff selection and recruitment, qualification, human resource allocation) within

the healthcare system. In every complex system at any given moment a certain amount of latent conditions are hidden. It can take years or even decades until such decisions have consequences for a patient. Until that day, nobody would call them "error" – in hindsight they seem to have been wrong from the beginning.

A substantial body of scientific evidence has made it apparent that latent conditions pose the greatest threat to the safety of a system. Healthcare organizations are especially vulnerable because they have to allocate resources to two distinct goals: production and safety. Because financial resources are finite, short-term conflicts of interest between production (i.e., patient care) and safety often are solved in favor of economic goals. So, the management decision to allocate only one anesthesia provider to every OR without having a spare professional to supervise less experienced staff (e.g., the resident physician) is a latent condition for the errors that trigger the critical situation in the case report. Another latent condition for that case – and probably for many others – is the design of the drug ampules that facilitates swapping.

3.3.5 Errors in Teamwork

Teamwork is an essential component of acute patient care. A close relationship exists between good teamwork and successful performance in a high-stakes environment (Wheelan et al. 2003), whereas poor teamwork and communication have emerged as key factors responsible for the occurrence of medical errors (Barrett et al. 2001; Morey et al. 2002). One of the consistently found reasons for poor team formation and teamwork is the lack of a shared understanding about necessity and forms of teamwork. As a result, emerging conflicts among team members and a breakdown in communication can impair collaboration and result in an underutilization of available resources and the creation of new problems. In addition, team members may not share the same situational model and may be reluctant to question actions of teammates even when serious concerns about the adequacy of a diagnosis or treatment exist. The fact that neither the surgeon communicated the application of epinephrine-soaked swabs nor the anesthesia resident inquired about any unusual procedures on behalf of the surgeon is an indicator of a poor or nonexistent teamwork concept in that particular hospital. Errors in teamwork are addressed in detail in Chap. 11.

3.4 The Dynamics of Accident Causation

The adverse consequences of latent conditions are not revealed until active failures occur. Latent conditions remain hidden within the system for considerable time until they combine with other factors and local triggering events (e.g., active failures of individuals) to breach the defensive barriers of the system. In order to breach defenses, an interaction of active and latent failures, the unlikely combination of several contributing factors on many levels within an organization is required. Unfortunately, the combination of these diverse events is usually unforeseen and unforeseeable. The most famous model of accident causation was proposed by James Reason (1990, 1995, 2001) who compared accident causation with a projectile which originates in latent decisions in the higher levels of an organization. In order to cause an accident ("ac-

cident opportunity"), it has to penetrate all layers, each of them representing an organizational, environmental, or personal defense (◘ Fig. 3.3), as follows:

- Latent failures at the organizational level (e.g., faulty management decisions, fallible organizational processes, absence of a safety culture) are transmitted along organizational and departmental pathways to the work place and create local conditions that can promote the occurrence of errors.
- Psychological precursors of unsafe acts are generated by local conditions, personality, and the "psycho-logic" of human action regulation (▶ Chap. 4).
- Unsafe acts can occur due to active failures (e.g., slips, lapses, mistakes) or violations and combine with the upstream conditions.
- "Defenses in depth" fail (e.g., technical and nontechnical skills, teamwork, technical safety systems), leaving the system vulnerable to the trajectory of accident causation.

If the projectile penetrates several defense layers but is then blocked before it can trigger an accident (e.g., if a healthcare provider notices an ampule

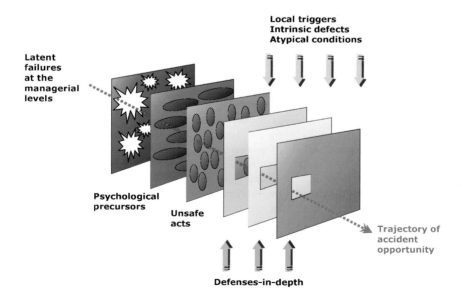

◘ **Fig. 3.3** The dynamics of accident causation. A complex interaction between latent failures, active errors, and a variety of local triggering events results in an accident. The trajectory of accident opportunity penetrates several layers in the defensive system. As all the loopholes have to overlay at a time for the accident to happen, the window of accident opportunity is very small. (Adapted from Reason 1990)

swap before he injects the wrong drug), an *incident* has occurred. Synonyms for incident found in literature are *critical incident* and *sentinel event*; thus, an incident is an unintended event which reduces, or could reduce, the safety margin for a patient. Incidents are like the basis of an iceberg, hidden below the surface (◘ Fig. 3.4). Accidents, in contrast, represent the tip of the incident iceberg: much more visible but much less in number than incidents.

Fortunately, few unsafe acts result in actual patient injury because system defenses can block the trajectory of accident opportunity. If each defense layer was impenetrable, an organization would have become error-proof. The reality, however, is different: Every single layer has loopholes which make the layer vulnerable. In addition, the defenses with their loopholes are not static but constantly in motion: At one time it is the healthcare professional who "has a bad day"; the next time equipment suddenly fails, etc. Due to this stochastic process, the overlay of loopholes is rendered possible and a limited window of accident opportunity is opened. All it then needs is an active failure by a healthcare professional and the accident will occur: For years the pharmaceutical company had produced two highly potent drugs with confusingly similar labels. For years the anesthesia department's policies allowed that both drugs could be placed next to each other in the anesthesia cart. Nothing ever happened. It was only when an inexperienced resident was unsupervised on duty, had a faulty treatment plan, worked under time pressure, and was inattentive that, in combination with these "upstream" factors, the accident occurred.

The remedial implication of the model is the notion that the psychological antecedents of unsafe acts (i.e., what goes on in the head of the healthcare professional) are extremely difficult to control. Distraction, inattention, forgetting, and loosing the big picture are entirely human reactions in a high-stakes working environment. Whereas active failures are unpredictable in their precise details and therefore hard to manage, latent conditions are, by definition, present within the organization before the incident or accident occurs. They represent the most suitable cases for treatment. Because nearly all incidents and accidents have organizational and systemic root causes, these latent factors are more amenable to diagnosis and remediation than the ephemeral tendencies of those working at the sharp end (Eagle et al. 1992; Gaba et al. 1987). Incidents, in addition, contain valuable information about latent failures within an organization. One of the major organizational responses in recent years has been to collect and analyze information from incidents and to take adequate measures in response. Incident-Reporting Systems (IRS) play a vital part in the quality improvement efforts of hospitals and healthcare organizations (► Chap. 15).

3.5   "The Nature of Error": in a Nutshell

- An error is a planned sequence of mental or physical activities that fails to achieve its intended outcome.
- Two distinct perspectives on error exist: consequential classifications ("What is the result?") and causal classifications ("Why did errors occur?"). The two perspectives give rise to two different approaches: the person-based approach and the system-based approach.
- Most cognitive scientists agree on the distinction of execution failure ("something was done wrongly") and planning failure ("something wrong was done").
- Errors are caused by execution failure and planning failure.
- Execution errors are usually skill-based errors. Planning failures can be rule-based errors as well as knowledge-based errors (errors in problem-solving).

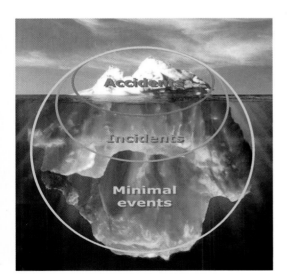

◘ **Fig. 3.4** The "incident iceberg"

- Violations are deviations from safe operating procedures, standards, or rules provided by the social context.
- Violations originate from regular psychological process: the choice between competing intentions.
- Errors committed actively by a person at the "sharp end" of the system are called "active failures." Errors created as the result of decisions far away from the actual patient encounter are called "latent failures" or "latent conditions."
- Latent conditions remain hidden within the system for considerable time until they combine with other factors and local triggering events to breach the defensive barriers of the system.
- An incident is an unintended event which reduces, or could reduce, the safety margin for a patient.
- Errors in teamwork occur as a result of poor team performance and inadequate communication.
- Whereas active failures are unpredictable in their precise details and therefore hard to manage, latent failures represent the most suitable cases for treatment because they are present within the organization before the accident occurs.

References

Barrett J, Gifford C, Morey J, Risser D, Salisbury M (2001) Enhancing patient safety through teamwork training. J Healthcare Risk Manag 21:57–65

Dekker S (2002) The field guide to human error investigations. Ashgate, Aldershot UK

Dekker S (2005) Ten questions about human error. A new view of human factors and system safety. Erlbaum, London UK

Dörner D (1996) The logic of failure. Recognizing and avoiding error in complex situations. Metropolitan Books, New York

Eagle CJ, Davies JM, Reason J (1992) Accident analysis of large-scale technological disasters applied to an anaesthetic complication. Can J Anaesth 39: 118–122

Freud S (1901) Psychopathology of everyday life. (Psychopatholgie des Alltagslebens) translated by A.A. Brill (1914), T. Fisher Unwin, London UK

Gaba DM, Maxwell M, DeAnda A (1987) Anesthetic mishaps: breaking the chain of accident evolution. Anesthesiology 66: 670–676

Kahneman D, Slovic P, Tversky A (1982) Judgement under uncertainty: heuristics and biases. Cambridge University Press, Cambridge UK

Morey JC, Simon R, Jay GD, Wears RL, Salisbury M, Dukes KA, Berns SD (2002) Error reduction and performance improvement in the emergency department through formal teamwork training: evaluation results of the MedTeams project. Health Serv Res 37:1553–1581

Norman D (1981) Categorization of action slips. Psychol Rev 88:1–15

Perrow C (1999) Normal accidents. Living with high-risk technologies. Princeton University Press, Princeton

Rasmussen J (1990) The role of error in organizing behaviour. Ergonomics 33:1185–1199

Reason J (1990) Human error. Cambridge University Press, Cambridge UK

Reason J (1995) Safety in the operating theatre, part 2: Human error and organisational failure. Curr Anaesth Crit Care 6:121–126

Reason J (1997) Managing the risk of organisational accidents. Ashgate, Aldershot

Reason J (2001) Understanding adverse events: the human factor. In: Vincent C (ed) Clinical risk management. Enhancing patient safety. Br Med J Books, London, pp 9–30

Senders JW, Moray NP (1991) Human error: cause, prediction, and reduction. Erlbaum, Hillsdale, New Jersey

Strauch B (2001) Investigating human error: incidents, accidents, and complex systems. Ashgate, Aldershot UK

Vaughan D (1997) The Challenger launch decision: risky technology, culture, and deviance at NASA. University of Chicago Press, Chicago

Wheelan SA, Burchill CN, Tilin F (2003) The link between teamwork and patients' outcomes in intensive care units. Am J Crit Care 12:527–534

4   The Psychology of Human Action

4.1   Case Study

It was 2 a.m. and two police officers were conducting routine traffic control. Suddenly, the driver of a van started to shoot at one of the police officers. Being protected by her bulletproof vest, the officer was shot only in right her arm. The second police officer immediately opened fire and shot the attacker in the chest and abdomen. Two ambulances and an emergency physician[1] were dispatched and arrived 8 min later at the shooting site. On arrival, EMS found a 28-year-old female police officer, alert and oriented, who was bleeding from the brachial artery. She complained of complete loss of sensation and strength in her right arm. No other injuries were found. The paramedics applied a pressure dressing and the bleeding stopped. The blood pressure was 95/50 mmHg and the heart rate was 90 bpm. Because the physician was busy inserting an intravenous line in the police officer, he asked one of the paramedics to evaluate the injured driver who was lying next to his car. The attacker was tachypneic, obtunded, and had weak peripheral pulses. At the physician's orders, an oxygen mask and an intravenous line were placed and volume resuscitation was initiated. The police officer was transferred to the ambulance and the physician was finally able to direct his attention to the attacker who had become unresponsive. On examination, he found several bullet entry points in the chest and abdomen. The central pulse was weak and fast. The patient was emergently intubated. No breath sounds were appreciated on auscultation on the side of the bullet holes. Cutaneous emphysema on the same side developed rapidly. The patient was positioned for emergency thoracocentesis and a chest tube was placed successfully. An outward rush of air and blood confirmed correct chest tube placement. By now, about 2000 ml of crystalloid solution had been infused but the blood pressure was still very low. Boluses of epinephrine were repeatedly administered to maintain circulation while the patient was being transported to the hospital. The patient continued to remain unstable despite aggressive resuscitation. On arrival to the Emergency Department, a hemopneumothorax and massive intraabdominal hemorrhage were diagnosed. De-

spite immediate surgical intervention, the patient died in the operating room. The police officer also underwent surgery during the same night. She recovered rapidly but maintained a neurological deficit in her right arm.

An emergency physician is confronted with two patients, one lightly and the other severely injured following a shooting: on the one hand, a hemodynamically stable female police officer with an arterial bleeding as a result of a perforating injury of the brachial artery; on the other hand, the male aggressor with a shock due to massive intraabdominal and intrathoracic blood loss. Against all medical urgency the emergency physician begins to treat the lightly injured person. Without having examined both of his patients and then treating them according to medical urgency, he spends almost a quarter of an hour with the police officer, delegating the treatment of the multiply injured patient to the paramedic before he takes care of that patient himself. At this time the physician knows about the injury pattern and the resulting vital threat for the patient. Nevertheless, he decides not to address this problem personally. Once he takes care he decides to spend additional time with the patient on site ("stay-and-play"). Patients with perforating injuries of the chest are one of the groups who might benefit from a rapid transport with a minimum of treatment done on site to the next trauma center ("scoop-and-run").

4.2   The "Psycho-logic" of Cognition, Emotions, and Motivation

The goal of all medical efforts is the safe treatment of patients. Right from its start modern medicine has claimed to be able to perform a rationally explainable therapy at any time. That claim implies a model of the "logic of behavior" in which behavior is always a reaction to the situational cues. Human behavior therefore would be exclusively determined by logical reasoning (◘ Fig. 4.1a). Problem-solving would aim at the best possible solution for the problem, nothing more. Apparently, the emergency physician's management in the case report does not follow this model: In obvious contrast to all medi-

---

1 The case report is taken from a European physician-based emergency medical system where a specially qualified "emergency physician" is brought to the site of accident and joins Emergency Medical Service in taking care of the patient.

cal necessity, he first and foremost takes care of the lightly injured person. We can only speculate about the reasons for his behavior. It might be because the patient was a victim of a shooting, because she carried a police officers uniform and was accompanied by a worried colleague, or simply because she was young and female. Whatever reason might be the true one, an uninvolved observer might get the impression that a couple of "illogical" factors governed the physician's behavior, and this impression indeed might be true: There is no human behavior exclusively governed by rational thinking. Human behavior always results from a complex interplay of cognition, emotions, and motivations; therefore, it seems more appropriate in this context to talk about a "psycho-logic" of human behavior (☐ Fig. 4.1b).

The "psycho-logic" of this interaction between reasoning, emotion, and motivation governs all our actions. It is Janus-faced, though: On the one hand, it enables humans to cope with complex and dynamic environments such as anesthesia, intensive care, and emergency medicine. Emotion-based decision-making is a valuable resource, especially under stress and time pressure (▶ Chap. 9). On the other hand, the "psycho-logic" helps to explain why the emergency physician did not stay "coolheaded" and did not stick to the ATLS protocol or any other medical guidelines: Unnoticed by himself, his decision-making was influenced by his emotions and his personal needs just as much as by rational reasoning. Simply to state that the physician's decisions were "illogical" or "irrational" and that he in-stead should have been guided by "mere facts" does not address the issue fully.

4.3 Principles of Human Behavior

In order to better understand the above roughly sketched "psycho-logic" of human emotion and motivation that we will explain in detail later in this chapter, we need to clear ground by introducing some basic presumptions about human behavior. These presumptions rely on the work of action psychologists (Dörner 1999; Hacker et al. 1982; Miller et al. 1960).

4.3.1 Bio-psycho-social Foundations of Behavior

Humans are *biological beings* who use their mind and body to meet biological needs. As a result of their mental capacities humans are "*psychological beings*" as well. They perceive their surrounding world in a subjective way and intend to meet their subjective psychological needs. In addition, humans are "*social beings*" who have to cooperate in communities in order to survive. The parallel evolution of biological, psychological, and social processes lead to a way of reasoning and acting ("action regulation") which is characteristic for the "bio-psycho-social-entity" human being (Kleinhempel et al. 1996; Brenner 2002):

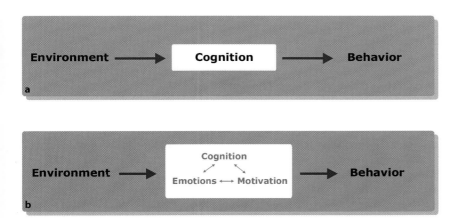

☐ **Fig. 4.1** Despite the widespread belief that logical reasoning alone guides human decision-making in response to environmental stimuli (**a**), reality favors the notion that the "psycho-logic" of an interaction between cognition, emotion, and intention has to be stressed (**b**)

- *Biologically* the human brain, the peripheral nervous system, and the human body as a whole are the medium of action regulation. Human behavior is based on the phylogenetically determined structure of neuronal processes, a fact which becomes quite obvious if, for example, perception (► Chap. 5) and the stress reaction (► Chap. 9) are considered.
- From a *psychological point of view* cognition and speech are the main tools for human behavior. Speech acts are the result of social relationships as well as the most important instrument to regulate these relationships. Furthermore, human cognition is irretrievably connected with emotions and motivations.
- The individual psychological development is inseparably connected to the *social* development, the sociogenesis. Human beings are essentially bound to living in groups; therefore, they are biologically oriented to charity and cooperation, psychologically to an information management by means of language and communication, and are socially dependent upon being integrated into a stable social community.

4.3.2   Action

Action is conditional on external demands and internal psychological processes. The range of possible options the emergency physician could have chosen was limited by characteristics of the emergency situation: the site of accident; the kind of injury; the pathophysiological state the patient was in; and the available technical and personal resources. They all were fixed determinants at the time the emergency medical team arrived on site.

At the same time, however, his behavior was also determined by his knowledge and also by the thoughts, feelings, and (hidden) intentions he brought with him or that he developed as a result of his first assessment of the situation. Because human action results from reasoning, emotions, and intentions in interaction with a given situation, we can speak of the "psycho-logic" of human action.

Action is intentional and goal-directed. Psychology understands action as a sequence of behaviors which are aimed at achieving a goal. An action in the psychological sense is "the smallest delimitable unit of consciously controlled activity" (Hacker 1986). Actions are goal-directed mental processes initiated and sustained by needs. In this broader sense actions are not only behavioral responses or a speech act by which we intend to influence our environment. Mental operations, such as planning or imagination, are regarded as actions as well if they aim at a goal.

Action can be described in terms of a control loop. Theoretical models of human behavior assume that mental processes can be described as control loops (Miller et al. 1960). Actions are oriented at an anticipated goal or set point: You keep on doing something until you have achieved your goal. Cognitive processes alternate between hierarchically structured goals (► Chap. 7). The mental structure the emergency physician developed when treating the severely injured patient showed one main goal (to keep the patient alive) which in turn could be divided into several partial or intermediate goals (to place i.v. lines, to intubate, to insert a chest tube). That way a hierarchical and sequential order of thought is built which is sustained until the main goal is accomplished (Hacker 1986).

Action is a result of information processing. The regulation of human action can be understood as information processing (Klix 1971; Dörner 1976). In this view, the concepts of motivation, emotion, and cognition all describe processes of information processing at different levels of the human cognitive system.

"Emotion," "intention," and "reasoning" constitute an autonomous system. Without being aware of the fact, the emergency physician's interaction with his environment is influenced by his emotions, intentions, and his thought processes. Our conscious self is not always aware of this influence. It even seems not to be necessary for the regulation of action; therefore, we can talk of an autonomous regulation of human action.

Human action is embedded in a social context. It is an essential characteristic of the psychological idea of "action" that individual actions always are "embedded" in a social context. Our individual goals always have a "social side." What we think or do serves our individual needs as well as our social relations. Keeping social relations stable and productive is a powerful social need. Maybe one of the reasons for the privileged treatment of the police officer was the desire to show respect to the executive powers of government.

Action can only be described on the level of visible behavior. The emergency management of the physician consists of a multitude of actions which we can observe and describe accordingly. We can make statements about what he did and when it happened. The external, visible organization of human action is called exactly that: organization of action.

Of course, we even can form our personal opinion about the appropriateness of some of his actions based on what we see; however, we cannot know why he did what he did. The internal powers which drive visible behavior stay hidden. So some of the more puzzling questions will have to remain unresolved: Why did he choose to handle the emergency the way he did? Did he know what he was doing? Did he realize he was violating existing treatment protocols? Of course, we can apply theory to reality and try to find answers to theses questions. The theory of human action regulation conceptualizes how cognition, motivation, and emotion are integrated in controlling human behavior in complex and dynamic domains of reality.

Action is a result of autonomous, internal information processing following control loops, embedded in social context, driven by the situation and internal needs. From these principles the following postulates can be derived which are helpful in understanding errors in an acute care setting:

– *Also errors follow the "psycho-logic" of human action regulation.* Every action is based on an intention, is done "on purpose" – even those that turn out to have been a mistake. From the medical point of view the physician has committed an error because he took care of the slightly injured police officer instead of the multiply injured patient; however, this does not imply that the physician explicitly wanted to harm this patient. Only the intentions governing his actions did not include the health and safety of the multiple injured patient. The delayed beginning of the medical management was caused by the fact that other intentions (such as caring for the police officer) were stronger. If there are competing intentions, the autonomous system has to choose between them. The main criterion for that choice is not necessarily an external one (the patient's injuries). Fulfilling internal needs (e.g., being friendly with a young woman) can be as important or more important for us. Of course,

the physician's decision was wrong from a medical point of view, yet this treatment error is caused by a regular psychological process – the choice between competing intentions.

– This fact can be broadly generalized: Errors do not originate from irrational or deficient psychological mechanisms but from useful psychological process. Errors and mistakes follow, just as correct actions do, the laws of the "psychologic" of human action regulation.

– *Errors can be avoided.* Despite being rooted in normal psychological processes, errors are not an inescapable fate which we humbly must accept. Circumstances which promote and enable error can be analyzed in advance (▸ Chap. 3). Working conditions as well as organizational structures can be designed to avoid errors. Conscious effort and efficient teamwork can overcome errors resulting from the "psycho-logic" of individual regulation.

Before we describe in greater detail those psychological processes which play a vital role in human action regulation, we summarize the characteristics of human action as follows:

– Human action can only be understood from the "psycho-logic" of human "action regulation."
– Human action is the sum total of biological, psychological, and social processes.
– Human action is influenced by the human history of development (phylogenesis), the individual development (ontogenesis) and the "cultural heritage."
– Human action is intentional and goal-directed.
– At the visible level human action can be described in terms of behavior and activities. The underlying "autonomous" processes (emotions, motivations, cognition) cannot be observed.
– Action can be understood in terms of information processing.
– Human action serves individual and social needs
– Erroneous decisions, too, are made in order to meet needs; therefore, they are not "irrational" but result from normal decision-making process.

4.4   Motivation

4.4.1   From Needs to Intention

4.4.1.1   Requirements, Needs, and Motives

Every human organism experiences differences between actual and nominal physiological conditions which it tries to balance. As soon as internal regulation mechanisms are no longer able to regulate the physiological requirements they are experienced as needs (❏ Fig. 4.2; Bischof 1985). Hunger is such a need and is based upon a requirement for nutriments which cannot be met by the body's own supplies. The perception of a need ("I'm hungry") triggers action. In analogy to the physiological needs, humans have social and "informational" needs as well (e.g., knowledge, proximity, safety; Dörner 1999). They are based on a need for information about the actual state of the environment, the need for social contact and acceptance by others and the need for being capable of influencing the environment.

A *motive* is a need in connection with a goal which is apt to meet this particular need (Bischof 1985). In other words, a motive is a need which knows about an adequate goal. However, for any need there may be several adequate goals from which we can chose, depending on the situation:

You can relieve your hunger by choosing to go to the cafeteria or by taking an apple out of your pocket.

All human activities arise from motives which in turn develop into behavior. In what follows the term "intention" is used as a collective term for all of the various terms used to denote action tendencies which are known colloquially as "wish," "aim," and "intention" (Dörner 1984; Heckhausen and Kuhl 1984).

4.4.1.2   Intentions

Intentions are a blend of different motives. When looking more closely at the satisfaction of needs it becomes apparent that people tend to meet several needs at the same time, and that therefore several motives must be active at the same time. For example, if you decide to go to the cafeteria you could be doing it because you indeed are hungry but also might want to go there because you want to meet colleagues, chat, and listen to relevant news. This kind of action goal ("to go to the cafeteria") which is determined by multiple motives is called an intention; thus, an intention is a "motive blend" that consists of many different motives (❏ Fig. 4.2). Intentions are permanently formed – depending on the actual physiological and psychological state

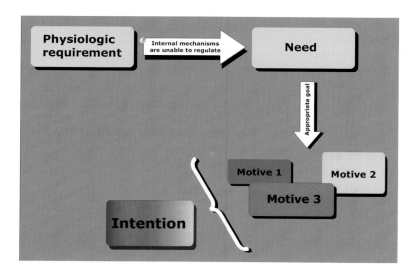

❏ **Fig. 4.2** From need to intention

of the organism – and compete with each other (Dörner 1999):

> — Humans have physiological and psychological needs.
> — Needs which are connected with an adequate goal are called motives.
> — Action goals which are determined by multiple motives are called intentions.

A Solution to the Competition of Intentions
Abraham Maslow (1943) proposed the well-known theory that needs are organized within a hierarchical structure. This structure he believed consisted of five successive layers of needs. Within this model, which can be depicted as a pyramid the most basic *physiological* needs lie at the bottom, whereas *psychological* needs (such as self-realization, concerns about safety) lie at the top. According to Maslow's theory these "higher" needs can only be met when the subordinate level successfully has been dealt with. If this is not the case, then there is always a danger that "lower" needs (such as the need to sleep) have a much stronger influence on decisions than, for example, considerations about patient safety. It is not a rare event in anesthesia that during nighttime the patient's "NPO time" is not waited for in order "to get on with the operation" and then be able to go to bed; however, this hierarchy of needs is not completely plausible: We all know of situations where we really were hungry or felt the urgency to go to a restroom but instead kept on going because the patient needed our full attention. At all times needs compete with each other, but the order of execution is not defined by their place in a hierarchy – a different mechanism comes into effect. For this mechanism (a) the selection in dependence from importance and chance of success, and (b) the idea of a shielding of the current intention has been advocated (Dörner 1999; Kuhl 1983): every intention is weighted in a multiplicative way by importance, on one side, and the subjective estimate of the manageability of the intention at a given time, on the other side. If something is completely unimportant or if there is no chance at all of being successful, no action will be initiated (weight = 0). It is always the intention with the highest weighting which will be executed. This way it is always one intention which comes out on top and inhibits other intentions. If there is only

a certain window of opportunity for the execution of an intention, its weight increases over time: urgency adds to the weight of an intention. Therefore, also less important intentions may get a chance, or they may permanently fall behind (Dörner 1999). The fact that seemingly unimportant tasks, such as phone calls, documentation, and other "trifles," constantly slip our mind has less to do with forgetting than with the dynamics of intentions: there are always some which are even more important. If this happens in everyday life, the consequences of this competition of intentions are merely annoying (for example, if you receive a dunning letter because you forgot to pay a bill). In critical situations, however, the weight of an intention can become a life and death issue. This is especially the case if non-case-related intentions, such as the maintenance of a feeling of competence, become stronger than the intention to solve the acute medical problem.

4.4.2 "Overall Competence Assessment" and the Need for Control

Every time an intention is executed specific motives are met. Parallel to this there is another strong and independent need which is embodied in every intention: the need to experience competence. Psychologists call that the need for control. This means that we have an existential need to be able to influence our environment according to own goals (e.g., Bandura 1977; Flammer 1990; Dörner 1999). We want to know with certainty what is happening around us, and we long for clarity of facts and certainty about future developments.

The internal overall competence assessment appears subjectively either as the feeling of measuring up to the situation, or as a feeling of helplessness and fear, as the case may be.

"Helplessness" as the subjectively felt incapability to influence the environment adequately poses an existential threat to the human psyche (Seligman 1975).

The current state of competence is perceived as a feeling of competence. Once this feeling starts to decrease because the impression of incompetence arises and one feels insecure and no longer capable, the motive of control is activated. Due to its inherent strength, it very often "wins" against other motives. In consequence, behavior is no longer governed by explicit patient-related goals but instead by the subconscious drive to regain the feeling of competence.

— The concepts of a motive of control and a need for competence describe the existential need of every human being to achieve clarity about the actual state of the situation, and certainty about future developments and the capability to influence the environment in accordance with one's own goals.
— The feeling of competence describes the perception of ones own capability to control circumstances.
— The need for competence becomes the driving force in decision-making when the feeling of competence is threatened by circumstances.
  Emergency situations in a high-stakes medical environments are examples of highly dynamic and opaque situations where people tend to have great difficulties in controlling their environment. Only few options are available. As a result of the perceived inability to control a situation, the feeling of competence can be threatened quite strongly. If this is the case, reducing the feeling of incapability and at regaining control will become an intention of its own. How successful this attempt will be depends on knowledge, skills, and confidence in one's own resources.
— Behavior in a complex and dynamic environment is also always directed at reducing indeterminacy by gaining control over the situation.

4.4.2.1 Wrong Assessment of Competence

The confidence in our own skills or capability is quite often misleading. Especially in complex situations, the subjective assessment of competence and the actual control over the situation can differ strongly. For example, if somebody *overestimates* his or her ability to cope with an emergency situation, he or she is more likely to take higher risks because of the (wrong) feeling of being up to the task. If someone *underestimates* the own competence, he or she will tend to act defensively and refrain from taking possibly helpful and necessary steps.

4.4.2.2 "Competence Protecting Rationality"

Complexity in combination with small prospect of success can diminish the feeling of competence and activate the need for control. Behavior will be directed upon quickly satisfying the competence motive: People start to do things they know well or which would be successful under comparable circumstances. But maybe they are busier regaining their feeling of competence than to actually solve the patient's problem. In such a state, people only want to receive information which does not confuse them further – doubt or contradictions would mean an additional threat to the feeling of competence. Therefore, only information which confirms the current model of the situation is taken into account ("confirmation bias"; ▶ Chap. 6).

If apparent failure adds to the uncertain situation, the protection of the feeling of competence will become the dominant motive. Actions are chosen not for the patient's sake but for our own defense. The examination of the critical situation on objective grounds becomes secondary. This *competence protecting rationality* (Strohschneider 1999) leads to "errors" – wrong actions from the patient safety perspective, "rational" with regard to a short-term protection of competence (◘ Fig. 4.3).

4.5 Emotions

In addition to motives, emotions play an important role in human action regulation.

4.5.1 What Are Emotions and Feelings?

The general understanding of "emotions" is that of something independent from rational thinking and experienced on a "gut" level. In some circles of academic medicine it even seems to be a worthy goal to strive for an "emotion-free" medical management; however, emotions can be conceptualized as a form of information processing, as a kind of "thinking alongside conscious thinking". In this perspective, emotions constitute a subconscious, rapid and holistic assessment of the current situation or event. This assessment is very quick and automated and can process much more information than conscious perception (▶ Chap. 5). This "integrated situational assessment" always includes a hedonic component (pleasure/aversion) and is accompanied by physiological activation (◨ Fig. 4.4; e.g., Scherer and Ekman 1984; Dörner 1999). The situational assess- ment (with activation and pleasure/aversion) is experienced as feeling.

If the emotional and cognitive assessment of a situation differ from each other, we tend to believe that our mind and our gut contradict each other.

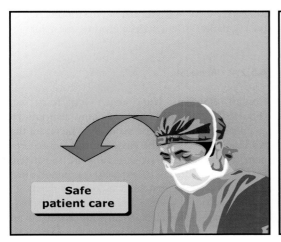
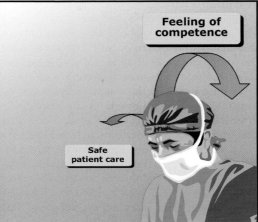

◨ **Fig. 4.3** Competence protecting rationality. Normally, safe patient care is the main focus of every healthcare provider (*left*); however, when faced with seemingly unsolvable problems (*right*), healthcare providers will try to protect or regain the feeling of competence by any means. As a result, the competence motive, rather than safe patient care, may become the dominant motive

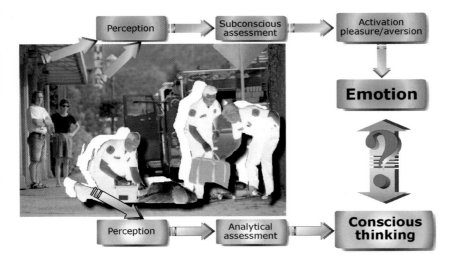

◨ **Fig. 4.4** Emotions as integrated situational assessment. Whereas conscious thinking assesses the emergency situation analytically, the emotional assessment processes more information and will provide the situation with its specific emotional "coloring"

But the reason is simply that emotions use different (and more) information than consciuous reasoning.

As soon as they are felt, emotions can be further processed just like any other perceptional data (▶ Chap. 5). The source of emotions can be analyzed and their intensity can be changed by means of self-instruction.

Feelings do not only accompany behavior, they also can become the goal of action. For example, a decision may be delayed because we want to avoid the feeling of failure or an action propagated because we already anticipate the feeling of success.

In situations were the cognitive ressources are overstrained humans switch to an emotionally driven style of action (Spering et al. 2005). It is characteristic for that regulation style that the emotional assesment is no longer cross-checked with conscious analysis of the facts. Swift and risky solutions are preferred and there is no room for reflection. The problem is oversimplified and solutions are considered satisfactory if they "feel good". This in turn leads to obviously inadequate decisions if the (subconscious) goal is the maintenance of a feeling of competence or the avoidance of negative emotions.

4.5.2   Emotions and Human Action Regulation

Apart from being holistic situational assessments, emotions can be further conceptualized as part of a regulation system which takes two relations of an organism to reality into account: the *unpredictability* of the environment (uncertainty) and the *estimated degree of efficiency* to tackle problems (competence; Belavkin and Ritter 2003). This regulation system modulates parameters which influence the selection of actions and their execution (Dörner 1999). Among the parameters influenced by emotions are:
— The general preparedness for action (arousal)
— The thresholds for selection of behavior and of perceptions
— The degree of resolution of a cognitive process
— The degree of externalization

It is an everyday experience that the way a task is performed greatly depends on the emotional state of a person: The execution of a task done even-tempered or angrily can look completely different. An "angry" mode of action therefore would be characterized by an increase in arousal, a decrease in the degree of resolution to guarantee quick action, little anticipation, an incomplete recall of possible modes of action, and a rough planning and hence a hasty action. In a way, emotions give cognitions their "coloring" – in both moods of the example, planning is the form of cognition, but the modulation of the regulation parameters determines the color.

4.5.2.1   Arousal

Certain emotions (e.g., anger, joy, fear) can "booster" people. This phenomenon, also known as unspecific sympathetic syndrome, increases the readiness to explore the environment and to prepare for action. The sense organs are sensitized, muscle tone is increased, and heart rate, blood pressure and breathing frequency increase (▶ Chap. 9). Other emotions, such as mourning or hopelessness, reduce arousal. Normally the chaos of an emergency situation is associated with an arousal.

4.5.2.2   Degree of Resolution

Depending on the emotional situation a cognitive process (e.g., perception, thinking) will run with a different "degree of resolution" and hence with varying accuracy. By "degree of resolution" we mean the level of differentiation and discrimination among dimensions of perception or cognition. "Judging the facts" can happen in a detailed, scrutinizing way or by simply taking in the most salient features of the situation. The resolution level is dependent on emotions (via the arousal), the importance of the situation, and (subjective) time pressure. The consequence for the clinician lies in the fact that the influence of our feelings can provide us with either a superficial ("over inclusive") or a detailed picture of the situation. For example, aversion against a task will reduce the degree of resolution; perception will be "coarse-grained" and the execution superficial.

4.5.2.3   Selection of Behavior: Concentration

Emotions influence the frequency of changes in intention and thus the intensity of action: A strong arousal increases the threshold of selection at which a motive can replace the leading motive and thus become the action-guiding motive. If the threshold for selection is high, people totally stick to a task without being distracted. If the threshold increases further, it can reach a point where people no longer are able to react to external triggers: neither monitor alarms nor requests from team members can penetrate this "wall of attention," and as a result "doc goes solo." The same can be seen in our case report: As long as his concern for the police officer was high, the emergency physician may have considered only her case and "forgot" the second patient for some time. As stated previously, however, this was not an issue of a faulty memory but of competing intentions. In contrast, when people feel helpless or have the impression that they are too incompetent to tackle a problem, the selection threshold is decreased. In the hope to bring about change they will try whatever comes to mind.

4.5.2.4 Externalization of Behavior

Emotions influence the extent to which attention focuses on external events or on internal cognitive processes (reflection, planning). This will have a major impact on how much a person is "driven" by events. For example, angry persons will focus on the stimulus of their anger (and how to get rid of it) rather than focus their thinking on a problem: Shouting at people instead of asking questions may be one result of externalization.

4.6 Thinking

"Thinking" encompasses all higher cognitive functions which govern human behavior at the level of planning, expectations, and decision-making. Although very powerful in its operations, thinking is a restricted resource because it basically uses language and thus operates in a sequential mode: People can only think one thought at the time.

4.6.1 Knowledge and Schemata

The material people use to think with is their knowledge; however knowledge is not stored in unrelated bits of information but instead in small meaning-ful entities, so-called schemata (Selz 1913; Bartlett 1932). Schemata are a cluster of structured data which are stored in the neuronal network of the brain. They basically contain information which is based on the regularity of the world and personal experiences with the environment (Cohen 1989). Schemata underlie every aspect of human knowledge and skills: They give structure to sensory impression (*sensory knowledge*), encode the generic information about our routine dealings with the environment (know-how; *procedural knowledge*), and represent concepts for the description of objects, facts, and procedures ("know what"; *declarative knowledge*). In addition, schemata can contain expectations about regularities or changes in the environment: we perceive a situation not only on the basis of momentary stimulus patterns, but also based on expectations we have about the possible developments of the situation (*horizon of expectations*; ► Chap. 8). Sometimes we even "see" or "hear" things that we expect, such as a confirmation of an order, just because we expect to see or hear it. Because schemata have this interpretative and inferential function, predictable biases in remembering can be expected: There is a strong tendency to bring presented material in accordance with the general character of previous personal experiences. This characteristic feature of schemata plays a vital role in the way human perception works (► Chap. 5).

> Schemata are high-order, generic cognitive structures that underlie all aspects of knowledge and skill.

The procedural knowledge which is encoded in schemata is the basis for any human behavior. It consists of "if-then" cycles which repeatedly are compared with expectations about the situation and outcome of actions (*action schemata*): "Given situation A, action B will be taken and situation C (or something similar to that) will be the outcome." If many action schemata are strung together, this is called a *behavioral program* or *script* (Schank and Abelson 1977). People store a range of successful cognitive and behavioral routines as behavioral programs. These are sequences of steps of perception, classification, assessment, and decision. The whole chain of a behavioral program can be "fired" effortlessly in a relevant situation, or the sequence of steps can be adapted and modified according to situational demands. Among typical behavioral programs common to clinicians, nurses and paramedics are the placement of i.v. lines and orotracheal intubation.

4.6.2   Memory

With this rough sketch of schemata we have already described a simple model of the human memory (overview in Dörner 1984; Dörner 1999): Knowledge always consists of schemata stored in neuronal networks. It operates through the interrelation of sensory perception with motor programs and motivation as behavioral program. The memory items are connected in an associative way which allows for a very quick retrieval of relevant information.

As a result of theses interrelations, the human memory is *active* and not like a computer, where information is stored on a hard disk and retrieved complete and unchanged whenever needed. Instead, the concepts stored in memory are constantly rearranged and re-organized depending on the actual needs and the general circumstances; therefore, memories are a reconstruction rather than a factual recall.

When and in which form information is recollected depends mainly on past interactions with the world, as well as on emotions and the current situation. Habits, too, can influence memory. Schemata which are activated more often are more readily available and can be faster reactivated.

Thinking is only possible if people can compare their current experiences with previous ones; therefore, they have to be able to access both the long-lasting information of the long-term memory as well as items of sensory perception which are only momentarily available. The memory items which are being active at a certain moment and with which thinking works are termed "working memory" (the previous term was "short-term memory"). The working memory is not a distinct functional entity but instead the description of the momentarily active schemata. In order to encode experiences in the long-term memory, humans are endowed with a "protocol feature" of the events. This protocol memory is more than a log file: It keeps track of the ongoing mental operations and filters out important and relevant details. "Important and relevant" is everything that is successful or pleasurable and everything unsuccessful and painful. With these main selection criteria

the memory, too, does not function in a machine-logic way but rather "psycho-logically": Only those events are transferred from the protocol memory to long-term-memory which were involved with the successful fulfillment of needs or a strong increase in the strength of needs. The selection by only those few criteria is sufficient to considerably broaden the human repertoire of experiences and actions. What is irrelevant is soon forgotten.

4.6.3   Thinking As Process

Thinking is the interpreting and order establishing processing of information (e.g., Selz 1913/22; Guilford 1967; Klix 1971; Dörner 1976, 1999). We see that in basic functions, such as recognition and identification (▶ Chap. 5), assessment, or conceptualization, the drawing of conclusions, planning, and decision-making, or, more generally stated: problem-solving. These cognitive operations are done with the help of schemata which are constructed, rearranged, amended, and brought intro relation.

Thinking without language can consist in the associative concatenation of schemata according to their emotional closeness. *Analytical* thinking, however, is dependent on language. As a consequence, analytical thinking is a slow, sequential working mode as only one thought at a time can be thought (▶ Chap. 6). In addition, attention is required (▶ Chap. 8), this source, too, being limited in a medical emergency. Language-based thinking operates with terms. The fact that knowledge can be broken down into higher-order and lower-order structures is essential for the organization of knowledge (Klix 1971). Often associative and analytical thinking work hand in hand, for example, when finding solutions to complex problems: An idea emerges from an association and is then analyzed.

4.6.4   Self-reflection: Thinking About Thinking

Thinking can be applied to itself: We can analyze and assess our own thought process. If the emergency physician from the case report asks himself after his mission in the field "How did I reach my decisions? Why did I manage the case the way I did?" he has the chance to clarify at least some of the motives for his actions. This might help him to gain insight into his very personal "psycho-logic" of decision-making and action. If he reflects on the strategy he applied to the initially successful (albeit delayed) management of the multiply injured patient, he could identify *successful* behavioral patterns. However, it is virtually impossible to attain complete and exhaustive self-awareness; therefore, clinicians will sometimes be surprised by their own reactions and behavior and will have to struggle with the painful question in the aftermath of an emergency: "What on earth drove me to behave that particular way?" This kind of thinking and reflection ("re-flecting thinking onto itself") is an essential learning opportunity in complex working environments where it may be too costly to learn by trial and error. Self-assessment (metacognition) enables people to better understand the basis on which good and bad decisions were made and to find starting points for change.

4.7 Hazardous Attitudes

One of the patterns which repeatedly can be found when accidents are analyzed for their root causes is the concurrence of a potentially dangerous initial situation with an inadequate attitude towards safety and risk on behalf of the acting subject. These attitudes illustrate quite accurately the above-mentioned "psycho-logic" of human behavior with its interaction of cognition, emotion, and motivation: Attitudes can be seen as a blend of situation assessment (cognition), emotional response (emotion), and an impulse for action (motivation; Hovland and Rosenberg 1960). The cognitions in an atti-

tude have strong emotional overtones which make it often difficult to verbalize them and as a result difficult to access for consciousness and reflection. Furthermore, they are driven by motives – certain attitudes do not come out of the clear blue sky but fit to our motives. Five typical hazardous attitudes can be distinguished which account for response patterns not guided by patient safety (Jensen 1995). Each of them emphasizes a different motive:

- The *macho-attitude*: courageous actions are supposed to strengthen the own feeling of competence (especially if other team members watch).
- If an *anti-authoritarian attitude* is adopted, people want to defy regulations because they cannot stand the feeling of being controlled by other people.
- *Impulsivity* as a dominating attitude is grounded in the inability to generate several options before taking action. To impulsive persons, "just do something, quick" seems superior to moments of inactivity and reflection.
- If somebody never has experienced an accident, they may tend to regard themselves as basically *invulnerable*. This in turn entails a tendency for risky decisions.
- A feeling of *resignation* makes people give up quickly when faced with difficulties. The feeling of competence is so low that no action is taken. Help is expected from others only.

▪ Table 4.1 shows the hazardous attitudes and some "antidote thoughts" meant to counteract them by introducing positive mental responses to each situation. The hazardous thought is "substituted" by the safe thought. Once people discover that they

▪ **Table 4.1** The five hazardous attitudes and their antidote. (From Jensen 1995)

Attitude	Thoughts in emergency situation	"Antidote"
Macho	I can do it, I'll show you!	Showing off is foolish
Anti-authority	Don't you tell me what I'm supposed to do	Stick to the rules, they are meant for everybody
Impulsivity	I have to act now – there's no time	Not so fast – think first
Invulnerability	Nothing will ever happen to me	It can happen to me
Resignation	What's the use of even trying?	I always can make a difference, so I'm not helpless

are having hazardous thoughts, they should say the antidote to themselves (Jensen 1995); however, the main limitation of this approach is that it demands self-reflection: It works only if people are able and willing to assess their own thoughts. Unfortunately, these hazardous attitudes most often come from a lack of reflective self-assessment. In this case patient safety can only be enhanced if other team members are in a position which allows them to address other persons' attitudes with constructive criticism (▶ Chap. 11). This may serve as an external trigger for reflection. As the attitude component of human judgment is highly responsive to training intervention, it should become part of a safety-oriented organizational culture to implement educational tools to foster the development of risk-avoiding attitudes (▶ Chap. 15).

4.8   "Principles of Human Behavior": in a Nutshell

- Human behavior does not strictly follow logical arguments but instead a "psycho-logic."
- "Psycho-logic" implies that the interaction with the environment can only be described as an interplay of cognition, emotion, and motivation.
- This action regulation is partly autonomous, i.e., a process without conscious decisions.
- Every action is motivated and is meant to meet one or several needs. Apart from basic needs that secure existence (physiological needs, safety), there are social (proximity, affiliation) and informational (competence, curiosity, aesthetics) motives for action.
- Emotions represent an integrated situational assessment. They are experienced as feelings. Emotions can be described as a modulation of the parameters of action regulation (arousal, selection, resolution level, and degree of externalization).
- Cognition is basically language-based operating with memory contents organized in schemata.
- Safety-relevant attitudes originate from an interaction of cognition, emotion, and motivation.

References

Bandura A (1977) Self-efficacy mechanisms in human agency. Am Psychol 37:122–147

Bartlett FC (1932) Remembering. Cambridge University Press, Cambridge UK

Belavkin RV, Ritter FE (2003) The use of entropy for analysis and control of cognitive models. Proc Fifth Int Conf on Analysis and Control of Cognitive Modeling. Universitaets-Verlag, Bamberg, pp 75–80

Bischof N (1985) Das Rätsel Ödipus [The riddle of Oedipus]. Piper, Munich Germany

Brenner HP (2002) Marxistische Persönlichkeitstheorie und die 'bio-psychosoziale Einheit Mensch' [Marxist personality theory and the bio-psycho-social entity man]. Pahl-Rugenstein Nachfolger, Cologne, Germany

Cohen G (1989) Memory in the real world. Erlbaum, London

Dörner D (1976) Problemlösen als Informationsverarbeitung [Problem-solving as information processing]. Kohlhammer, Stuttgart Germany

Dörner D (1984) Memory systems and the regulation of behavior. In: Hoffmann J, van der Meer E (eds) Knowledge aided information processing. Elsevier, Amsterdam

Dörner D (1999) Bauplan für eine Seele [Blueprint for a soul]. Rowohlt, Reinbek Germany

Flammer A (1990) Erfahrung der eigenen Wirksamkeit. Einführung in die Psychologie der Kontrolle [Introduction to the pychology of control]. Huber, Bern

Guilford (1967) The nature of human intelligence. McGraw-Hill, New York

Hacker W (1986) Arbeitspsychologie: Psychische Regulation von Arbeitstätigkeiten [work psychology. Psychological regulation of working activities]. Huber, Bern

Hacker W, Volpert, W, Cranach M von (1982) (eds) Cognitive and motivational aspects of action. Deutscher Verlag der Wissenschaften, Berlin

Heckhausen H, Kuhl J (1985) From wishes to actions: the dead ends and short cuts on the long way to action. In: Frese M, Sabini J (eds) Goal directed behavior: psychological theory and research on action. Erlbaum, Hillsdale, New Jersey, pp 134–159

Hovland CI, Rosenberg MJ (eds) (1960) Attitude, Organization and Change: an analysis of consistency among attitude components. Yale University Press, New Haven

Jensen RS (1995) Pilot judgement and crew resource management. Ashgate Publishing, Vermont

Kleinhempel F, Möbius A, Soschinka HU, Wassermann M (eds) (1996) Die biopsychosoziale Einheit Mensch. Festschrift für Karl-Friedrich Wessel [The bio-psycho-social entity man. Hommage to K.F. Wessel]. Kleine Verlag, Bielefeld

Klix F (1971) Information und Verhalten. Kybernetische Aspekte der organismischen Informationsverarbeitung [Information and behavior. Cybernetic aspects of organismic information processing]. Hans Huber, Bern

Kuhl J (1983) Motivation, Konflikt und Handlungskontrolle [Motivation, conflict, and action control]. Springer, Berlin Heidelberg New York

Maslow AH (1943) A theory of human motivation. Psychol Rev 50:370–396

Miller GA, Galanter E, Pribram KH (1960) Plans and the structure of behavior. Holt, New York

Schank RC, Abelson R (1977) Scripts, plans, goals, and understanding. Erlbaum, Hillsdale, New Jersey

Scherer K, Ekman P (eds) (1984) Approaches to emotion. Erlbaum, Hillsdale, New Jersey

Seligman ME (1975) Helplessness. On depression, development and death. Freeman, San Francisco

Selz O (1912/13) Über die Gesetze des geordneten Denkverlaufs [On the laws of the structured thought process]. Spaemann, Stuttgart

Spering M, Wagener D, Funke J (2005) The role of emotions in complex problem-solving. Cogn Emotion 19:1252–1261

Strohschneider S (1999) Human behavior and complex systems: some aspects of the regulation of emotions and cognitive information processing related to planning. In Stuhler EA, de Tombe DJ (eds) Complex problem-solving: cognitve psychological issues and environmental policy applications. Hampp, München, pp 61–73

II Individual Factors of Behavior

Problematic situations demand a different extent of conscious thinking, planning, and decision-making. Whether or not action routines can be applied or new solutions to problems have to be found depends mainly on two factors:
- How *complex* is the emergency situation?
- Has the clinician *experience* with comparable situations?

The less experience a clinician has with a critical situation and the more complex and dynamic the emergency is, the more necessary it becomes for him or her to switch from the application of rules to creative problem-solving.

Conscious problem-solving behavior in anesthesia, intensive care, and emergency medicine can be subdivided into several consecutive steps, the so-called organization of behavior. Against the background of the "psycho-logic" of cognition, emotion and intention, and the awareness of the fact that errors will always happen, we look at them in closer detail in part II. The following chapters focus on the factors that influence the individual. The team decision-making process and teamwork are the subject matter of part III.

The steps involved in the organization of behavior are as follows (Dörner 1996):
- Information processing and building of mental models
- Formation of goals
- Planning
- Decision-making

The chapters corresponding to the respective step within the organization of behavior are framed by chapters dealing with the unconscious processes which govern behavior and thus can impair it. These processes are:
- Perception
- Control of attention
- Stress

5 Human Perception: the Way We See Things

5.1   Case Study

At the end of an uneventful operation maintained by a total intravenous anesthesia (TIVA) a patient started to buck against the endotracheal tube prompting the anesthetist to switch the anesthesia machine from a mandatory to a spontaneous breathing mode. He did this by first selecting the new ventilation mode from the software menu and then pressing a button to accept the chosen value. While doing so the anesthetist turned his attention briefly to a concurrent problem. Shortly after, the anesthetist returned his attention to the patient and all signs indicated adequate spontaneous breathing: chest excursions were regular; the capnography curve displayed a regular pattern; the expiratory minute volume was adequate; and the saturation was at 100%. Again, the patient started to buck against the tube and the anesthetist decided to extubate the patient. Shortly after the extubation, the saturation began to drop and the patient became cyanotic. The anesthetist then realized that the ventilator was still working in the volume-controlled mode and had not been switched into the spontaneous breathing mode as he initially thought. He began to mask ventilate the patient until the patient started breathing spontaneously a few minutes later.

An anesthetist decides to extubate his patient and therefore tests the patient's ability to breathe spontaneously. Because of a handling error, the anesthesia machine is not switched into a spontaneous breathing mode but instead continues to mechanically ventilate the patient. In the wrong conviction that the patient is breathing on his own, the anesthetist interprets his clinical observation and the information gathered from his monitor as signs of adequate spontaneous breathing: The regular and deep chest excursions, the flawless pattern of the capnography curve and an expiratory minute volume close to what he would expect for his patient all reinforce his conviction that the patient can now be safely extubated. However, as other problems demand his attention he does not realize that his monitor displays additional ventilation curves which actually contradict his current assumption (e.g., the pressure/time curve and the flow/time curve). Because he accepts his perception as not being in conflict with his working hypotheses of a spontaneously breathing patient, a critical re-examination of the situation does not occur until the patient has serious problems.

Human perception has one primary task to fulfill: It has to provide adequate information about that particular part of the external environment on which human survival depends. On the basis of this information we can find our way in unknown territory, avoid danger and are able to meet our needs. Sensory information enables humans to see "where food can be found and dangers abound". Thus, human perception was never meant to accurately and flawlessly reproduce an image of the environment. The widespread analogy of human perception with the information processing of a computer is therefore wrong. The eyes are *not* camcorders or digital cameras which scan the original image and then store the gathered information on a cerebral hard disc. Quite the contrary is true: The original image is not completely scanned at all and the resulting information which human sense organs provide from "outside" or from within the body is being filtered, evaluated, and reorganized all the time. Although the nature of these environmental stimuli includes a wide range of stimuli (acoustic, visual, olfactory, gustatory, haptic, nociceptive, and vestibulocochlear), only a small set of common principles underlie all sensory processes. Thus, herein the functional features of perception are exemplified by the visual and acoustic system. This is done for educational purpose only; all relevant mechanisms apply to other sensory processes as well.

The process of visual perception, to start with, can be subdivided into three distinguishable (albeit not sharply) steps. An example might be the path from the information content of a capnography curve on the monitor display up to the thought, "This patient shows sufficient spontaneous breathing" (◘ Fig. 5.1).

5.2   From Stimulus to Sensation: Sensory Physiology

Environmental stimuli (e.g., sound, light, heat, smells, tastes, tactile stimuli) are "detected" by sensory receptors, specific biological structures that "transduce" small amounts of environmental energy into the generation of cellular action potentials. After the reception of the sensory stimulus, the generated sensory signal is encoded and transmitted via different neural pathways to specific regions of the spinal cord and the cortex. The interpretation of the sensory input by the central

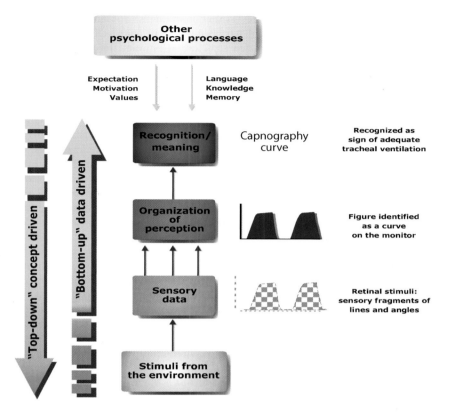

Fig. 5.1 Multistage process of perception (after Zimbardo and Gerrig 1996). Top-down (concept-guided) and bottom-up (data-guided) processes interrelate in a complex and mostly unexplained way

nervous system (CNS) depends on the pathway it takes to the brain, the representation of information in specific areas of the brain, and networking between functional areas of the CNS; however, this process of sensation describes only the first few steps in the far more complex process of *perception*, in which sensory information is integrated with previously learned information and other sensory input, thus enabling humans to make judgments about the quality, intensity, and relevance of what is being sensed.

In their entirety, human sensory organs work like an evolutionary developed filter: They reduce the abundance of possible sensory inputs but give humans access to the sector of reality relevant to them. This is the main reason why humans cannot see ultraviolet light, cannot orient themselves by means of the terrestrial magnetic field, and cannot espy a mouse from a bird's perspective of

100 m above ground. Instead, human sensory organs have naturally optimized their response to those environmental stimuli which have to be perceived for an effective exploration of the environment (Goldstein 2006; Klix 1971; Ramachandran and Blakeslee 1999; for a detailed description of the sensory physiology see Goldstein 2006).

Most sensory organs respond preferentially to a single kind of environmental stimulus. This specificity is due to several features that match a receptor to its preferred stimulus. For the reception of the matching stimulus every receptor has a relative and an absolute threshold. Relative thresholds describe how much two stimuli have to differ from each other in order to be distinguished. The difference can be in duration, strength, wave length, etc. The stronger the prevailing stimulus, the greater this difference has to be; the increment threshold to the background is a constant (Weber's law). So when people work in a noisy environment (e.g., resuscitation room, trauma management on scene), the beeper volume or a monitor's audio alarm has to be set so that it is much louder than the environment if it should be heard. If the same alarm is set in a quiet environment (e.g., OR with a routine operation), it is enough if the alarm is a little louder than the environment.

Absolute thresholds determine the range within which an environmental stimulus (e.g. light, sound) can actually be detected. Sensory thresholds are not fixed during a lifetime. They can be permanently altered as a result of nerve injury (e.g., trauma, aging – elder people tend to become hard of hearing). Short-term alterations in sensory thresholds can be the result of adaptation as well as the result of motivational processes which regulate attention (▶ Chaps. 4 and 8). Short-term adaptation allows the fine-tuning of perception processes to the changes in the environment (adaptation to darkness and light). Short-term adaptation also prevents "sensory overload," thus allowing less important or unchanging environmental stimuli to be partially ignored. A continuous tone will "die away" to our brain and smells will loose their sweet or penetrating quality within minutes. When a change occurs, however, the initial response pattern will reemerge and the sensory input will become temporarily more noticeable. On the level of sensory receptors adaptation and fatigue are the two relevant neurophysiological mechanisms which account for perceptive errors.

5.3 "Gestalt" Theory and Meaningful Patterns: the Organization of Visual Perception

The first functional step in the process of perception happens at the level of the sensory organs: Chemical or physical stimuli are converted into neuronal activity. This neuronal activity is forwarded via different neuronal pathways to higher cerebral centers. At this level relevant impressions are filtered from the sensory input and undergo an active process of reduction, simplification, addition, combination, and organization. The perceived result is a meaningful whole, the so-called Gestalt (Wertheimer 1923, 1925, 1959; Metzger 2006; Eysenck 1942; Koehler 1992; overview in Hartmann and Poffenberger 2006). The German word "Gestalt" has no

direct translation in English but refers to "the way a thing has been placed or put together" and an "organized structure". Common translations include "form" and "shape," but science has always used the original term. For Gestalt psychologists *form* is the most basic unit of perception: We do not perceive sensory impressions as fractional particles in disorder, but instead as well-organized coherent patterns, as a meaningful "Gestalt." What is "meaningful" or relevant for a person is partially predetermined by evolutionary development and partially the result of experience and a lifelong learning process; thus, when humans perceive, they will always pick out form, and the whole of this form will be more than the sum of its parts: The perception process adds experience and inborn processing patterns to sensory inputs. Moreover, the meaning of a part depends on the particular whole in which it occurs. This fundamental feature of perception is not restricted to the visual mode.

A Gestalt can be "transposed" into other realms and remains identifiable even if crucial parts are altered (Vulkovich 2000): From the rhythmical beeps of a patient monitor we "hear" the heart beat and we can "see" a patient breathing in a colored, bell-shaped form on the display of the anesthesia machine. Once we know what to expect, we actually can "see" biological organs behind the various kinds and levels of physical energy which stimulate our sense organs.

However, perception neither "reveals" objects and events of the physical world nor is there such thing as "mere reality" which we could directly access via our sensory systems. Instead, the human brain "constructs" reality by means of an interplay of inherited neuronal mechanisms and learned processes of pattern recognition. This reconstruction happens as soon as a few sensory inputs have reached the brain. The result is that an object does not have to be completely scanned before it is perceived as a whole. The reason lies in the characteristics of Gestalt perception: it follows the so-called Gestalt rules which describe the way in which the perceptive system decides which sensory stimuli belong together and to which Gestalt this would correspond. Once "the whole" has been determined, humans can orientate in physical space, can distinguish figures from a background and can receive the general impression that what they see actually "makes sense". The Gestalt rules describe in detail the two basic features of Gestalt perception:

- There are always only a few possible "Gestalten" (the plural of "Gestalt") which are selected from a variety of theoretically possible interpretations of sensory impressions.
- The interpretation of sensory impressions tries to give them as good a Gestalt way as possible (the law of "Praegnanz" – *good form*). If the configuration of stimuli allows for alternative interpretations, it will always be the one with a good Gestalt which will prevail. In this sense "good" can mean regular, orderly, simplistic, symmetrical, etc.

This law of Praegnanz can be further concretized in different laws. They all describe different aspects of the form-forming capability of our perception.

Every human sensory experience is transformed through this constructive activity into a meaningful whole that is well structured and clearly distinguished from the background. This is even true for sensory stimuli which "objectively" seem to be without order. In this case, too, a Gestalt will be constructed from the available information. This is the neuropsychological basis for all kinds of optical delusion. From a functional point of view this constructive activity enables a rapid and sufficient orientation in the external environment. An example of the law of Praegnanz is given in ◘ Fig. 5.2, where a cube can be seen which is actually only defined by the white parts of the other figures – the tendency to build good Gestalten is so strong that we even "see" nonexistent white lines on the white ground.

The focal point of Gestalt theory is the tendency to interpret a visual field or a problem by means of "grouping" similar or proximate objects. The grouping of the stimuli, the viewing of an "organized whole," follows the laws of organization (Wertheimer 1923; Metzger 2006), with its main factors being the following:

- Figure and ground: We tend to organize our perceptions by distinguishing between a figure and a ground.
- Proximity: Elements tend to be grouped together according to their proximity.
- Similarity: Items similar in some respect tend to be grouped together. The similarity depends on relationships constructed about form, color, size, and brightness of the elements.
- Closure: Items are grouped together in a way that they complete patterns. Missing pieces of the total are simply added through extrapolation in the generative process of perception.
- Continuity: Figures are perceived as combination of meaningful lines. If there are crossing lines on the monitor (or voices "crossing" each other), we perceive them as pattern of several continuing lines.
- Simplicity: Items are organized into simple figures according to symmetry, regularity, and smoothness.

The laws of organization do not seem to operate independently; instead, they appear to influence each other, so that the final perception is the result of all Gestalt grouping laws acting together. Gestalt theory applies not only to perception and problem-solving but also to all other aspects of human learning.

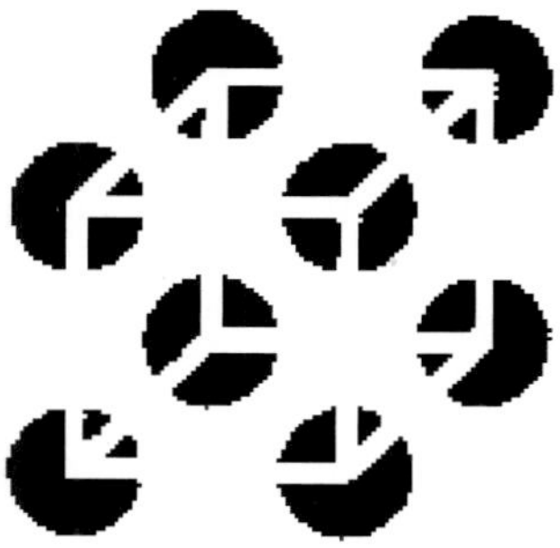

5.3.1 Hypothesis-Based Perception

The powerful nature of perception exceeds the ability to group elements and amend an incomplete or partially obscured object: Even the perception of completely presented objects remains incomplete. Already the first sensory input is aligned with the memory and a hypothesis is formed (unconsciously) as to which object this could be (hypothesis-based perception; Bruner and Postman 1951). The hypothesis with the highest probability for success, which is the memory item with the greatest facilitation, is further pursued (Dörner 1999). An expectation is formed about what ought to be seen at a certain point in the visual field and this expec-

◘ **Fig. 5.2** The law of "Praegnanz" (good form) facilitates the identification of incomplete objects. Human perception does not scan objects but instead "constructs" reality through pattern recognition and its form-forming capability

tation is then checked. This cycle is repeated until a sufficient number of hits allow for the conclusion that the object indeed has been identified: The process is terminated even though the object has only been scanned in part and the missing rest will be added to the picture – in a way "hallucinated." Because expectations are a very powerful drive of human perception, we normally only see what we (subconsciously) want to see or are used to seeing; and we hear what we expect to hear, e.g., the name of an often-used drug. Errors thus can occur if a doctor orders a different but similar-sounding drug and the nurse "hears" the expected (but wrong) drug simply because he or she is used to hearing it.

Once a hypothesis has been advanced and a perception seemingly has affirmed this assumption, it takes deliberate effort to reevaluate the underlying data and to strive for a new interpretation.

5.3.2 Hypotheses Are Knowledge Dependent

The hypotheses which guide the process of perception are based mainly upon knowledge. Common objects are more rapidly identified than unknown ones; a familiar sight is more readily recognized than an unfamiliar one: Due to his clinical experience, the anesthetist rapidly detected the cyanosis and interpreted it as a clinical sign of insufficient spontaneous breathing. A layperson would have seen nothing but a dark-blue face. Besides implicit knowledge based on experience it is also logical

reasoning which can generate a hypothesis that will guide perception. Sometimes it is only the explicit knowledge about what is to be expected that actually enables "seeing" (◘ Fig. 5.3).

This mechanism of hypothesis-based perception accepts errors. A multitude of optical illusions readily underscores the fact that our perceptive system can easily be fooled. Nonetheless, the phrase "likely things are likely to happen" is not only a good diagnostic rule for common medical problems; it also seems to be the selection rule par excellence our cognitive system applies. From an evolutionary point of view, the ability to rapidly produce workable patterns of the environment seems to have been advantageous compared with a 100% scanning of the surroundings, which would have been error-free albeit very slow. Last but not least, the aforementioned optical illusions occur far more infrequently than sudden changes in the immediate vicinity, which could signal imminent danger. This cognitive default mode of an expectation-based perception which never completely scans the object in question can only be altered by means of attention control (► Chap. 8): It will always take a conscious effort to question present assumptions and to scrutinize the obvious. The unexpected cyanosis was an external trigger for the anesthetist to redirect his attention to the seemingly breathing patient – before he had actually "seen" the patient breathe because he expected him to do so.

The mechanism of hypothesis-based perception also explains why medication errors have a strong tendency to occur during critical situations in a

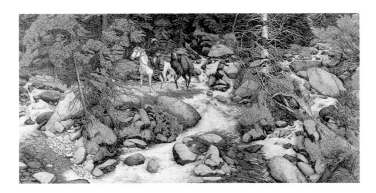

◘ **Fig. 5.3** Example for a hypothesis-based perception: Bev Doolittle's painting "The Woods Have Many Faces" (1985). At first the trees and rock formations are seen as trees and rocks; however, as soon as people are told to look for faces, the individual elements of the picture are re-interpreted differently. A total of 13 faces are "hidden" in the picture

high-stakes environment: time pressure reduces the interval until a hypothesis is accepted as fact. If ampoules of highly potent drugs have a similar appearance, and if people expect them in a certain tray of the anesthesia cart, the drug is taken out without a second look at the label. If stress further impairs conscious action control, the mistake will go unnoticed with potentially disastrous consequences for the patient. For over a decade a European pharmaceutical company produced two potent drugs, namely Beloc (metoprolole) and Xylocain 2% (lidocaine), with an almost identical labeling. More than one patient suffered harm as a result of a clinician mistaking the drugs (compare case report in Chap. 3; ◘ Fig. 5.4.).

The laws of Gestalt, however, are not only useful in explaining action errors. From the knowledge of the laws of Gestalt, major ergonomic requirements for monitoring engineering and the software development can be deduced. If these are considered, information can be displayed more legibly and will be easier to interpret.

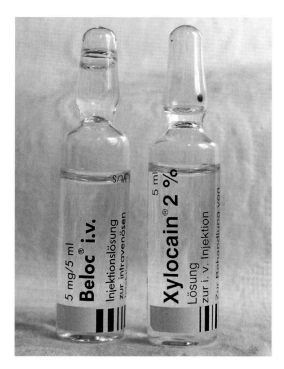

◘ **Fig. 5.4** For a long time the two cardiovascular drugs, Beloc (metoprolole) and Xylocain 2% (lidocaine), had an almost identical labeling which resulted in several drug errors

5.4 Recognition and Creating Meaning

In the third step of the perception process the visual patterns are identified and interpreted, i.e., given a meaning. The sensory data, already selected and processed, is identified by comparing it with small meaningful entities, so-called schemata, and thus classified into our knowledge categories. If what a person experiences is familiar, the perception is named. It is at this level that perception receives its meaning and can be placed into a broader context: Visual stimuli turn into a capnography curve on the monitor and the thought arises "this patient breathes spontaneously" (◘ Fig. 5.1). Only after this last step took place with the information having been filtered and processed several times does perception enter consciousness for the first time. However, for the subject himself these processes go unnoticed: Despite the multilevel processing of sensory data, perception always appears to be objective and to capture nothing but mere facts. In other words, we believe that what we actually see, hear, and feel is reality, is "just the way things are." Because perception almost always feels real, it is contra-intuitive for us to actually question it. This sense of objectivity makes it difficult to actually apply the knowledge about the fallibility of sensory impressions to daily life and not just acknowledge it intellectually.

That's so typical! Expectancies. The identification and categorization of perceptive data is substantially alleviated by mental precepts and expectancies (mind sets): Because some perceptions are more probable to occur within a certain context than others, they are preactivated neuronally. "More probable" means in this context that in one's personal experience a certain perception has occurred more often in combination with a corresponding sensory impression and therefore has been typical up to now. A dark-blue face during emergence from anesthesia is more likely to be a sign of inadequate ventilation than the result of venous congestion of the face or of intravenous methylene blue. Thanks to the neuronal preactivation, the recognition and identification becomes faster and shows less error; however, unexpected information has to be looked at longer and in greater detail before it is recognized beyond doubt.

Thus, the preactivation is an experience-dependent phenomenon: Knowledge defines what is probable in a certain situation and what is not; however, if past experiences are the main interpretative frame for new sensory information, the danger is great that we then will only see what we have always seen and that it is virtually impossible to "think outside the box." Furthermore, we might only see what we want to see: Because motivational forces (e.g., needs) are potent trigger for this preactivation (Dörner 1999), humans tend to select and interpret sensory information in a way which enables them to have their needs met. If an anesthetist wants to extubate the patient as quickly as possible because dinner is waiting in the cafeteria, or because it is 2 a.m. in the morning and he or she is dead tired and wants to go to bed, then he or she will tend to interpret the capnography curve as a sign of sufficient spontaneous breathing. The *wish* determines the thought.

With the subsumption into categories and the classification as "something," perception enters consciousness and is available for the rational thought process (▶ Chap. 6).

5.5 Perception and Emotion

The perception of events in critical situations is not restricted to its cognitive aspects. Human perception is always accompanied by emotions (Scherer and Ekman 1984): The reason therefore lies in the fact that every single time people are exposed to environmental changes a "holistic" emotional assessment of the situation on the basis of all perceptions will take place – even if the results of this assessment do not readily surface to conscious processing (▶ Chaps. 4 and 8.). Instead, these emotions are very often quite vague and people usually have difficulty in recognizing and articulating them. Because emotions result from a subconscious perceptive process, they are difficult to analyze on a rational basis. Nonetheless, they are based on perceptions and therefore should be taken seriously: They are like "smoke signals" for a fire which burns "beyond

the horizon" of conscious perception. To have an "uneasy" feeling could always mean that the situational assessment "there's something wrong" has been made, on the basis of whatever information. It is always worthwhile to reflect upon the question as to why this feeling arose under these particular circumstances. Maybe they signal imminent danger of which, up to this moment, a person was completely unaware. Emotions come to the surface of consciousness just like any other perceptive content. That is why people experience them as an external event and not like an internal construction. For the adequate response to emotions one aspect is crucial: It is never the event per se which generates an emotion but instead the subjective assessment of this event and the meaning it has for the subject (◻ Fig. 5.5). Once a patient restarts spontaneous breathing at the end of anesthesia, the anesthetist does not only see the capnography curve, he also experiences "relief" regarding the meaning he ascribes to this sensory impression: The patient soon will be completely awake and therefore the anesthesia application was successful.

To see emotions as the product of a subjective situational assessment, instead of as something events or people do to us, might be helpful in situations where strong emotions surface: be it the response to behavior or remarks of other team members, or the coping with feelings of helplessness, or even panic. Most of the time these situations receive their burdening component through the interpretation which subjects give to the behavior of their counterpart or to the meaning of a fact. Very often it is possible to "see things differently" and thereby "take some of the emotional pressure" out of a situation.

5.6 Tips for Clinical Practice

The following are tips for clinical practice:
− Perception is always subjective. Rely on four eyes rather than two if the matter is of importance.
− Always be prepared that your perception might actually deceive you; therefore, increase the level

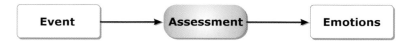

◻ **Fig. 5.5** Relationship between external events and the onset of emotions. Not the event itself but rather the subjective assessment of the meaning the event has for a person will generate the feelings

of resolution in critical situations – better look twice and pay close attention so that you may discover errors.

- Perception is guided by expectations. Be aware of your expectations; this can enable you to have a less biased approach to a situation.
- Use as many sensory modalities as possible if you want to get a precise picture of the situation –*hear*, *see*, *smell*, and *feel* how the patient is doing.
- A situation cannot cause emotions, but your interpretation of the situation can; therefore, take emotions seriously and look for possible causes. Remember when strong and unpleasant emotions arise that you are not a victim of emotions because you always have at least one other option as to how you can see the situation.

5.7   "Perception": in a Nutshell

From all the above-stated information the following principles can be derived, which apply to all levels of human perception:

- Perception is the process by which sensory information is integrated with previously learned information and other sensory inputs, enabling humans to make judgments about the quality, intensity, and relevance of what is being sensed.
- Perception enables humans to orient themselves in their environment. Perception does not strive for truth but for practicability (i.e., viability). Humans construct from incompletely perceived sensory impressions the relevant sector of reality which is necessary for their survival.
- Perception happens in three consecutive and interrelated steps: processing of sensory stimuli in the sense organs; organization of perception (Gestalt perception and meaningful patterns); and the recognition and assignment of meaning. These three processes influence each other and are dependent on knowledge and experience.
- Perception is limited by absolute and relative thresholds. Some of these thresholds are biologically determined; some can be influenced by motivation and conscious control of attention.
- Perception is hypothesis based: Expectancies about what ought to be there control the perceptive process and in part replace the factual scanning of the environmental objects. The human cognition is unable to distinguish between real and constructed data. The underlying

hypotheses are based on previous experience and motivation.

- Perception accepts the possibility of error to achieve efficiency and speed: The hypotheses-based organization of sensory impressions serves a quick, unambiguous, stable, and therefore reliable orientation in the external environment; therefore, the susceptibility for optical delusions and errors is an inherent feature of human perception – the "downside" of having a brain.

References

Bruner JS, Postman L (1951) An approach to social perception. In: Dennis W, Lipitt R (eds) Current trends in social psychology. University of Pittsburgh Press, Pittsburg

Dörner D (1996) The logic of failure. Recognizing and avoiding error in complex situations. Metropolitan Books, New York

Dörner D (1999) Bauplan für eine Seele [Blueprint for a soul]. Rowohlt, Reinbek bei Hamburg, Germany

Eysenck H (1942) The experimental study of the "good Gestalt": a new approach. Psychol Rev 49:344–364

Goldstein EB (2006) Sensation and perception, 6th edn. Wadsworth, Belmont California

Hartmann GW, Poffenberger AT (eds) (2006) Gestalt psychology: a survey of facts and principles. Kessinger, Whitefish, Montana

Klix F (1971) Information und Verhalten. Kybernetische Aspekte der organismischen Informationsverarbeitung [information and behavior. Cyberbetic aspects of organismic information processing]. Huber, Bern

Koehler W (1992) Gestalt psychology: the definitive statement of the Gestalt theory. Liveright Books, New York

Metzger W (2006) Laws of seeing (originally published 1936) Translated by L. Spillmann, S. Lehar, M. Stromeyer, and M. Wertheimer. MIT Press, Cambridge

Ramachandran V, Blakeslee S (1999) Phantoms in the brain: human nature and the architecture of the mind. Fourth Estate, London

Scherer K, Ekman P (eds) (1984) Approaches to emotion. Erlbaum, Hillsdale, New Jersey

Wertheimer M (1923) Laws of organization in perceptual forms. First published as "Untersuchungen zur Lehre von der Gestalt". Psychol Forsch 4:301–350. Translation published in: Ellis W (1938) A source book of gestalt psychology. Routledge and Kegan Paul, London, pp 71–88

Wertheimer M (1925) Über Gestalttheorie [on Gestalt Theory]. Verlag der philosophischen Akademie, Erlangen. Reprint: Gestalt Theory 7:99–120

Wertheimer M (1959) Productive thinking (enlarged edition). Harper and Row, New York

Vukovich A (2000) Christian v. Ehrenfels: "Über 'Gestaltqualitäten'" ["on Gestalt qualities"]. In: Schmale H (ed) Hauptwerke der Psychologie. Kröner, Stuttgart

Zimbardo G, Gerrig RJ (eds) (1996) Psychology and life, 14th edn. Harper Collins, New York

6 Information Processing and Mental Models: World Views

6.1   Case Study

At 10:35 in the morning two ambulances were sent to the site of a rural two-car traffic accident. The first unit that arrived at the scene confirmed that two cars were involved and three people were injured. According to the eyewitnesses' accounts of the event, the driver of one of the cars had lost control of his vehicle and collided frontally with the second car. The two occupants of the second vehicle had only minor injuries, but the driver who had caused the accident was already comatose. After assessment and triage, the second EMS team focused on the two mildly injured occupants, of which one was complaining of paresthesia likely secondary to a whiplash injury. The unconscious victim had been quickly removed from his vehicle by the first team and transferred to the ambulance. He received oxygen via face mask and two large-bore intravenous lines were inserted. A normal blood-sugar finger stick ruled out hypoglycemia as a cause for the unconsciousness. Volume resuscitation was started and the patient was intubated. As the victim showed no external injuries, the working diagnosis at this point included deceleration injury with severe internal bleeding, injuries to major intra-abdominal organs, and severe head injury. After 2000 ml of crystalloid solution had been infused without any effect on the arterial blood pressure, an epinephrine drip was started. The jugular veins were noted to be markedly distended, which suggested the possibility of a pneumothorax; however, the chest auscultation revealed bilateral breath sounds, and on chest palpation no rib fractures or subcutaneous emphysema were appreciated; therefore, the diagnosis of pneumothorax was ruled out. On arrival at the emergency department, the patient continued to be hemodynamically unstable. The ultrasound scan showed no intraabdominal organs injuries or free intraperitoneal fluid. The chest X-ray revealed adequately ventilated lungs, marked perihilar congestion, normal aortic arch, and significantly enlarged cardiac silhouette. Up to this point, 3500 ml of crystalloid solution had been infused and the rate of the epinephrine drip had reached 5 mg per hour. A transesophageal echocardiography was performed which revealed a dilated left ventricle, with severe inferior and apical akinesia. The patient died shortly after his admission to the ICU as a result of severe cardiogenic shock.

A team of paramedics is confronted with a routine rescue operation: a motor vehicle accident with two lightly injured patients and one severely injured patient. The medical treatment of the patient with the clinical signs of volume depletion is routine: oxygen via face mask; the placement of several i.v. lines, and volume resuscitation; however, the emergency situation does feature some noteworthy exceptions from "the routine MVA" which are not realized by the EMTs: Neither the unclear circumstances of how the accident happened, nor the missing signs of injury, nor the sternotomy scar which could indicate previous cardiac surgery (e.g., CABG) receive appropriate attention; therefore, the initial assumption of volume loss as reason for the arterial hypotension is never questioned. A non-traumatological cause, such as an acute myocardial infarction, is not considered. Available information is not searched for nor taken into account during the entire rescue operation.

This "blindness to the obvious" is not an unusual phenomenon in clinical medicine. How can it be explained that none of the team members were able to see during the management that the external circumstances of the accident could be interpreted quite differently? This question leads to the way human information processing works.

Human thinking processes information which is presented by perception and memory (▶ Chaps. 4 and 5); however, memory items – our knowledge – are not available in the same way as information which can be read from a computer's hard disc. The selection of relevant memory contents underlies the same principles as perception. Items are classified as "relevant" and thus are more easily and faster retrieved from memory if:

- They are common
- They meet the expectation horizon and therefore are preactivated
- They are important
- They have a strong emotional component
- They are related in some way to other activated items (associative retrieval)

Conscious thought processes, such as judgment, planning, generation of analogies, or prognostic statements about the anticipated development of events, are based on a multitude of subconscious steps of information processing. In this respect thinking is analogous to perception, in which a multitude of subconscious processes precede the conscious perception. Basic cognitive processes which run on the basis of the architecture of memory are, for example, as follows (Lompscher 1972; Selz 1913):

- Identification and classification of objects and events
- Assessment
- Association
- Linking
- Imagination

From the memory retrieval conditions mentioned above, and the basic cognitive processes, fundamental principles of information processing can be deduced. These principles explain both the enormous performance of human cognition as well as many errors in thinking.

6.2 The Organization of Knowledge: Schemata and Mental Models

All human knowledge – sensory, procedural, and concept knowledge – can be conceived as a network of sensory and motor schemata, and of the concepts of language (▶ Chap. 4). Schemata are chunks of information, "knowledge packages," encoding either generic concepts (e.g., "everything that is needed for starting an i.v. line") or familiar episodes or scenarios ("how to puncture a peripheral vein"), also known as *scripts* (Schank and Abelson 1977). Schemata exhibit the following fundamental aspects (Bartlett 1932; Anderson 1983):

- They are unconscious mental structures. People are unaware of the fact that both the encoding and storage of information, as well as the recall and perception of reality, is guided by meaningful high-level knowledge structures and not by atomistic bits of information.
- These high-level knowledge structures are composed of knowledge and past experiences: People try to integrate new material into established knowledge structures; thus, we can only recognize and classify items similar to what we have already experienced.
- Schemata are stored in a hierarchical system with primary rules for solving problems on the top and secondary rules and exceptions for the rules further down in the hierarchy. Whereas novices have only a limited number of schemata, mostly of primary rules, the expert problem solver has

stored a multitude of secondary rules and exceptions along with the primary rules.

- A recall of long-term memory actively reconstructs past experiences and not merely reads the unaltered data from the brain's "hard disk." As a result, certain predictable biases in remembering can be expected because people tend to interpret presented data in keeping with their own expectations and established habits of thought.
- The recall of schemata follows the principle of economy, which attempts to achieve its goal with the least possible effort: "effort after meaning." What makes a schema strong is how recently and how frequently it has been used. This law of economy can actively be overcome by conscious effort and investment of time, both scarce resources in an emergency situation.

The fact that the regularities of the world, as well as our routine dealings with them, have been represented internally as schemata explains the inferential and interpretative function of human cognition which goes beyond the given information; thus, in almost any given situation (e.g.,"induction of anesthesia") data can be:

- Identified and assessed ("the patient has lost consciousness and can be ventilated by mask. Everything goes as intended")
- Explained ("the unconsciousness is the effect of thiopental")
- Predicted ("once thiopental is injected, the patient will become unconscious")

The entirety of the schemata which refer to a certain area of reality is called a mental model (Johnson-Laird 1983). Behind this term stands the idea that we build from our experience a picture of the situation – a model of a part of the world in our mind. Mental models organize knowledge in a stable way and thus provide a basis for planned actions. Mental models encompass an interpretation of the current situation which is integrated into our previous knowledge. Extensive work in naturalistic decision-making has been able to confirm that expert individuals rapidly analyze situations by pattern matching against their mental library of prior experience (Klein 1992). Because these mental models contain knowledge derived from past personal interactions with the world, they will always differ between different people. In an emergency situation this requires communication as a

6.3 · Are We Too Lazy to Think? Economy, Competence, and Safety

71 **6**

means of aligning the mental models of each team member. If this is not accomplished, the odds are high that every team member will act upon different prerequisites (▶ Chap 11).

Handling New Information. Whenever possible, new information is added to preexisting mental models (assimilation). Learning in this case means that mental models are enlarged without the need of a structural change. An arterial hypotension in relation to a traffic accident "fits" as extension into the basic model "volume depletion"; however, new information can conflict with already available data. In this case it cannot simply be integrated into an already existing model: Mental models have to be rearranged and have to undergo a structural change in order to fit the new circumstances (accommodation; Piaget et al 1985). Learning thus means that the world has to be conceived differently and hitherto existing approaches have to be changed. As humans are creatures of habit and generally prefer to maintain existing mental models, the internal resistance to this learning process can be very high – under stress, we ignore information rather than change our image of the world.

6.3 Are We Too Lazy to Think? Economy, Competence, and Safety

Many mistakes originate from false knowledge or an inadequate application of correct knowledge (▶ Chap. 3). Although it would be possible to describe many mistakes in information processing, there are three basic principles which form the basis of these mistakes:

— Resource protection (principle of economy)
— Guarding the feeling of competence
— Search for order

These factors all interact with each other (◘ Fig. 6.1).

6.3.1 Too Lazy to Think: Resource Protection

Conscious thinking, the very "tool" we need to deal with unknown realities, functions slowly and is not capable of processing many different pieces of information at any one time. It has limited capacity and prompts us to use our scarce resources

as efficiently as possible. We therefore avoid conscious thinking whenever possible and instead take shortcuts or rely on automated cognition. Many failings in our thought process are an expression of this tendency to economize. In everyday life this principle of economy does make sense: Every time we think that we already know something, we can restrict ourselves in data gathering and hypothesis formation; it is "business as usual." The same is true for emergency situations: A traffic accident then becomes just another one of "these motor vehicle accidents" and an arterial hypotension must be caused by volume depletion, as so many times before. What people perceive and think is greatly influenced by what they already know and therefore expect. So, only part of the situation is actually scanned and assessed, and if it fits into a mental model, the gaps are completed by existing knowledge. This principle of completion indeed leads to an economical application of thinking, but it causes errors if (a) our knowledge is not consistent with reality because it is wrong or inappropriate, or (b) the matching with reality was too superficial, so things are not what they seem to be at first glance.

In everyday life this mode of behavior is not faulty at all but is instead the prerequisite for successful action. A strategy that uses only a limited amount of information can indeed lead to good results and is effective most of the time (Hertwig and Todd 2001; Gigerenzer 2000); however, once stress or emotional pressure increase, the principle of economy can start to deform the thought process: The agreement of the mental model with reality becomes even more superficial, and the probability for errors, such as overlooking, confusing, and mishearing, increases (▶ Chap. 9).

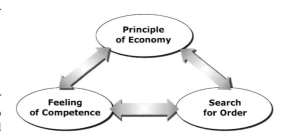

◘ **Fig. 6.1** Three basic factors which influence each other in the construction of mental models

6.3.2 Beware of Drowning! Guarding the Feeling of Competence

In order to be able to act efficiently, people need a stable mental model which sufficiently explains the current situation. This is best achieved by clinging to an image of reality as long as possible. As long as this picture is in place, present assumptions do not have to be questioned and the course of action can remain unaltered. So, "my mental model is wrong" means "I have to think anew before I can act." However, the notion of "not knowing" also seems to have direct impact on one's feeling of competence. Most human beings prefer not to be confronted with errors or unexpected changes in situation but instead prefer to maintain their mental models in order to guard their own feeling of competence (Dörner 1996).

This strong tendency to guard one's own feeling of competence does not only explain the stability of mental models but also the form they tend to take: straightforward and simple models. They create a feeling of safety and personal intelligence, whereas complex and differentiated explanations only raise doubt and increase insecurity. Therefore, whenever possible, people tend to simplify complex and opaque situations and focus solely on the predominant problem (Dörner 1996). To a certain extent this approach to reality does make sense, as someone who considers himself to be incapable of acting will hardly act: The motivation to protect one's feeling of competence is an important part of our internal regulation. However, in the attempt to maintain a high opinion of one's own competence in problem-solving, people do the following:

— Fail to take notice of data which indicate that they are wrong ("fixation error").
— Do not turn to the possible developments and long-term consequences of a critical situation. Subjects prefer to attend to a single problem *they have* rather than bother about possible problems they do *not yet have* ("predominance of current problems").
— Do not check the effects of their actions and therefore act "ballistically": They "fire" their measures like cannon balls, never controlling the further course of events ("ballistic action"; Dörner 1996).

In critical situations the urge to guard the feeling of competence can become the all-dominant motive for action: "Saving face" suddenly becomes more important than saving a patient's life, and an adequate treatment of the patient's medical problem becomes secondary to the control of one's own feelings (of course, we hardly ever notice that in ourselves).

Self-reflective examination and critique of one's own way of acting would be the essential means of preventing the hazardous impact of the guarding motive in critical situations. Unfortunately, it is precisely in these situations that self-reflection is dispensed.

6.3.3 Certainty and Order: the Avoidance of Ambiguity

Mental models do not simply summarize our knowledge of the world in some form or fashion: They instead give "structure" to the world by merging similar experiences and ascribing significance to perceptual data, thereby creating a consistent image of reality. Mental models tend to be cohesive and stable. This enables us to explain the present and extrapolate into the future. For this reason people tend to strive for clarity and to avoid ambiguity and uncertainty whenever possible (ambiguity aversion; Camerer and Weber 1992; Heath and Tversky 1991; Curley et al 1986).

Structure and order are important because they provide a feeling of certainty, but for the memory and cognitive processes, too, structure is a central feature: Structured data can be more readily memorized and retrieved easier. If humans are forced to process a greater amount of data, this is only possible if these data are somehow structured. Thinking, therefore, can be described in sum as a process whereby humans give structure to their environment (Selz 1913/1922). In an acute care setting this need for a structure in thinking becomes most obvious in the search for an unambiguous diagnosis. This unambiguity is necessary for both, the treatment of the patient and the thinking of the physician.

6.4 Wishful Thinking and Reality: Distortion of Information

In the effort not to question their knowledge, people subconsciously tend to warp information until it fits into their mental model of the situation. This inadequate processing of information can follow different routes (☐ Fig. 6.2).

6.4.1   Biased Search for Information

Those pieces of information are searched for which reinforce present knowledge or hypotheses (confirmation bias; Kahneman et al. 1982). Data which would question present assumptions about a problem have to be presented with more emphasis than those which reaffirm the prevailing mental model. If someone would have mentioned to the EMS team that the patient had complained about retrosternal burning pain prior to the accident, the diagnosis most probably would have been different; however, without an external prompting people seldom actively search for information which would contradict the present assumption: The EMS team was no exception to this rule. The only way to avoid this kind of wishful thinking is a deep-rooted skepticism about the appropriateness of any initial diagnosis: The odds are high that some information was overlooked and we indeed did not yet get everything right.

6.4.2   Distortion and Suppression

If critical situations are experienced as a threat to one's feeling of competence, then the need to maintain the current mental model can become overwhelming: Ambiguous information is reinterpreted in a way that corroborates present knowledge. This can go so far that people no longer are able to hear or see unpleasant information but instead completely block it out.

6.4.3   Minimum Acquisition of Information

The guarding of a feeling of competence is not the only reason why an adequate model of reality is affected. The same is true for the way information management is handled. The abundance, interrelatedness, ambiguity, and uncertainty of the perceptual data (► Chap. 2) jointly create a situation of excessive demand for the cognitive system. Once subjects have reached the limits of their cognitive capacity, they try to decrease the cognitive workload by reducing the acquisition of information to a minimum. Decisions are then based on an insufficient "database" and a diagnosis is made on the first cue. Once a decision has been reached, it probably will not be reevaluated later in the light of new data.

6.5   Illusions: Inadequate Mental Models

Resource protection, the guarding of a feeling of competence, and the avoidance of ambiguity are responsible for many mistakes. Other mistakes occur because humans have an innate difficulty in handling probabilities and frequencies. Neverthe-

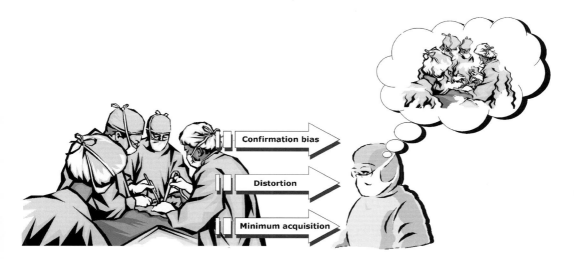

Fig. 6.2 Distortion of information leads to inadequate mental models

less, all of them have one feature in common: The picture someone has in his or her mind does not correlate with reality as displayed in data and seen in retrospect. It was only after the rescue operation that the EMS team from our case study realized that they had "bet on the wrong horse" and actually had not realized the true problem. The amount of literature on faulty decision-making seems to be on overload; therefore, we restrict ourselves to a discussion of those forms of error which impact decision-making in the acute care setting.

6.5.1 Fixation Error: Maintaining Mental Models Despite the Evidence

In critical situations the guarding of competence and an imminent excessive cognitive demand can lead to a situation in which the wish for a stable mental model rules all behavior. Once a situation assessment has been made, people tend to stay fixed on it even if there is sufficient data pointing in the opposite direction. People develop a cognitive tunnel vision. This error of fixation (DeKeyser and Woods 1990; Gaba 1992) is characterized by a tendency to search for confirming information and to distort data so as to fit the current mental model (◘ Table 6.1). This becomes most apparent when a certain possibility is rejected at all costs ("everything but this"). Besides the necessity to protect one's mental models, the main motive remains the need to control the situation: If this situation really is "it," then one would indeed have to deal with a serious problem and possibly would be helpless; therefore, what is not *supposed* to be simply *cannot* be.

6.5.2 Too Simple Mental Model About Complex Problems

When humans are faced with everyday problems, they find an appropriate solution by applying simple mental models. Complex problems, however, demand a complex understanding of the situation and the surrounding conditions, if an appropriate solution is to be found. Because simple models have paid off countless times in everyday life, humans continue to use them even when they are faced with unusual, opaque, and complex problems (Dörner et al. 1983; Dörner 1996; Sterman 1994). If thinking is made easy in such a way, then:

- The whole extent of a problem will be underestimated.
- Too simple assumptions about the chain of causation will be made.
- Interrelations will be ignored and single aspects of a problem will be treated as being independent. This will cause unwanted side effects.
- The dynamics of the development will be misjudged. People tend to anticipate the development of variables by means of linear extrapolation. When they suddenly are confronted with a nonlinear development, such as sudden "catastrophic" situations, they will be taken by surprise.

6.5.3 Knowledge Errors

It is not always the case that people will create a completely faulty mental model about a certain problem. Sometimes it is not the entire model but only a part thereof which is affected: The person has a particu-

◘ **Table 6.1** Fixation errors. (From DeKeyser and Woods 1990)

Fixation error	Meaning
"This and only this"	Persistent failure to revise a diagnosis or plan despite sufficient evidence to the contrary
"Everything but that"	Persistent failure to address a serious problem. Every possible explanation for a situation, with exception of a real emergency, is taken into account
"Everything's OK"	Persistent belief that there is no danger despite sufficient evidence to the contrary

lar "knowledge," but it is actually incorrect given the context. The *knowledge* is recalled correctly but the *application* under the given circumstances is inappropriate: An intensive care physician might diagnose an ECG rhythm correctly but then may err in the selection of the antiarrhythmic drug, because the pharmacological profile of this drug is not appropriate in treating this specific dysrhythmia.

It seems to be the case much more often that the person has correct knowledge that eventually winds up being useless because it does not help to solve the particular problem at hand. Healthcare providers can fall into this error trap very quickly if they are accustomed to acting before they have spent sufficient time on creating an adequate mental model of the situation. In this case familiar action schemata are triggered by only a few characteristics of a situation (►Chap. 4): An aggressive volume replacement is usually indicated in a severe hypovolemic shock following a motor vehicle accident; however, the underlying – and unquestioned – assumption is that the shock has been caused by volume loss and not by a global cardiac failure. Interestingly, it is experienced clinicians who are especially vulnerable to this kind of misjudgment. Decades of clinical practice have provided them with a wealth of clinical strategies which they can apply following a salient cue. Because these behavioral patterns clearly have proven to be successful in past experience, the danger is great that the initial situational assessment will not be questioned. A behavior which pays attention to the peculiarity of every single case is replaced by the "methodism"(Dörner 1996; "cognitive conservatism", Reason 1990) of the "experienced" caregiver. Methodism – seeing new situations in terms of old, established patterns of action that need only be set in motion – is far more economical than considering in each individual case what the specific local conditions would demand as an adequate way of responding. In many complex situations, considering a few "characteristic" features of the situation and developing an appropriate course of action is not the essential point. Instead, the most important thing is to consider the specific, individual configuration of those features and to develop a "customized" sequence of actions.

The third way knowledge errors can occur is when people do not reevaluate a situation and therefore do not adapt the management accord-

ingly: "One's knowledge was correct about something, but now things have changed." In other words, assumptions about therapeutic options were initially right but then became wrong in the course of the treatment. Because critical situations can change dynamically, the prerequisites for successful action may change as well. Nitroglycerine will be the first-line treatment for a patient with stenocardic complaints caused by a myocardial infarction; however, if ischemia increases and contractility is further impaired, the resulting arterial hypotension will then be a strong contraindication for the same drug. Failing to regularly take the blood pressure would lead to a potential fatal treatment error. Situation awareness (►Chap. 8; Endsley 1995) – the knowledge about where exactly one *is* within a critical situation and about the validity of current assumptions – is a critical ability which healthcare providers need in order to prevent errors of fixation and to correct faulty mental models of a situation.

6.6 What Is likely? The Handling of Uncertain Information

Estimations about frequency and probability play a vital role on every level of information processing. Perception is based in large part on the selection of the most probable hypothesis or schemata (► Chap. 5). In order to be able to assess a situation, diagnose a problem, select a therapy, and take a risk, however, probabilities have to be estimated and judged. This subjective assessment of probabilities happens mostly subconsciously. For the delivery of acute medical care information given in numerical form is of less importance than the fact that many diagnostic and therapeutic decisions are based on beliefs concerning the likelihood of uncertain events. "Probability" in the psychological sense can be defined as subjective conviction that an event will take place or a statement is true, given all the information available (Kahneman et al. 1982).

6.6.1 Assessment of Probability: Rules of Thumb for Everyday Life

When faced with the task of judging probabilities and predicting values, people generally experience great difficulties. That is the reason why people generally use a limited number of rules of thumb (heuristics) to simplify these judgmental operations. In general, two heuristic principles are applied which are very useful in everyday life but which sometimes can lead to severe and systematic errors (Tversky and Kahneman 1974):

- *Representativeness:* Items are judged to be similar based on how closely they resemble each other. Assessment of resemblance relies on prototypical features rather than on close analysis.
- *Availability:* People assess the frequency or the probability of an event by the ease with which instances or occurrences can be brought to mind (i.e., retrieved from memory).

6.6.1.1 Representativeness

The assessment that the patient from the case study suffers from a severe volume loss is based on "typical" features of the schema "trauma victim following motor vehicle accident." If a situation contains some representative evidence of a certain category, then people assume that the situation indeed belongs in this category. The categorization of the present emergency situation into the category "motor vehicle accident with multiple casualties" happens on the basis of the similarity with a prototype (similarity matching; Reason 1990). What sounds rather abstract is nevertheless clinically relevant: If the diagnosis "shock resulting from significant blood loss" is derived solely on the basis of weak peripheral pulses in combination with the mechanism of injury without any further detailed examination, then precious time is won and volume resuscitation can begin immediately; however, this shortcut seduces people into concentrating on only a few characteristics of the situation and neglecting others. The heuristic of representativeness can become even more misleading if it is applied in reverse: "What does not look like a typical myocardial infarction cannot be one." As past experiences had taught the medical team that patients with a myocardial infarction "typically" await them at home, they were unprepared to meet this medical condition under these unusual circumstances: That a patient with an acute myocardial infarction actually can cause a traffic accident is indeed improbable. What is typical for a situation depends on knowledge and experience. The more differentiated a mental model of a situation is, the more features can be included in the assessment.

6.6.1.2 Availability

The assessed likelihood of an event depends on the ease with which schemata can be retrieved from memory: That what people can remember most easily determines the picture of the situation. Lifelong experience has taught us the following:

- Instances of frequent classes are recalled better and faster than instances of less frequent classes.
- Likely occurrences are easier to imagine than unlikely ones.
- Associative connections are strengthened when two events frequently occur (Tversky and Kahneman 1974).

Because the availability of schemata depends on the *frequency* with which they are used, this heuristic is effective most of the time; however, other factors as well influence the likelihood of memory recall:

- Conspicuity/distinctiveness/salience
- Importance
- Time since last recall

The fact that many anesthesiologists suspect or at least consider a case of malign hyperthermia as soon as an abnormal increase in end-tidal CO_2 is detected is due to the importance of an early diagnosis and treatment, and not to the general incidence of the disease itself. Furthermore, if a healthcare provider has just finished reading an educational article about a certain clinical problem, he or she will be prone to presume exactly this and no other problem behind any compatible clinical pattern he or she will encounter in the near future.

6.6.2 Problems in Dealing with Probabilities

The inability to deal with probabilities does not only stem from the reliance on judgmental heuristics, nor is it attributable to motivational effects alone or to the economy of mental models: Most people simply disregard some basic principles of statistical reasoning which would enable them to estimate probabilities correctly. In the field of healthcare this is relevant whenever decisions are based on data, such as the choice between different treatments or when taking side effects into account (▶ Gigerenzer 2000 for a collection of examples from healthcare). Even when probabilities are not expressed in numbers, but instead verbally, there are nevertheless pitfalls within this process of assessment and judgment which can lead to serious errors:

- Beware of "felt likelihood": The emotional assessment of probabilities is highly erroneous especially when two probabilities are interconnected (this may even lead to contraintuitive results).
- Beware of "pseudo-accuracy": If there is a general lack of information, you have to draw assumptions about basic probabilities of certain risks. If you then start calculating with these numbers, though, you will receive "exact" results in the end; however, this number only reflects personal assumptions and presumptions. Beware if approximations are multiplied with each other.
- Beware of confounding cause and correlation! The joint occurrence of two events does not allow any statement about their causal relationship ($a \rightarrow b$, $b \rightarrow a$, or both, are caused by a third variable c).
- Beware of reverse conclusions: If $a \rightarrow b$, this does not automatically imply that if a is not given, then b cannot be (e.g., "if a myocardial infarction does not happen within a 'typical setting,' then it cannot possibly be a myocardial infarction").
- Beware of the base-rate fallacy when dealing with test results: You have to know the base rate in the population *and* the error rate of a test if you want to determine the probability that a test result is correct. People tend to neglect the base rate and use only the data on test reliability.
- Where there is an α-error, there is a β-error, also known as false-negative or false-positive result. It is (for logical reasons) impossible to reduce both at the same time. Tests which are highly sensitive and therefore include all relevant cases lead to false alarms (false positives) more often than those tests which fail to detect some of the cases and therefore are less sensitive (false negative). Whether it is worse to overlook a diagnosis or to wrongly diagnose a disease (which means to commit an α- or β-error) is a decision the physician has to make.

6.6.3   No Risk, No Fun? How to Deal with Risk

As complexity will always include uncertainty about the result of an intentional action (▶ Chap. 2), risk is an unavoidable component of healthcare; therefore, the question for healthcare providers can never be, *if they actually are willing* to take risks in their actions but rather *under which circumstances* they will do so and for which reason. Judgment of risks is based on perceived risk, not on objective facts; therefore, risk assessment is always subjective and prone to error. For actions in an acute care setting an absolute estimate about risk assessment is often impossible ("How dangerous is option X?"), not like the relative assessment when comparing two treatment options ("Is option X more risky than option Y?"). Whenever a decision between two actions in a critical situation has to be made, this should never be done spontaneously. On the contrary, in risk assessment for treatment options, the following three questions should be applied to every option in order to minimize the risk of every action:

- How high is the probability of unwanted events?
- How high is the probability that I will be unable to cope with the situation I am about to create?
- How high is the price the patient and/or I will have to pay if I am unable to cope with this situation?

The safety of the patient depends in large part on the ability of the caregivers to make a controlled decision when accepting risk. Which risk the decision will bring for the patient will depend, in the end, on the caregivers' (a) awareness of and knowledge about dangers, (b) experience with comparable situations, and (c) actual competence.

6.6.3.1   Motivation

It is not uncommon that motives other than patient safety guide medical decisions. The avoidance of boredom ("no risk, no fun"), the desire to make autonomous decisions irrespective of safety standard ("man, don't you tell me!"), or the desire to become a "hero" by spectacular actions ("now watch me doing this!") can all lead to an underestimation of risk. The key for successful risk management lies in the realistic assessment of one's own competence and in the control of those motives which favor a risky decision; therefore, the basic working philosophy should always be to avoid working near your performance limit because then the safety of the patient cannot be ensured. Team members are a valuable resource in addressing the issue of taking unnecessary risks.

6.6.3.2 Heuristics

As the identification of an acceptable level of risk constitutes a probabilistic assessment, it is done by means of heuristics. The most relevant heuristic for risk assessment is the *rule of availability* (see above). The likelihood of a complication is estimated by the ease with which it comes to mind. The imaginative drive can stem from own experience, from discussions with colleagues, or from a recently read educational article. The risk for a complication is *overestimated* if one happened to talk about a similar case just yesterday or if one still has lively memories about an incident which happened not too long ago. A risk is *underestimated* if one never has experienced a certain complication or if risky behavior has received positive feedback: In both cases one simply cannot imagine why this patient should be an exception to that rule, and that such a complication actually could happen right now.

6.7   Tips for Clinical Practice

Both, the individual and the team, can avoid being trapped by the law of economy and the protection of competence if they intentionally direct the perception and processing of information. The following ideas are basically easy to put into practice; however, they require a conscious effort to redirect personal thinking habits. This can be strenuous and sometimes very unpleasant!

6.7.1   Information Processing and Mental Models

- "Wipe the slate clean." Avoid thinking about any medico-legal or social implication and direct all attention to the problem. It is of fundamental importance that you start from scratch. Never assume that any single item of your current mental model is a given fact.
- Critically reevaluate your first hypothesis: The probability that your initial diagnosis has been made by means of heuristics is high. It is possible that critical aspects of a situation have been neglected; therefore, you should always actively search for information which contradicts and disproves the initial diagnosis. This questioning of an initial diagnosis is all the more important

in a critical situation, as there will be only few external corrective aids. As stress further impairs the ability to search for contradictory data, it should become a habit of thought in clinical routine to ask oneself these questions:
  - Did I overlook facts?
  - Do new data fit my initial assumptions?
  - Has there been any relevant developments recently?
  - Is there any reason why the initial assumption could be wrong?
- The ability to make allowances for incomplete and incorrect information and conclusions is an important requirement for dealing with complex situations.
- Generate Alternatives. You can avoid fixation errors best by making it your habit to explicitly name several possible differential diagnoses or alternative actions every time a first idea comes readily to your mind. If newly found evidence indeed favors an alternative explanation for the clinical problem, then always remember: The ability to admit mistaken assumptions and to revise an initial diagnosis or decision is a sign of wisdom and competence, not of weakness.
- Appreciate that the path to incidents is paved with false assumptions.

6.7.2   Probabilistic Risk Assessment

- Always be extremely cautious if you have to make a decision about an irretrievable action. If you want to take the patient's ability to breathe spontaneously by giving a muscle relaxant, or if the patient is supposed to be extubated, then you should always ask yourself: "Do I really want to do that now?"
- "As an overall philosophy, it is wise to use good judgment to avoid, whenever possible, situations in which superior skills must be applied to ensure safety" (Hawkins 1987).
- Civil aviation has taught the principle of deliberate risk taking with the acronym "CAREFUL": **C**onsciously **A**ccept **R**isks **E**valuated with **F**orethought, **U**nderstanding, and **L**ogic.
- Always deliberately set a minimum safety level for everything you do – and *never* go below it. Remember: If it is not worth doing safely, it is not worth doing!

6.8 "Information Processing and Mental Models": in a Nutshell

- Conscious thinking is based upon several basic, subconscious levels of information management processing.
- Knowledge is organized into schemata (e.g., schemata of events, of expectations, of conceptual knowledge) and mental models. They allow for the recognition, interpretation, and extrapolation of events.
- Many errors originate from basic features of information processing: cognitive economy; protection of the feeling of competence; and the avoidance of ambiguity.
- Common problems of information gathering are the selective search for confirming information ("confirmation bias"), distortion of information, the suppression of unwanted information, and reduced acquisition of information.
- Mental models can be inappropriate for a given problem. Fixation error, too simple models, knowledge errors, and methodism of the experienced caregiver can affect the problem-solving.
- The handling of uncertain information and of probabilities is difficult for most people; therefore, people use heuristics, such as *representativeness* and the *rule of availability*, in order to assess the likelihood of risk. Despite their usefulness in everyday life, they can be misleading in critical situations. Mental operations with probabilities often lead to erroneous results because probability calculations are often contraintuitive.
- Risk taking is unavoidable in anesthesia, intensive care, and emergency medicine. Risks can be over- or underestimated depending on motivation and the heuristics applied.
- The ability to admit mistaken assumptions and to revise an initial diagnosis or decision is a sign of wisdom and competence, not of weakness.

References

Anderson JR (1983) The architecture of cognition. Harvard University Press, Cambridge, Massachusetts

Bartlett FC (1932) Remembering. Cambridge University Press, Cambridge UK

Camerer C, Weber M (1992) Recent developments in modeling preferences: uncertainty and ambiguity. J Risk Uncertainty 5:325–370

Curley SP, Yates JF, Abrams RA (1986) Psychological sources of ambiguity avoidance. Organ Behav Human Decis Process 38:230–256

DeKeyser V, Woods DD (1990) Fixation errors: failures to revise situation assessment in dynamic and risky systems. In: Colombo AG, Bustamante AS (eds) Systems reliability assessment. Kluwer, Dordrecht

Dörner D (1996) The logic of failure. Recognizing and avoiding error in complex situations. Metropolitan Books, New York

Dörner D, Kreuzig H, Reither F, Stäudel T (1983) Lohhausen. Vom Umgang mit Unbestimmtheit und Komplexität [Lohhausen. Dealing with uncertainty and complexity]. Huber, Bern

Endsley MR (1995) Toward a theory of situation awareness in dynamic systems. Hum Factors 37:32–64

Gaba D (1992) Dynamic decision-making in anesthesiology: cognitive models and training approaches. In: Evans DA, Patel VL (eds) Advanced models of cognition for medical training and practice. Springer, Berlin Heidelberg New York, pp 123–48

Gigerenzer G (2000) Adaptive thinking. Rationality in the real world. University Press, Oxford

Hawkins FH (1987) Human factors in flight. Ashgate, Aldershot, UK

Heath C, Tversky A (1991) Preference and belief: ambiguity and competence in choice under uncertainty. J Risk Uncertainty 4:5–28

Hertwig R, Todd P (2001) More is not always better: the benefits of cognitive limits. In: Hardman D (ed) The psychology of reasoning and decision-making: a handbook. Wiley, Chichester, UK

Johnson-Laird PN (1983) Mental models. Towards a cognitive science of language, interference, and consciousness. Cambridge University Press, Cambridge

Kahneman D, Slovic P, Tversky A (1982) Judgement under uncertainty: heuristics and biases. Cambridge University Press, Cambridge

Klein G (1992) A recognition-primed decision (RPD) model of rapid decision-making. In: Klein G, Orasanu J, Calderwood R, Zsamboka E (eds) Decision-making in action: models and methods. Ablex, Norwood, New Jersey, pp 138–147

Lompscher J (1972) Theoretische und experimentelle Untersuchungen zur Entwicklung geistiger Fähigkeiten [Theoretical and experimental studies on the development of mental abilities]. Volk und Wissen, Berlin

Piaget J, Brown T, Thampy KJ (1985) Equilibration of cognitive structures: the central problem of intellectual development. University of Chicago Press, Chicago

Reason J (1990) Human error. Cambridge University Press, Cambridge

Schank RC, Abelson R (1977) Scripts, plans, goals, and understanding. Erlbaum, Hillsdale, New Jersey

Selz O (1913/1922) Über die Gesetze des geordneten Denkverlaufs [On the laws of structured thought processes]. Spemann, Stuttgart

Sterman JD (1994) Learning in and about complex systems. Syst Dyn Rev 10:291–330

Tversky A, Kahneman D (1974) Judgment under uncertainty: heuristics and biases. Science 185:1124–1130

7   Goals and Plans: Turning Points for Success

7.1   Case Study

After emergency surgery, an obese patient with multiple injuries was transferred from the operating room to the surgical intensive care unit (SICU). His diagnoses included open fractures of the forearm and the femur, blunt chest trauma, a mild head injury, and multiple lacerations. The chest X-ray showed evidence of a lung contusion without any signs of fractured ribs or of a pneumothorax. On admission to the SICU the patient was adequately ventilated and his initial hemoglobin concentration was 11.5 g/dl. After 2 h of an uneventful course, the patient suddenly developed increasing peak airway pressures. Despite increasing the inspired oxygen concentration to 70%, the saturation continued to decrease and the patient remained hemodynamically instable. The resident physician in charge examined the patient and auscultated the lung and found decreased chest motion and decreased breath sounds over the right hemithorax. He assumed a pneumothorax and decided, without confirming his diagnosis by additional examinations and studies (e.g., chest X-ray), to perform a tube thoracostomy at once through an anterior axillary line incision. Because he had never performed this procedure and because the anatomy of the patient was less than favorable for an exact identification of anatomical landmarks, he accidentally perforated the liver with the trocar. There was an initial blood return through the chest tube that he interpreted as a result of intrapleural bleeding. Despite his intervention, the oxygenation did not improve and the peak airway pressure did not normalize. Drawing no further conclusions from these facts, no additional interventions were performed at this time by the resident. Over the next 20 min 1500 ml of blood drained from the chest tube and the arterial blood pressure began to drop. The resident inserted two large-bore intravenous lines and rapidly infused crystalloid and colloid solutions. At the same time, he asked the nurse to prepare an infusion pump with epinephrine, to check the arterial blood gas, and to request packed red blood cells (PRBCs) and fresh frozen plasma (FFP) from the blood bank. The resident finally called for his attending physician, but before he arrived in the SICU, the patient went into cardiac arrest. Cardiopulmonary resuscitation (CPR) was immediately started and spontaneous circulation returned. From the location of the thoracostomy site and from the clinical course

the attending physician assumed intraabdominal bleeding from a perforated liver and planned for an emergency exploratory laparotomy. Following a massive volume resuscitation of blood products and crystalloid, the patient was stabilized and transported to the operating room. Laparotomy confirmed the diagnosis of a massive hemorrhage from a laceration to the liver. With an aggressive operative approach the bleeding was controlled and the blood pressure improved. As a result of the massive transfusion of blood products, the patient developed transfusion related lung injury (TRALI) and required mechanical ventilation for several weeks. An intraoperative bronchoscopy revealed a large blood cloth which had almost completely obstructed the right mainstem bronchus as the cause for the initial problems. After removal, the saturation and airway pressures normalized rapidly.

An intern is confronted with a ventilatory problem in an intensive care patient. He interprets the presenting constellation of symptoms (increased airway pressure, absent breath sounds over the right lung, a slowly decreasing saturation) as diagnostic signs of a tension pneumothorax. Although there would have been several more differential diagnoses for this symptom constellation, and although the patient is in no vital danger, the intern starts to act following his first assumption. He neither searches for alternative causes for the clinical problem, nor does he request a second opinion. As he performs thoracostomy without supervision by an experienced colleague, he obviously does not take the possibility of a complication into account. When the complication indeed occurs he does not recognize it as such. The clinical course leads to the patient's cardiac arrest and cardiopulmonary resuscitation is started. Because of a massive replacement with volume and red blood cells, CPR is successful. As a result of this massive transfusion, the pulmonary situation of the patient deteriorates and he develops a full-blown ARDS. The actual trigger for the situation, a blood cloth in the right main bronchus, could have been removed bronchoscopically without any danger for the patient. Because the intern prematurely formulated the goal "inserting a chest tube" and because he subsequently planned for this action poorly (if at all), he put the patient's life at risk. *Setting goals* as well as *planning actions* did not adequately take place.

Goals and plans are thoughts about the future – anticipated events, developments, and actions.

Although goals are part of the planning process, the elaboration of goals nevertheless poses cognitive demands different from those of planning. Also, different mistakes occur during the formulation of goals and during the process of planning; therefore, goals and plans are treated separately here.

7.2 Setting and Elaboration of Goals

To think about goals seems at first an unnecessary task for any person involved in acute and emergency healthcare. Why bother about formulating goals if the obligation to maintain and regain vital functions is more than obvious? Goals that point in a certain basic direction, such as "to normalize ventilation" in the adipose multiple-injured patient, are called general goals. There is seldom doubt or conflict about this kind of goals when treating a patient. But at a more concrete level, when general goals have to be translated into specific goals and plans of action, things can change quickly: This is where, in our case study, uncertainty arises for the intensive care physician: Quite obviously the patient has a medical problem, which could lead to many different treatment goals. On the one hand, the symptoms could be caused by a tension pneumothorax. This is a life-threatening condition which would be best treated by a rapid decompression of the intrapleural air. A specific goal would then be the immediate decompression of the tension pneumothorax. On the other hand, several other, less rapidly progressing causes could be responsible for the symptoms. A specific goal here would be "analysis of causes." In order to identify and reflect upon possible differential diagnosis the physician would have to spend time, which might not be available if the clinical condition is indeed deteriorating rapidly. If his goal is to act immediately and therefore to insert a chest tube all by himself, then this procedure can cause complications, especially when performed by an inexperienced person. If he sets the goal "maximum patient safety" and therefore calls an experienced colleague for help, he might fail to satisfy his educational goal "gaining experience with invasive emergency procedures." The intensivist has to balance all these diverse goals.

The need to pursue multiple goals (▶ Chap. 2) is one of the main problems of setting goals in an acute care setting. This plurality of goals means that people have to attend to many factors and satisfy several criteria at once when they act. In addition, these goals can be negatively linked: If one criterion is satisfied, one will necessarily fail to satisfy the other (and vice versa, if the dependency is reciprocal). This dilemma of a plurality of goals is intensified by the *intransparence of reality*. An increased airway pressure, irregular breath sounds and a slowly declining saturation signal are alterations which may have several different causes. Our case study is one of countless examples which demonstrate that the data which physicians and other healthcare workers take to formulate goals are incomplete and opaque; however, if people do not know what exactly the problem is, they have difficulty in defining a final goal. The vague setting of goals is not only in this case study a source of error. In addition, the intensivist, like all physicians, did not only have *explicit* goals like the well-being of the patient. At the same time he was pursuing *implicit* goals as well, intended to meet very personal needs (▶ Chap. 4): To feel competent, to try something new (e.g., the insertion of a chest tube), to protect self-esteem, to be successful – all these motives subconsciously influenced the formation of goals and hence the intensivist's decision for or against a certain procedure. The fact that personal motives influence decisions is unavoidable and actually not bad. It only leads to problems if, as in the case study, those non-issue-related motives start to uncontrollably govern behavior. Non-issue-related goals become apparent when actions lead to medical problems or other errors.

7.2.1 What is a Good Goal?

To have a goal means to accomplish some end with our activity, to have certain needs met. Goals tell us which way to go; they serve as "beacons for our actions" (◾Fig. 7.1; Dörner 1996). Good goals are those goals which help to satisfy as many concurrent needs as possible without creating new problems. The goals of the intensive care physician did not meet these criteria. Whenever one is confronted with a complex problem (see Frensch and Funke 1995 on complex problem-solving), the task of formulating an adequate goal should not be underestimated. Sometimes this even turns out to be the central cognitive task which greatly impacts any further planning and decision-making (Dörner 1996); however, "good" in this context does not

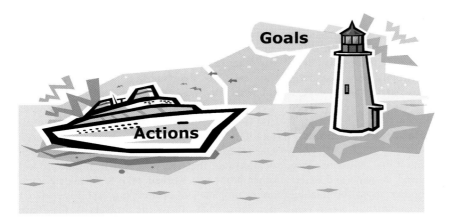

Fig. 7.1 Goals as beacons for action

imply an ethical assessment of its content but rather the ability of a goal to successfully direct action.

Good goals therefore fall into clear criteria (von der Weth 1990), which are:

— Formulated as a positive goal: Goals should be formulated as a positive goal whenever possible: Simply to avoid something, to want to make a situation "different" – these goals lack specificity and are inadequate as guideposts for planning and action. With a positive goal, however, we want to achieve some definite condition.

— Clearly specified: A specific goal is defined by many criteria and can be described and conceptualized very precisely. Those criteria can be numerical values ("given a F_iO_2 of 0.7 the saturation shall rise above 95%") or qualitative statements ("the airway pressures shall lie within the range of normal").

— Structured: General goals always consist of multiple specific goals. For example, in order to achieve normal airway pressures (general goal), certain changes have to be envisaged (change in lung physiology, respirator settings). Moreover, goals can be further subdivided into partial goals, which become increasingly specific until they can give rise to action.

— Prioritized: Goals need to be prioritized according to content and time. Which goal do we want to achieve under all circumstances; what should be avoided at all costs (normocapnia vs. peak airway pressure)? What are we willing to sacrifice?

— Checked for conflicts and contradictions: Which goals are mutually exclusive? This is especially important if side effects should be avoided: To experiment with a new invasive procedure and at the same time to ensure patient safety are mutually exclusive. One should not realize only in hindsight that reaching one goal has made it virtually impossible to satisfy the other.

— Allow for flexibility: The development of a situation very often is fairly unpredictable. Not to define rigid goals too early in the course of action allows for a flexibility which seizes opportunities as they emerge.

> Characteristics of good goals are as follows:
> — They are formulated as a positive goal.
> — They are clearly specified.
> — They are structured.
> — They are prioritized.
> — They are checked for conflicts and contradictions.
> — They allow for flexibility.

7.2.2   Problems with Setting Goals

The conscious formulation of goals is rarely exercised in everyday practice. In critical situations this missing habit can have unpleasant consequences, because a faulty formulation of goals may result in ineffective action. Experiments to elucidate the problems of goal setting have identified several critical issues (e.g.; Dörner and Pfeifer 1993; Dörner 1996; Dörner and Schaub 1994; Schaub 1997), as given below.

7.2.2.1 No Formulation of Goals: Action Counts

The formulation of goals should serve to gain or regain control over a critical situation; however, if the level of stress experienced by an individual or a team exceeds their coping capacity, these demands can become overwhelming and one starts to act inconsiderately. Without having set a goal, spontaneous ideas will be the basis for all plans and actions: To be able to do something gives a good feeling in a difficult situation. As a result, the process of planning is not guided by goals which should be achieved but by the awareness of the effects of one's actions. People tend to demonstrate their competence with actions that look powerful. Especially teamwork suffers from the fact that goals are not clearly communicated; only general goals are shared. What the goals are seems to be quite obvious for everyone while working on a common task. It is often only in hindsight that we realize that everybody had acted on their own account.

7.2.2.2 No Priorities Set

Complex and time-critical situations will always create more than one goal which has to be addressed. These goals can conflict with one another, either because the variables relating to them are negatively linked (which basically means that by achieving one goal you may be unable to succeed with the other), because a given time frame allows only for one goal to be pursued, or the resources (e.g., personal, material) are inadequate to meet all demands of a situation. Therefore, as it is impossible to solve all the problems at once, a way has to be found to organize the list of problems according to their importance and urgency. This has to take place before actions are planned, delegated, and executed. If, as usually happens, the team leader eases the task of dealing with multiple problems by delegation, he or she will need to distinguish between "delegating problems" and "dumping responsibility" for them onto others. It is not an uncommon phenomenon that a physician who is unclear about

the priorities of his or her tasks may thrust a multitude of orders on medical assistance staff. It is then up to each team member to decide which of these many orders are tackled first. Their priorities, however, may be governed by many different motifs: They may decide to solve the problems on the basis of competence or personal preference; or they might do what was said last or what brings them out of this particular situation as quickly as possible. All of these selection criteria may not help to solve the most important or urgent problem.

Poor analysis of problems and inefficient setting of priorities will sometimes lead to "repair-service behavior" (Dörner 1996). Like a plumber who runs from one leaking pipe to the next, we address problems according to urgency and awareness only. The main consequence of repair-service behavior is that the wrong problems are solved: Criteria such as obviousness or personal competence determine the selection of a problem. We wrongly imagine ourselves to be in charge of a situation and to be accomplishing good for the patient. We also fail to see that circumstances more or less randomly generate the list of actions and that we remain "captives" of the moment. Repair-service behavior is, in its very nature, a reactive behavior, and it therefore will always stay behind the game. If problems are not addressed adequately, they may go unnoticed for a long time, starting small and then developing with increasing speed. Unless we anticipate such problems, they will take us by surprise. As repair-service behavior does not take the future development of a situation into account, it is unsuitable to deal with the dynamics of complex systems.

7.2.2.3 Unawareness of Conflicting Goals

As complex situations are characterized by the interrelatedness of many system variables (on-scene situation, pathophysiology of the patient, main motives of the different professional groups involved), there will be some goals which are in themselves justified but which are mutually exclusive – be it the parallel technical and medical rescue operation on site or the side by side of diagnostic and therapy during resuscitation of a trauma patient in the emergency room. There is always the possibility of conflicting goals which can only be resolved by compromise or the setting of one clear priority. If those conflicting issues are not addressed appropriately, the solution to a problem will be left to chance, to hierarchy, or to time pressure.

7.2.2.4 Lack of Clarity

The most frequent problem which occurs in setting goals is that the process itself is abandoned too early. As a result, goals will remain unclear and will be inadequate as guideposts for planning and action. Furthermore, unclear goals lack a criterion by which we can decide with certainty whether progress is in fact being made, or whether the goal has been achieved. Sometimes this might even be what people subconsciously intend: If the achievement of a goal cannot be verified, we still can feel competent even in the face of the most difficult problems. Lack of specificity creates an atmosphere of teamwork where it remains unclear what exactly should be done by whom exactly; however, teams willingly accept unclear goals as they hardly ever create conflict. Setting goals in such a manner is more a strategy for conflict avoidance than an adequate preparation for planning.

7.2.2.5 Insufficient Partial Goals

Basically it is clear in which direction the patient's status should evolve. Concretely, however, one has not deliberated much about the question as to how the different steps on the way to the "big goal" might actually look. Partial goals help in planning concrete steps of action. If they are missing, the action sequence can easily become random and aimless.

7.2.2.6 Missing Awareness About "Nonfactual" Goals

Explicitly formulated medical goals are very often only the ostensible drive for action. At the same time there will always be motives and implicit goals such as protection of competence, control, personal status, fear of failure, competition, or simple convenience. It lies in the "psycho-logic" of human behavior that there are no "mere factual" decisions: In everything we do self-regulation (how to take care of oneself), social regulation (how to connect and communicate with other people), and

the principle of economy (how to use the resource "thinking" as economically as possible) play a vital role. If a subject remains unaware of his or here "nonfactual" goals, they can develop a life on their own and secretly govern decision-making. Often these implicit goals remain hidden from ourselves and are only detected in hindsight, but they may be more readily detected by team members at the time of their influence.

7.2.2.7 Early Adoption of Final Goals

Once a final goal has been set it will not be revised, even if new information actually would make this necessary. In our case example, the obvious facts that neither peak airway pressure nor oxygenation improved upon the insertion of a chest tube did not make the resident doubt the adequacy of his goal. One reason for that may be the belief that to change an opinion might mean to lack competence in the mind of the professional. A lack of competence, however, is something most people do not easily admit. Because doubts are not allowed to arise, behavior becomes rigid and the person is no longer open to the developments of the situation.

7.2.2.8 Fixation on Negative Goals

By setting negative goals (what should be avoided) instead of positive goals (what should be achieved), people often try to defuse a critical situation ("the oxygenation should not deteriorate further"). Unfortunately, with this approach, what should actually be achieved remains unrealized, and planned action becomes virtually impossible. Furthermore, the intensive mental occupation with the negative goal may precipitate the unwanted event in the first place.

Frequent mistakes in setting goals are:
- No clear formulation of goals
- No priorities set
- Unawareness of conflicting goals
- Lack of clarity
- Insufficient partial goals
- Missing awareness about "nonfactual" goals
- Early adoption of final goals
- Fixation upon negative goals

7.3   Planning

Planning is a mental activity. It is "probationary action" (Freud 1911), in a way an imagined approach to a desired goal (Funke and Fritz 1995). Planning means (Hacker 1986; Strohschneider 1999):

- To identify available options
- To assess these options (risks and benefits, possibility of execution, framework requirements)
- To string individual actions together and schedule each step (who, when, where)

In planning we do not do anything but instead just consider what we *might* do. We think through the consequences of certain actions and see whether those actions will bring us closer to our desired goal. We reflect upon the question, under which *circumstances* a measure could "work," which *consequences* an action would entail, which *alternatives* exist, and what the *risks* of this actions would be. Planning has one big advantage: It is absolutely safe because it is not real. It is like sending up mental "trial balloons": Even if they pop, nobody will suffer harm. However, the disadvantage of planning is exactly this: It is not real. You only know with hindsight whether or not a plan worked out even!

A plan can refer to an isolated action or to a sequence of actions. In any case the planning sequence would comprise the three elements "*condition* for task X – *action* X – *result* of action X": "If it is possible to insert another i.v. line in this adipose patient, he will immediately receive 250 cc of a hypertonic saline–dextran for small-volume resuscitation and then his blood pressure will increase." If a certain action may lead to not just one result but to different results, a plan can branch out in different directions: "If it is possible to insert another i.v. line in this adipose patient, then we can start volume therapy. If we do not succeed, then we will try the other arm or proceed with a central venous catheter." A plan can follow different paths depending on circumstances (◻ Fig. 7.2). Because the precise sequence of actions cannot be determined in advance in an acute care setting, the consistent planning of all possible branching would soon result in an unmanageable tree; therefore, it would be wise not to predefine too many steps in advance, but instead plan ahead up to the most important partial goals and then wait and see how things actually develop ("muddling through"; Lindblom 1959).

Planning does not only consist of one planning process originating in a starting point right at the be-

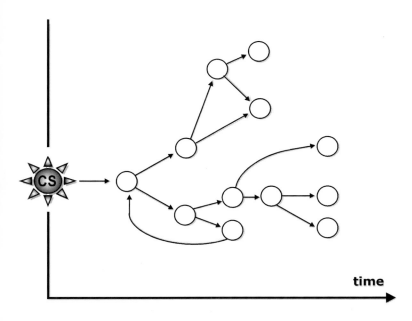

time

◻ **Fig. 7.2** Branching structure of a planning process (after Dörner 1999). The starting point where the plan originates is a critical situation (*CS*). *Arrows* represent actions. The *circles* indicate the goals subjects hope to achieve with those actions

ginning and moving toward a final goal. In fact, we can distinguish between two kinds of planning: forward planning and "reverse" planning (Dörner 1996).

In forward planning, we begin at the beginning and think from the momentary situation: This is the current state of the patient; how do we proceed from here? In some sense this is the "natural" form of planning to take. We plan the way we will actually act.

To plan in "reverse" means to plan with the goal as starting point: What conditions would have to prevail just prior to the desired goal in order for us to achieve that goal by means of specific action? For reverse planning it is crucial to have a clear goal in mind and then to develop adequate intermediate goals. If the goal is foggy and unclear, we will not have a solid frame of reference for the preceding steps, which might be the main reason why people show little spontaneous enthusiasm for this kind of planning. Many clinical problems require both kinds of planning, shifting back and forth between the forward and the reverse mode.

An additional requirement for the planning process emerges from the fact that the medical treatment of critically ill patients is given in an interdisciplinary setting: Not only does the own treatment plan has to be kept in mind; it also has to be adjusted to the plans of the other professional groups involved. The implications with regard to conflicting goals and solutions to this problem are treated in detail in Chap. 11.

7.3.1 Appropriate Planning in Complex Situations

Complex problematic situations in acute care medicine are characterized by intransparence and high internal dynamics (► Chap. 2): Just like the resident in the case study we often simply do not know enough about the patient to be able to plan "adequately." Furthermore, the situation develops independently while we are still busy reflecting upon the problem. The consequences of one's own actions are not so easily identified: For quite a long time the resident was convinced that he had successfully placed a chest tube. All these characteristics lead to the fact that it is virtually impossible to develop a comprehensive and long-term plan which would include all the eventualities that can occur in a planning process; therefore, planning here cannot mean to predefine the entire path from the current

situation to the final goal in all its details. It will always be necessary to adjust plans according to the patient's condition or the development of the situation. Even if flexibility is one of the central requirements for planning in complex situations, it nevertheless is possible to formulate some basic rules for good planning: Good planning in the context of acute care medicine is absolutely necessary.

7.3.1.1 "Branches Out Moderately"

The complexity of a critical situation is not reduced by propagating one single path that works from the starting point to the final goal. Instead, good plans consider alternatives. For that predetermined "hyphenation points" are necessary, where a decision has to be made whether or not the present proceeding has proved effective. If intermediate goals have been formulated, they can serve as such a hyphenation point: If a particular intermediate goal has not been reached, the entire plan should be reconsidered. In our case study such an intermediate goal could have been the normalization of ventilation parameters following chest drainage. The fact that they remained unchanged should have made him think again.

7.3.1.2 Checked for Side Effects and Long-Range Consequences

As our actions are planned towards a goal, we often are satisfied and stop planning when we see a way to reach that goal; however, every treatment contains the risk of unwanted side effects and long-range consequences. One main requirement for successful planning is therefore not only to envisage the treatment path, but also to reflect on the unwanted consequences of our action which may only arise with great delay. Quite obviously, in the case study the side effects and long-range consequences of actions were not considered when planning for a thoracostomy.

7.3.1.3 Planned with Sufficient "Buffer"

Because critical situations constantly change, it is necessary to plan a buffer for anything that may interfere. It is quite probable that situations will develop differently then planned, although it is unclear in advance what this change will be. Buffer in the acute care setting are first and foremost manpower and material resources; however, in a time of scarce economical resources in the health system it is exactly those buffers which seem to be decreased. Planning without buffer increases the risk for severe accidents and incidents, as a deviation from the initial plan cannot be reversed.

> The characteristics of good planning are that it:
> — "branches out moderately",
> — is checked for side effects and long-range consequences,
> — is planned with sufficient buffer.

7.3.2 Mistakes and Problems with Planning

Complexity and dynamics restrict the possibility to plan for the future. Common mistakes in the planning process are given below (Dörner 1996; Dörner and Schaub 1994; Schaub 1997; Strohschneider 1999; Strohschneider and Weth 2001).

7.3.2.1 Missing Planning: Methodism

If a clinical rule has been employed successfully in the past, there is an almost overwhelming tendency for healthcare providers to apply it again and again; thus, past experiences can lead to rigidity in rule-based problem-solving, to *methodism* (Dörner 1996; Reason 1990 uses the term "cognitive conservatism"). It is foremost the experienced healthcare professional who will succumb to methodism: "I know this kind of situation, I have experienced it many times before, I know what to do!" By acting on the basis of what has proved successful in the past the planning process is skipped and established patterns of actions are activated. What can happen is that such rules, though perfectly adequate in certain circumstances, may be misapplied if the situation differs slightly, but in important features, from previous situations. Because these unobtrusive but important details are missed – or even not looked for – the resulting behavior will take the form "strong but wrong" (Reason 1990). The erroneous behavior was more in keeping with past practice than the current situation demanded.

7.3.2.2 Planning without Alternatives, with Only One Emphasis

The decision maker only considers one single action without taking branching or alternatives into account. The course of action in the case study following the assumed successful puncture of a pneumothorax shows in an almost classical way as to how one completely has to restart the planning process once an idea has proven to be unsuccessful if the plan contained no alternatives. Sometimes this has to be done under great time pressure.

7.3.2.3 Planning without Considering Side Effects or Long-term Consequences

It is important to understand the links among goal criteria. "You cannot do only one thing" – what may sound like a truism nevertheless contains a deep truth for the management of complex situations. Every action has unwanted side effects and long-term effects which should be taken into account before acting. The prize for treatment should not be higher than that of the disease; however, this maxim is frequently disregarded as it leads to doubts about the appropriateness and consequences of one's treatment options and it will, like other forms of reflection, cost time and additional mental effort. But if we act without this kind of planning and unwanted side effects occur, we will be surprised by them.

7.3.2.4 Not Enough Planning

To subdivide a general plan into many partial goals requires a lot of mental capacity. Because this resource is scarce in complex situations with high demands, the plans are preferably formulated on a vague level. Within certain limits this is indeed a sound approach; however, many options seem to be possible only as long as we do not think about the concrete realization. "Under-planning" brings us into danger of following a path of action that turns out to be a dead end.

7.3.2.5 Over-Confidence in Planning

As soon as wishful thinking starts to prevail and failure no longer is thought of as a serious option, then excessive optimism about our plan will govern behavior: "The insertion of the chest tube will go well because it has to go well." The perception of feedback from the system (e.g., bleeding, unchanged ventilatory situation) will be selective; one chooses to see what one wants to see because one presumes to know already that the plan will be successful. The most serious variant of unjustified confidence in planning is the complete disregard for the option that complications (e.g., the perforation of the liver) or other critical situations could actually arise. In case of a complication, we are then totally surprised and have not only to build new plans (then under time pressure), but also to cope with our failure.

> Common mistakes in planning are:
> — Missing planning: Methodism
> — Planning without alternatives
> — Planning without considering side effects or long-term consequences
> — Not enough planning
> — Over-confidence in planning

7.4 Tips for Clinical Practice

7.4.1 Goals

— Set realistic goals! Always remember that a decision is only good insofar as there is actually time and possibility to put it into practice.

— Focus on clarifying your goals and the criteria by which you can decide with certainty whether the goal has been achieved.

— Prioritize your goals *before* you address your medical assistance.

— Be self-critical about any nonmedical motive or goal which might govern your actions.

— Whenever possible, restate a negative goal as a positive goal. Which state you want to achieve is important and not which state you want to avoid.

— Always remember that you can never do just one thing, never can focus on just one isolated goal. Always expect conflicting goals.

— Use communication about the treatment goals as a chance to improve teamwork: Shared goals are a prerequisite for joint action.

7.4.2 Planning

— Hope fort he best but prepare for the worst! If you implement a "worst-case" scenario into your planning process, unexpected developments will not catch you off guard.

— Always remember: It can happen to you, too! The fact that even the most experienced healthcare worker will suffer from inadequate planning has more to do with the nature of planning in complex situations than with personal incompetence.

— Always plan with alternatives and sufficient buffer (time, resources, staff).

— Take unwanted side effects and long-term side effects into account. Ask yourself: If I choose this action, what could possibly happen down the road?

— Never forget that planning is a mental *activity*. It requires strength and can become tiresome; therefore, a minimum of rest and energy is vital, even in critical situations. Wherever possible, the most experienced person should delegate all manual activities to team members to have his or her mind free for planning.

7.5 "Plans and Goals": in a Nutshell

— To have a goal means to know how certain needs can be met. Good goals are those which can satisfy many needs at the same time without creating new problems.

— Goals tell us which way to go, they serve as "beacons for actions"

— Good goals are set as general, intermediate, and partial goals, and they are prioritized and checked for conflicts. They are formulated as a positive goal, clarified, and have criteria by which a decision can be made, whether or not a goal has been achieved. Flexibility in dynamic situations which can help the person to seize opportunities as they emerge is an important demand.

— Common problems in setting goals are actionism, lack of prioritizing, unclearness about conflicting goals, missing specification and structuring, too rigid definitions of final goals, and fixation upon negative goals.

- Nonmedical goals may have a great influence on our actions. Most notably protection of competence can govern behavior in critical situations.
- Planning is an imagined approach to a goal. To plan means to search for and assess options for action and then to plan for concrete steps.
- Under the terms of complexity in acute and emergency healthcare comprehensive and long-term planning is impossible. Good planning under such circumstances would be moderately branched, would include sufficient buffer, and would be checked for side effects and long-term consequences.
- Common problems in planning are methodism, planning without alternatives, planning without considering side effects or long-term consequences, underplanning, and overconfidence in planning.

References

Dörner D (1996) The Logic of failure. Recognizing and avoiding error in complex situations. Metropolitan Books, New York

Dörner D (1999) Bauplan für eine Seele [Blueprint for a soul]. Rowohlt, Reinbek bei Hamburg, Germany

Dörner D, Pfeifer E (1993) Strategic thinking and stress. Ergonomics 36:1345–1360

Dörner D, Schaub H (1994) Errors in planning and decision-making and the nature of human information processing. Appl Psychol Int Rev 43:433–453

Freud S (1911/1961) Formulierungen über die zwei Prinzipien des psychischen Geschehens [two principles of psychological regulation]. Gesammelte Werke, Band VIII. Fischer, Frankfurt am Main

Frensch PA, Funke J (eds) (1995) Complex problem-solving: the European perspective. Erlbaum, Hillsdale, New Jersey

Funke J, Fritz A (1995) Über Planen, Problemlösen und Handeln [On planning, problem-solving, and action]. In: Funke J, Fritz A (eds) Neue Konzepte und Instrumente zur Planungsdiagnostik. Deutscher Psychologen Verlag, Bonn, pp 1–45

Hacker W (1986) Arbeitspsychologie [work psychology]. Deutscher Verlag der Wissenschaften, Berlin

Lindblom CE (1959) The science of muddling through. Public Admin Rev 19:79–88

Reason J (1990) Human error. Cambridge University Press, Cambridge UK

Schaub H (1997) Decision-making in complex situations: cognitive and motivational limitations. In: Flin R, Salas E, Strub ME, Martin L (eds) Decision-making under stress. Emerging Themes and Applications. Ashgate, Aldershot, pp 291–300

Strohschneider S (1999) Human behavior and complex systems: some aspects of the regulation of emotions and cognitive information processing related to planning. In: Stuhler EA, deTombe DJ (eds) Complex problem-solving: cognitive psychological issues and environment policy applications. Hampp, Munich, pp 61–73

Strohschneider, S, Weth R von der (eds) (2001) Ja, mach nur einen Plan: Pannen und Fehlschläge – Ursachen, Beispiele, Lösungen [Problems in planning – examples, causes, solutions]. Huber, Bern

Weth R von der (1990) Zielbildung bei der Organisation des Handelns [elaboration of goals in action regulation] Peter Lang, Frankfurt a.M.

8   Attention: in the Focus of Consciousness

8.1   Case Study

A resident physician was finishing his last night shift at the end of a week of night calls. It was 5 a.m. and the last few hours had been particularly straining because of several unstable patients. The resident was feeling very tired, but he decided to do rounds one more time on his patients before getting some rest. While evaluating a patient whose hemodynamic status had recently worsened, he was emergently called for another patient who had been inadvertently extubated during positioning. When the resident arrived at the bedside, the patient's oxygen saturation was 85%, and he was being mask ventilated by a nurse. The physician took over the ventilation and asked the nurse to prepare for reintubation. Because the patient was agitated and resisted mask ventilation, the resident decided to give him a bolus of fentanyl and midazolam from the infusion pump. Immediately after the injection, the patient became severely tachycardic and hypertensive. The heart rate was 180 bpm and the blood pressure rose to 260/150 mm Hg. A quick glance at the infusion pump labels made the resident realize that he had mistakenly delivered a bolus of epinephrine instead of fentanyl. Upon recognition of the error, the patient's hemodynamic response was rapidly controlled with boluses of nitroglycerin, and soon after, his vital functions returned to normal. The patient was then uneventfully intubated.

After 1 week of night shift on an ICU, a fatigued physician is faced with an emergency. The call for help reaches him in a moment when his attention is focused on another problem. Tired and still immersed in thought, he has to manage an emergency situation where he has to concentrate on successful mask ventilation and at the same time prepare for reintubation. When he manually wants to give a bolus of an analgosedative drug to the patient he accidentally manipulates the wrong infusion pump and applies a high dose of a catecholamine. Due to an immediate intervention with a vasodilating drug, further patient harm from an excessive increase in both hearth rate and arterial blood pressure can be prevented.

8.2   The Control of Action: Attention, Vigilance, and Concentration

Human thinking, perception, and action can be consciously controlled and influenced. This conscious control is vital for successful problem-solving and for any action which requires precision and permanence. The relevant central resource, the process by which we focus our awareness, is called attention. It enables humans to be completely present in a certain task. Attention, however, is also a vulnerable resource: If it decreases or, like in the case study, is defective due to fatigue, then people often suffer from a loss of control over their behavior. Mistakes are more readily committed.

Human-factors research has proposed (a) phasic and tonic activation, permanent attention, and vigilance as *characteristics of attention*, and (b) tiredness, fatigue, and monotony as *disturbance of attention*.

8.2.1   Attention

Due to a brief moment of inattention, an intensive care physician injects a bolus of a wrong drug. It is not until monitor alarms make him aware of a dangerously high blood pressure and heart rate that he notices his mistake. Although he is completely present in the emergency situation, one part of his actions escapes his attention, namely the injection of the drug. How then should we conceptualize "attention"? "Every one knows what attention is," the psychologist James stated as early as 1890. "It is the taking possession by the mind, in clear and vivid form, of one out of what seem several simultaneously possible objects or trains of thought. Focalization, concentration of consciousness are of its essence. It implies withdrawal from some things in order to deal effectively with other" (James 1890). Despite this obvious explanation, there is no clear definition to the present day (e.g., Eysenck and Keane 2000). Instead, several metaphors are used to describe certain aspects of attention (Zimbardo and Gerrig 2007). The three most distinct metaphors are those of a spotlight, a filter, and a bottleneck.

8.2.1.1   Metaphors of Attention

The spotlight metaphor visualizes: *Not everything that is present in the environment is consciously perceived by humans.* We can only look at, listen to, and reflect upon that which is in the focus of attention. The "spotlight attention" is intimately connected with consciousness; however, information which is not in the focus of attention is not lost; it still can enter perception, be processed, and then become apparent as emotions. This happens in a cryptic form as emotions are flash-like, holistic summaries of situational assessments and as such do not explain themselves (▶ Chap. 4).

The metaphor of a filter emphasizes the fact that *not everything that humans perceive actually enters consciousness* (▶ Chap. 5). The most popular conceptualization of this theory is Broadbent's metaphor of a bottleneck (Broadbent 1958): As attention is a limited resource, every piece of information which is not consecutively processed on a conscious level, and hence passes through the bottleneck, will be lost. The modified version of this theory is empirically supported by neurophysiological findings: Although the conscious processing of information depends on attention, other sensory inputs, although not perceived consciously, will be partially analyzed (◻ Fig. 8.1). This is accomplished through neuronal networks other than the cortex: They check perceptive data which has not been filtered by attention with respect to relevance and fit them into existing schemata (Ramachandran and Blakeslee 1999). If a perception is judged to be "relevant," an involuntary orientation towards the source of the sensory stimulus occurs (*orientation response*; Sokolov 1963). The monitor alarm caused by a violation of the upper blood pressure limit is such a source of a sensory stimulus which causes a

reorientation of the resident's attention. For him the sound of the alarm is a relevant perception.

8.2.1.2 Physiology of Attention

The physiological correlate for attention is the activation of the central nervous system. According to the quality of activation, two basic forms of attention can be discerned: a tonic and a phasic arousal.

Tonic arousal describes the wakefulness of a person. This arousal is not accessible by conscious control but regulated by the circadian sleep/wake rhythm and impaired by sleep deprivation. At the moment the emergency occurs the tonic arousal of the resident is low.

Phasic arousal describes the increase in CNS activation which follows a stimulus (e.g., alarm) signaling imminent danger. The physiological consequence of phasic arousal is an increase in heart rate and blood pressure, dilated pupils, and increase in skin resistance. When the resident is told about the emergency in the patient box his attention undergoes a phasic activation.

In contrast to the central nervous activation, the other aspects of attention, namely vigilance, selective attention, and shared attention, can at least partly be consciously controlled.

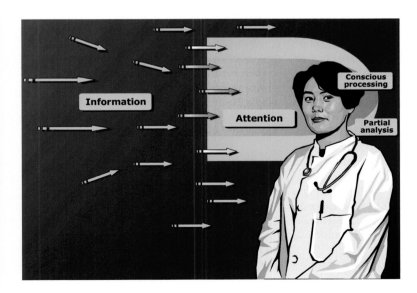

◻ **Fig. 8.1** Modified bottleneck metaphor of attention: As attention is a limited resource ("the bottleneck"), every piece of information has to be processed on a conscious level or it will be lost; however, there is some information which, although not perceived consciously, will be partially analyzed

8.2.2 Vigilance

Vigilance is the ability to remain alertly watchful for extended periods of time and to react to rare and accidentally occurring stimuli. Vigilance is controlled by consciousness (Mackworth 1970). Vigilance in the acute and emergency healthcare setting is important for the observation of monitors, a fact that some societies of anesthesia have accommodated by integrating "vigilance" into their societies maxim ("vigila et ventila"; stay vigilant and ventilate). In carrying out a lengthy vigilant surveillance task, one can anticipate performance decrements. These decrements manifest as decreases in reaction time and a drop in visual or auditory alarm detection probability (Krueger 1994). During lengthy surgeries, vigilance decrements can become a problem for anesthesia providers who must continuously monitor patient vital signs, monitor variables, and administer drugs or for surgical residents who may have to perform monotone tasks. Vigilance is one of the critical key characteristics in the successful prevention of critical situations (Howard and Gaba 1997). Performance shaping factors which increase (e.g., stress) or reduce (e.g., sleepiness and fatigue) the level of activation will both impair vigilance.

8.2.3 Concentration

Concentration is the permanent focus of attention on a specific, consciously selected segment of reality (Zimbardo and Gerrig 2007). Concentration depends on the ability to pay *selective attention* by which disturbing stimuli can be blocked out and a conscious selection from all possible perceptive stimuli is made. In order to be able to fully concentrate on one aspect of reality, the actual motive has to be guarded from concurrent motives which strive to be activated (Chap. 4). In addition, concentration demands an increase in the perception thresholds so that other stimuli cannot distract us. So, concentration means as much the inhibition of unwanted stimuli and motives as the continuous maintenance of a chosen focus.

8.2.4 Divided Attention

The term "divided attention" is used if someone has to tackle two or more tasks at the same time (Ey-senck and Keane 2000). Most people are unable to consciously process data in a parallel manner. They can only execute several tasks if only one of them demands conscious thinking and all the others can be processed automatically (Schneider and Shiffrin 1997). The intensive care physician from the case study is no exception to this rule: His attention is focused on successful mask ventilation, and the preparation for reintubating the patient. The bolus application of the assumed analgosedative drug, however, is done automatically without looking closely at the infusion pump. If a task such as the bolus application is executed automatically, then attention will only turn toward the automatism at certain "control points" to check the correct execution. The remaining time, his attention is focused on mask ventilation, and the planned intubation as these tasks demand conscious thinking; however, as the intensive care physician is tired, these tasks demand more of his attention than usually necessary. As a consequence, he misses "control points" of the drug administration and allows the automatism of manipulating the pump to be executed without control. This leads to the above-described situation. To deal with several tasks simultaneously without a loss in efficiency is more easily possible if different sensory modalities are involved. The physician can give orders and at the same time listen to the signal of the pulse oximeter. Analytic thinking, in contrast, would require his full concentration and therefore shielding of his attention from all other tasks.

The necessity to divide attention between multiple concurrent tasks is not only characteristic for certain medical emergencies but also for the task environment of acute medical care provision as a whole: Healthcare professionals are often "interrupt driven" in their task performance and have to manage many "break-in tasks" (Chisholm et al. 2000).

8.3 Open for News: Background Control and the Horizon of Expectations

An essential precondition for most tasks in acute and emergency healthcare is the ability to completely focus on the actual intention: Only the current activity counts; however, this concentration on one task should never become absolute – otherwise, it would be impossible to detect both good opportunities for other intentions and imminent complications and dangers. Background control is the mechanism by which the human cognitive system tries to avoid this pitfall (Dörner 1999). This term conceptualizes the phenomenon that people tend to scan their environment on a regular base for relevant and new clues. This is done by letting attention scan the environment and then having it return to its primary task.

Background control happens without conscious planning. If a task is very important or if the stress level rises, background control is reduced or completely abolished. Background control is also influenced by the feeling of competence. If someone feels incompetent, they will either start to control their environment less in order to prevent threatening events from being discovered ("encapsulating"), or they will start to control quite frequently (volatility and unfocusedness).

The extent to which people control the background depends on the safety of the environment, the difficulty of the current task, and the expectations about the future progress of events ("horizon of expectations"; ◘ Fig. 8.2). The horizon of expectations is a prognosis about the expected, an extrapolation of the present into the future. The physician's horizon of expectations consists of continuing the unproblematic preparation for reintubation. The moment the horizon of expectation breaks (because the increase in heart rate and arterial blood pressure trigger an alarm) he is astonished and possibly even frightened. Attention is focused toward the infusion pumps (orientation response) and he reflects on the situation: What happened? Why are things not going on as expected?

The horizon of expectations is necessary for the regulation of attention: Events which are expected with certainty are not consciously controlled. Occasional controls are enough to refresh the situational picture. Events, however, which cannot be

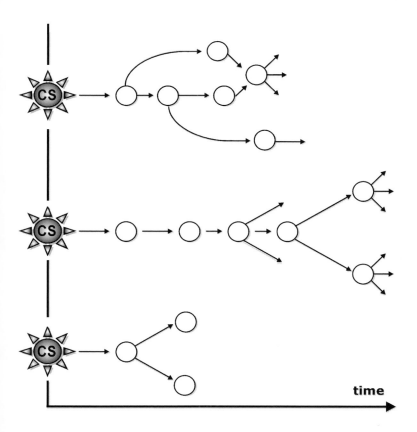

◘ **Fig. 8.2** Horizon of expectations (after Dörner 1999). Every critical situation (CS) is extrapolated into the future. *Circles* represent events, the arrows alternative actions or developments. The further away from the present an event is, the more options are thinkable and expectations become increasingly imprecise

predicted with certainty have to be tracked more closely. The greater the uncertainty about expectations concerning the future (uncertain horizon of expectations) the more often people have to control the background.

8.4   Situation Awareness

Human-factors research recently has rediscovered the importance of situation awareness as one central factor for error reduction in complex technical systems. Situation awareness denotes that people always have to be oriented in the entirety of their environment in order to be able to control it (Endsley 1995, 2000; Carskadon-Banbury and Tremblay 2004). Situation awareness includes the ability to know:

- What actually happens and which items are present in the actual situation
- What the actual events signify
- In which directions the situation could evolve

In order to develop and maintain situation awareness, people first have to construct an image of the current situation by detecting all objects, parameters, and events which might be relevant for this situation. In order to keep the image up to date and to maintain a high degree of situation awareness, two processes have to be in operation:

- The situational image has to be updated regularly. This is done by the above-described process of background control. For the build-up of situation awareness this control has to be done consciously by allocating attention.
- The perceived elements have to be assessed with respect to their relevance. This demands clarity about goals in this particular situation, as relevance can only refer to goals.

Situation awareness depends on the lay-out of a working place as well as on the way in which necessary information is presented. If the cognitive system of the user and behavioral processes are taken into account, intelligent design of monitor alarms, and integrated graphical displays will support situation awareness (e.g., Drews and Westenskow 2006; Edworth and Hellier 2006; Michels et al. 1997).

Another valuable source for an adequate situational model are team mates. One of the main tasks in team formation is the creation of a shared situational awareness, a shared mental model of the situation. Developing shared mental models for a problem will create a context within which decisions can be made and the cognitive resources of the entire team can be exploited (Stout et al. 1997). Such shared knowledge enables each person to carry out his or her role in a timely and coordinated fashion, helping the team to function as a single unit with little negotiation of what to do and when to do it (► Chap. 11).

8.5   Disturbances of Attention

Conscious control of actions can be impaired by many factors. Some disorders, somatic as well as psychiatric (e.g., depression, schizophrenia), change the regulation of attention. Furthermore, some people habitually show an insufficient regulation of attention (cognitive failure; Broadbent et al. 1982). This appears to be a relatively stable personality trait. In the context of this chapter acute alterations in attention due to tiredness, fatigue, monotony, and "encapsulation" are examined. These impairments have in common that they decrease general performance and may cause mistakes.

8.5.1   "Rien ne va plus": Fatigue

The term fatigue describes the diminished ability to perform both cognitive and physical tasks which are caused by excessive mental or muscular work. Fatigue is a protective physiological function which signals that the margin of effective performance has been reached. Fatigue appears as a reversible reduction in the physical and mental performance and is accompanied by feelings of physical exhaustion (muscular fatigue) and by the subjective feeling of tiredness (mental fatigue). In contrast to monotony, the effects of fatigue can only be compensated for by rest, not by a change in activity. Fatigue has various effects on physiological outcomes and on both mental and behavioral performance (Zimbardo and Gerrig 2007; Dinges 1995; Rosekind 1995), among others:

- Alertness (tonic activation) and attention/vigilance are reduced. People become unable to concentrate on a task for a longer period of time.
- Reduced motor performance (fine motor skills and eye–hand coordination) with a decrease of motor tasks (speed–accuracy trade-off).

- Prolonged reaction time and decision-making. In order to reduce effort, rule-based decisions are preferred over knowledge-based decision-making (principle of economy; ▶ Chap. 6).
- Impaired memory function with a reduced ability both to learn and to recall items.
- Motivational alteration of the thinking process: people become careless in the formation of opinion, increasingly tolerant of their own mistakes, and prone to hasty decisions.
- Change in social behavior with disrupted communications, uncontrolled affects, and a reduced willingness to share information with team members.
- Alterations in visual perception ranging from changes in the sensitivity threshold of the eye to perceptual disorders (illusions, hallucinations) in the case of prolonged severe sleep deprivation. In addition, the degree of resolution of perception can decrease which may lead to important details being missed out by the tired individual.
- Somatic symptoms with an increase in heart rate, shallow breathing, a reduction in muscular tone, and an increase in oxygen consumption albeit an unchanged level of work.

Fatigue and its recovery follow exponential curves, albeit reciprocally: The decrement in psychomotor performance begins slowly and becomes more manifest the longer a mental or physical strain is sustained. In contrast, the recreational effect of a break or a short nap is strongest right at the beginning and will then take a long time until complete recovery; therefore many short breaks are more effective than a single long one.

There is a significant discrepancy between subjective reports of fatigue and alertness and objective measures of physiological status (Howard et al. 2002). The feeling of tiredness is perceived much later than the actual decline in the physical performance or mental capability starts. Physicians seem to be especially prone to this kind of misjudgment. In contrast to other professional groups (e.g., pilots, nurses), physicians often believe that they can perform flawlessly even when fatigued (❏ Fig. 8.3; Flin et al. 2003, Helmreich and Merritt 1998).

Because the feeling of tiredness is no reliable indicator of the actual effect of fatigue, people often react to this feeling only when their performance has already decreased. This is one of the reasons why breaks are often taken too late. Recovery will then take much more time compared with situations when breaks are taken early. With respect to patient safety, it is important to obtain sufficient and timely breaks.

8.5.2 I'd Rather Be in Bed: Sleepiness

Fatigue is caused by physical and cognitive work or by prolonged stressful situations and demands rest. Sleepiness, however, is caused by the need to sleep and prompts people to go to bed and thus to recover. Sleepiness is part of the natural sleep/wake cycle which is synchronized to a 24-h circadian rhythm. This circadian rhythm, with its timekeeper located in the suprachiasmatic nucleus (SCN) of the

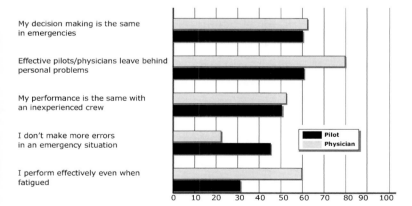

❏ **Fig. 8.3** Percentage of physicians and pilots who had an unrealistic attitude toward their performance limit. Two of three physicians denied any detrimental effect of fatigue on their performance. (From Helmreich and Merritt 1998)

human brain, is biphasic with a state of increased sleep tendency at night and during early afternoon (circadian lulls) and periods of maximal alertness during the late morning and the late evening hours. Among other factors which increase sleepiness, a decreased quantity or poor quality of sleep and the use of certain medications known to disrupt normal sleep structure (e.g., caffeine, ethanol, and certain antihistamines) are relevant to the practice of safe healthcare. The most obvious effects of failing to obtain adequate sleep is sleepiness at times when working time collides with the personal circadian rhythm (e.g., during night shift) and at times when a person should be awake but suffers from a sleep deprivation from the previous night(s) (daytime sleepiness; Monk 1991).

Sleepiness negatively impacts the physiological and cognitive performance in a variety of ways. Fatigue-related performance decrements in psychomotor function are further aggravated by the effects of total sleep deprivation (e.g., no sleep during the entire night shift). In a study, following 17 h of wakefulness the performance in psychomotor tests was comparable to the effect of a blood alcohol concentration of 0.5°/oo. After 24 h of sustained wakefulness, the psychomotor ability further decreased to a performance comparable to that of a person with a blood alcohol concentration of 1°/oo (Dawson and Reid 1997; Arnedt et al. 2005). Men seem to perform more poorly after night calls than women and may be especially prone to accidents when driving home after a night on call (Ware et al. 2006).

In addition, healthcare workers can be physiologically sleepy near to pathological levels without being aware of this fact. As with fatigue, the objective evidence of sleep, too, differs from the subjective ability to determine whether one actually has fallen asleep: In an experimental setup every second subject in whom EEG/EOG measurements showed that they had fallen asleep still believed that they had stayed awake throughout the entire study period (Howard et al. 1995). Besides its effect on psychomotor performance, sleepiness also impacts motivation: The urge to go to sleep can become so overwhelming that we try to get our job done as quickly as possible so that we finally might be able to go to bed. Besides having a major impact on the ability to perform adequately, sleepiness also interferes with personal lives during training programs (e.g., residency programs), leaving many personal and social activities and meaningful personal pleasures deferred (Papp et al. 2004).

Errors During Nighttime. If healthcare workers suffer from fragmented sleep because they have to get up from bed several times during on-call duty, they will experience partial sleep deprivation. More often even these short periods of rest are denied as resident physicians may have to work up to 36 h or longer. In combination with a weekly working time of 100–120 h performance, alertness and mood are severely impaired as a result of the massive sleep deficit and the disrupted circadian rhythm which has been acquired (Howard et al. 2002; Samkoff and Jacques 1991; Wilker et al. 1994). Chronic sleep deprivation is a system problem in healthcare. A multitude of research has been done on the impact of night services and on-call duties on the performance and the susceptibility to error of physicians (see Howard et al. 2002; Samkoff and Jacques 1991 for overview). Recent research on the performance of surgeons (Taffinder et al. 1998; Grantcharov et al. 2001), anesthetists (Howard et al. 2002), and residents (Barger et al 2006) following sleep deprivation were able to demonstrate that the incidence of errors increased as a function of sleepiness. Although there is no clear-cut correlation between sleepiness and a direct harm to patients, surveys support this assumption: In an interview with anesthetists more than half of the group was able to remember one or more clinical errors which they thought they had committed as a direct result of extreme sleepiness (Gaba et al. 1994; Gravenstein et al. 1990). Similar results have been reported from other medical areas (Baldwin and Daugherty 2004).

As healthcare professionals try to "treat" their disruptive sleep pattern by the use of sleep aids, the use of pharmacological sleep aids has increased among physicians: In a recent study every second emergency resident reported regular use of alcohol, antihistamines, sleep adjuncts, and benzodiazepines to help them fall or stay asleep (Handel et al. 2006).

8.5.3   Nothing to Do: Monotony

Monotony is a state of reduced mental and physical activity (Ulich 2001). This condition arises when people in an environment with few relevant stimuli frequently have to repeat uniform tasks which demand their attention. These tasks cannot be automated but they do not demand hard thinking either. In contrast to fatigue (which demands recovery), monotony disappears as soon as the task is altered: "seconds of terror" dispel the "hours of boredom." Monotony is best addressed by a change in tasks, through music and through physical exercise; however, monotony is a rare phenomenon in the context of acute and emergency healthcare. Tasks such as monitor surveillance may be boring but do not create monotony; instead, they demand vigilance.

8.5.4 Tightly Focused: Too Much Concentration and Missing Background Control

Up to now we have described how too little arousal impairs attention. But the contrary can be true as well: excessive concentration on a task can interfere with an appropriate distribution of attention. If people are too preoccupied with a task, then the occasional scanning of the environment for relevant information (background control) will be omitted. We then are no longer open for other relevant clues and are unable to notice when another problem becomes more important than the one with the momentary focus: This is like wearing blinders (▶ Chap. 9 on the influence of stress).

8.6 Tips for Clinical Practice

— Take the effects of fatigue seriously. The feeling of wakefulness can be deceptive. Do not wait until you feel tired before you get some rest. Take scheduled breaks.
— If you are unable to work safely, you should take measures to go home.
— If you work in a team, you can avoid fatigue by relieving each other from time to time.
— Before you appoint a task to someone, make sure that the person is paying attention.
— Ensure that important actions can be performed without interruption.

8.7 "Attention": in a nutshell

— Attention is the conscious focus of perception and thinking on an object.
— Besides being the focus of attention, information can enter consciousness via a second, indirect way: the preconscious processing and test for relevance which is experienced as emotion.

— Relevant stimuli lead to an automatic orientation of attention.
— Vigilance is the ability to maintain attention for extended periods of time and to react to rare and accidentally occurring stimuli.
— Concentration is the permanent focus of attention on a specific, consciously selected segment of reality. Concentration includes selective attention, guarding from concurrent motives, and an increase in the perception threshold.
— The "horizon of expectations" is a (subconscious) prognosis about the expected and an extrapolation of the present into the future.
— The horizon of expectations is necessary for the regulation of attention: Events which are expected with certainty are not consciously controlled. An occasional control suffices to refresh the situational picture.
— Situation awareness is the ability to perceive and assess a situation and anticipate the future development.
— Fatigue is a reversible reduction in the achievement potential. Its effect can only be counterbalanced by rest, not by a change in activity.
— Tiredness is caused by the need to sleep and is a natural function of the circadian rhythm.
— Feeling fatigued does not correlate with the actual physiological impairment of fatigue. People often experience fatigue only when the achievement potential has already decreased.
— After 24 h of continuous wakefulness, the psychomotor ability of a subject decreases to a performance comparable to that of a person with a blood alcohol concentration of 1°/oo.
— Physicians are prone to misjudgment about their achievement potential. They often believe themselves to be unimpaired even when fatigued.
— Monotony is a state of reduced mental and physical activity.

References

Arnedt TJ, Owens J, Crouch M, Stahl J (2005) Neurobehavioral performance of residents after heavy night call vs after alcohol ingestion. J Am Med Assoc 294:1025–1033
Baldwin DC, Daugherty SR (2004) Sleep deprivation and fatigue in residency training:results of a national survey of first- and second-year residents. Sleep 27:217–223
Barger LK, Ayas NT, Cade BE, Cronin JW, Rosner B, Speizer FE, Czeisler CA (2006) Impact of extended-duration shifts on medical errors, adverse events, and attentional failures. PLoS Med 3:e487

Broadbent DE (1958) Perception and communication. Pergamon Press, London

Broadbent DE, Cooper PF, Fitzgerald P, Parkes KR (1982) The Cognitive Failures Questionnaire (CFQ) and its correlates. Br J Clin Psychol 21:1–16

Carskadon-Banbury S, Tremblay S (2004) A cognitive approach to situation awareness:Theory and application. Ashgate, Aldershot

Chisholm CD, Collison, EK, Nelson DR, Cordell WH (2000) Emergency department workplace interruptions:are emergency physicians "interrupt-driven" and "multitasking"? Acad Emerg Med 7:1239–1243

Dawson D, Reid K (1997) Fatigue, alcohol and performance impairment. Nature 388:235

Dinges DF (1995) The performance effects of fatigue. In: Proc Fatigue Symposium. National Transportation Safety Board/ NASA Ames Research Center, 1–2 November

Dörner D (1999) Bauplan für eine Seele [Blueprint for a soul]. Rowohlt, Reinbek

Drews FA, Westenskow DR (2006) The right picture is worth a thousand numbers: data displays in anesthesia. Hum Factors 48:59–71

Edworthy J, Hellier E (2006) Alarms and human behaviour: implications for medical alarms. Br J Anaesth 97:12–17

Endsley MR (1995) Toward a theory of situation awareness in dynamic systems. Hum Factors 37:32–64

Endsley MR (2000) Situation awareness and measurement. Erlbaum, Mahwah, New Jersey

Eysenck MW, Keane MT (2000) Cognitive psychology, 4th edn. Psychology Press, Hove

Flin R, Fletcher G, McGeorge P, Sutherland A, Patey R (2003) Anaesthetists' attitudes to teamwork and safety. Anaesthesia 58:233–242

Gaba DM, Howard SK, Jump B (1994) Production pressure in the work environment: California anesthesiologists' attitudes and experiences. Anesthesiology 81:488

Grantcharov TP, Bardram L, Funch-Jensen P, Rosenberg J (2001) Laparoscopic performance after one night call in a surgical department: prospective study. Br Med J 323:1222–1223

Gravenstein JS, Cooper JB, Orkin FK (1990) Work and rest cycles in anesthesia practice. Anesthesiology 72:737

Handel DA, Raja A, Lindsell CJ (2006) The use of sleep aids among emergency medicine residents:a web based survey. BMC Health Serv Res 19:136

Helmreich RL, Merritt AC (1998) Culture at work in aviation and medicine. National, organizational and professional influences. Ashgate, Aldershot

Howard SK, Gaba DM (1997) Human performance and patient safety In Morell R, Eichhorn J (eds) Patient safety in anesthetic practice. Churchill Livingstone, London, pp 431–466

Howard SK, Gaba DM, Rosekind MR (1995) Evaluation of daytime sleepiness in resident anesthesiologists. Anesthesiology 83:A1007

Howard SK, Rosekind MR, Katz JD, Berry AJ (2002) Fatigue in anesthesia: implications and strategies for patient and provider safety. Anesthesiology 97:1281–1294

James W (1890) The principles of psychology. Henry Holt, New York

Krueger GP (1994) Fatigue, performance and medical error. In: Bogner M (ed) Human error in medicine. Erlbaum, Hillsdale, New Jersey, pp 311–326

Mackworth JF (1970) Vigilance and attention. Penguin Books, Hammondsworth

Michels P, Gravenstein D, Westenskow DR (1997) An integrated graphic data display improves detection and identification of critical events during anesthesia. J Clin Monit 13:249–259

Monk TH (1991) Sleep, sleepiness and performance. Wiley, Chichester, UK

Papp KK, Stoler EP, Sage P, Aikens JE, Owens J, Avidan A, Phillips B, Rosen R, Strohl KP (2004) The effects of sleep loss and fatigue on resident-physicians: a multi-institutional, mixed-method study. Acad Med 79:394–406

Ramachandran V, Blakeslee S (1999) Phantoms in the brain: human nature and the architecture of the mind. Fourth Estate, London

Rosekind MR (1995) Physiological considerations of fatigue. In: Proc Fatigue Symp. National Transportation Safety board/ NASA Ames Research Center, 1–2November

Samkoff JS, Jacques CH (1991) A review of studies concerning effects of sleep deprivation and fatigue on residents' performance. Acad Med 66:687–693

Schneider W, Shiffrin RM (1977) Controlled and automatic human information processing: I. Detection, search, and attention. Psychol Rev 84:1–66

Sokolov E (1963) Perception and conditioned reflex. Pergamon, Oxford

Stout RJ, Salas E, Fowlkes JE (1997) Enhancing teamwork in complex environments through team training. Group Dyn 1:169–182

Taffinder NJ, McManus IC, Gul Y, Russell RC, Darzi A (1998) Effect of sleep deprivation on surgeons' dexterity on laparoscopy simulator. Lancet 352:1191

Ulich E (2001) Arbeitspsychologie [Work psychology]. 5. Vdf, Zürich/Schäffer-Pöschel, Stuttgart

Ware JC, Risser MR, Manser T, Karlson KH (2006) Medical resident driving simulator performance following a night on call. Behav Sleep Med 4:1–12

Wilker FW, Bischoff C, Novak P (Ed) (1994) Medizinische Psychologie, Medizinische Soziologie (2.Auflage) [Medical psychology and medical sociology]. Urban and Schwarzenberg, Munich

Zimbardo P, Gerrig R (2007) Psychology and life, 18th edn. Allyn and Bacon, Boston

9 Stress

9.1   Case Study

The emergency department of a local hospital was notified by the emergency dispatch center that an ambulance had just responded to a trauma scene in which a pediatric patient had fallen from a window. About 15 min later, the ambulance team arrived in the resuscitation room with a 15-month-old male. The patient was handed over to a trauma team comprised of an emergency physician, a surgeon, a radiologist, and two nurses. Due to a case of illness on that day, there was no anesthesiologist available to join the team. Hospital policy mandated that the emergency resident physician assume the role of the team leader. Unfortunately, he had limited experience with trauma patients of this age. An initial assessment of the trauma victim revealed an unresponsive and tachypneic infant with severe facial and head trauma and weak central pulses. The EMT reported that the child had fallen from an open third-floor window without any obvious external influence. While one of the nurses provided mask ventilation the emergency physician made several attempts to place a peripheral i.v. line into the chubby extremities of the infant, but his efforts were unsuccessful. During this period the ECG showed two episodes of bradycardia. It was not until the second nurse mentioned an intraosseous needle that the physician considered changing his plan. Although he had no experience with this technique, the emergency physician nevertheless succeeded in establishing an intraosseous access on the first try. General anesthesia was induced with atropine, midazolam, and ketamine to maintain spontaneous ventilation. The intubation was more difficult than expected because blood and secretions had obstructed the pharynx, but after several attempts the infant was intubated. Immediately after the intubation, however, the saturation began to drop. Because a clearly inflated abdomen suggested an esophageal intubation, the endotracheal tube was withdrawn and the infant mask ventilated until the saturation improved. The infant was reintubated, this time successfully. Auscultation revealed bilateral breath sounds and discrete rales, most likely due to an aspiration of blood and mucus, but peak airway pressures remained above normal and the saturation did not rise above 89%. Following the insertion of an orogastric tube and suctioning of gastric contents, the abdomen deflated and the saturation returned to normal. Forty minutes after presenting to the emergency department and the initial resuscitation, the patient was transported to the CT scanner for further diagnostic evaluation.

A small trauma team has to render care to a seriously injured infant. The physician with a leadership role is an emergency medicine resident who has no experience with the management of this group of patients. This means that the emergency situation is a huge medical challenge. The fact that his patient is a toddler adds additional emotional strain on the physician. Both factors combined put the physician under enormous stress. The stress is further increased by the fact that he has difficulty in performing time-critical procedures such as inserting an i.v. line and intubating the infant. Due to the prolonged initial resuscitation phase, it takes almost an hour before the patient is sufficiently stable to be transported into the CT.

9.2   What is Stress?

For the young physician the treatment of the pediatric trauma patient is pure stress! He is confronted with a situation that brings him to the brink of his skills and clinical competence as well as his emotional resilience. In this case the cause for the acute stress is obvious: the clear knowledge about a discrepancy between a perceived state and a desired state: his own capabilities and the available resources, and the situational demands for a successful treatment of a pediatric trauma patient. In addition, factors such as the sight of a severely injured infant, the consecutive experience of failure, the race against time, and the responsibility for life and death all add to this great discrepancy. But there might have been several other factors which contributed to his limited ability to manage the situation adequately (e.g., trouble at home, recent illness, long working hours, many nights on-call with insufficient sleep, a never-ending flood of paper work, keen competition among colleagues, insufficient support from his supervisors). All of these permanent strains cumulate to chronic stress, which can impair human performance on a long-term level.

Generally, stress is a state of physical and psychological activation in reaction to external demands. These demands require an immediate change in, or adaptation of behavior, from the subject involved. The resulting state of activation prepares the organism for a goal-directed action. The term "stress" in its original meaning is not restricted to a negative connotation (Selye 1936; Semmer et al. 2005); it simply describes bodily activation and mental arousal. For the young physician, however, the stressful situation is accompanied by strong, unpleasant emotions. He experiences the demand for change in behavior as a threat, because he feels that there is an imbalance between the demands of the emergency situation and the available resources.

9.2.1 When Does Stress Start? It's a Matter of Assessment!

9.2.1.1 Situational Assessment

One of the central features of acute and emergency healthcare is the fact that people are faced with an unknown situation from one moment to another. For the physician, the pediatric trauma is a situation he has never experienced before. Everything that people perceive within the first few moments of a new situation is assessed in a rapid, subconscious, and holistic way. The assessment may surface as emotion (▶ Chap. 5.3). In a new situation, the primary situational assessment is: "Does this situation threaten my goals or is it neutral or even favorable?"

Essential for the assessment "this situation is threatening" is the subjective view of the situation and not the situation itself. Whether or not a situation is attended to by "threatening" depends a lot on the skills, knowledge, and resources a person

has available, as well as his or her ethical values and world views, and the physical and emotional condition in which the person is. Because the physician has no experience at all with pediatric emergencies, this situation threatens him; however, he comes to this conclusion even before he first sees the patient: As soon as he is called to the emergency department and learns about the patient, he anticipates the forthcoming events in the light of his missing clinical experience. Already the *anticipation* of excessive situational demands is enough to create stress (Ulich 2001; Semmer 1997). An experienced physician who is confronted with the same situation might come to quite a different assessment.

If people have the impression that a situation is a threat, they instantaneously know that things cannot stay the way they are: Either the situation or the acting person himself or herself has to change, and even the anticipation of a need for change may be enough to create stress (Lazarus and Folkman 1984; Semmer 2003; Ulich 2001).

A second assessment, equally holistic and subconscious, follows the first. This time it comprises a comparison of all available resources with the situational demands: "Will I be able to manage this critical situation"? Depending on how this assessment turns out, different strategies will be applied to deal with the stressful situation (◻ Fig. 9.1).

The physician can only manage this situation if his personal resources (e.g., experience, skills, equipment, team members) exceed the demands of the pediatric emergency. But another subjective

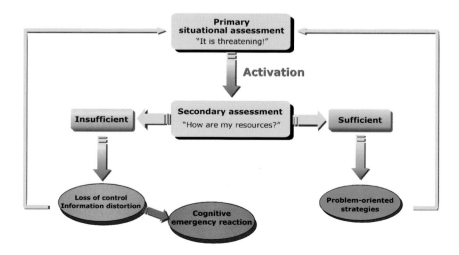

◻ **Fig. 9.1** Primary and secondary assessment of a situation (after the model of Lazarus 1991)

factor enters the equation: Whether or not available resources suffice for the management of a certain situation depends highly on the goal which is pursued in this situation (▶ Chap. 7). If the aim of his emergency management consisted merely of getting the multiple-injured infant somehow out of the ER as quickly as possible, the physician might be much more confident that he could achieve his goal than if he wanted to treat his small patient flawlessly according to Pediatric Advanced Trauma Life Support guidelines.

In addition, the extent to which goals become explicit and to which they are further broken down into intermediate goals, the more probable it will be that one or several of these goals are threatened. If the physician had made the plan "I will have an i.v. access within 2 min, then I will be able to intubate the child on the first try and we will be in the CT within 10 min," he certainly would have failed on every single goal. Unfortunately, it will cause stress if goals are threatened. Goals in question can range from goals concerning *identity* ("I want to be

an excellent physician in every possible situation") over *global* goals ("I want this child to survive") to *explicit* goals ("I want to intubate this child"). If stakes are high, as in the case of a patient's life, goals are especially important to the person and a lot of stress is caused if they are threatened.

9.2.1.2 Stressors

Whether or not a factor actually will cause stress is first and foremost a very subjective matter. Nevertheless, certain factors have been identified which increase the likelihood for the development of stress (Lazarus and Folkman 1984; Semmer 1997). Such risk factors for the development of stress are called *stressors*. Stressors are events which most people will experience as a threat for important goals or for physical integrity. Some of these stressors only appear in critical situations (acute stressors); others are a constant part of the working environment (chronic stressors; ◻ Table 9.1).

◻ **Table 9.1** Acute and chronic stressors in an acute care setting

Acute stressors	Chronic stressors
Acoustic alarms, dropping frequency of the saturation signal	Excessive working hours
Time pressure, production pressure ("surgery has to start right now")	Chronic sleep deprivation
Complexity of the work environment (▶ Chap. 2)	Constant economic production pressure (e.g., fast changing of patients in the OR)
High-stakes environment; responsibility for a patient's life	Bureaucracy
Not enough professional skills	Missing support by supervisors
Errors committed	Dependence on goodwill of supervisors (necessary procedures for specialty training)
Fatigue	Competition among colleagues
Constant interruptions of routine procedures	Professional identity: inadequate error culture and unrealistic dogmas ("no patient shall ever die on the table")
Working in a bad team climate	Constant confrontation with death and suffering
Unclear distribution of competence	
Fear of medico-legal consequences	

Acute and chronic stressors have an additive effect (◘ Fig. 9.2). One of the immediate consequences is the fact that health care workers who are constantly exposed to chronic stressors tolerate less acute stress before they become overstrained than people who experience very little chronic stressors. So, reducing chronic stressors is essential for dealing with acute stress appropriately, too.

9.2.1.3   Resilience

Some people quite obviously can tolerate more stressors than others. Several characteristics can be identified which are responsible for this resilience. People who show resilience:

— Have the feeling that successful actions depend on their own capabilities (internal locus of control) and are not dictated by external factors (external locus of control).
— See stressors as a positive challenge and not as another unwelcome burden.
— Generally express a positive attitude towards life without being naïve.
— Are highly devoted to their goals without becoming rigid. They are flexible enough to adapt their goals to the circumstances when needed.
— Accept failure and errors as a normal part of life and do not see them as a confirmation of their own inability (Semmer 2003).

9.2.2   The Stress Response: Fight or Flight

The stress response (Cannon 1928; Selye 1936) is a stereotypical physiological response of the human organism to different external challenges or threats. The purpose is physical integrity and survival. When the external balance is challenged, the organism changes its internal balance accordingly. Whenever an organism is confronted with a threat, the high physiological arousal which is part of the stress response rapidly provides resources to deal with the threat by either fighting it (if the danger is perceived as weaker than one's own strength) or by running away (if an attack seems futile; *fight-or-flight response*). This threat does not necessarily have to be another living being: Any sensory stimulus which is perceived as dangerous for the physical integrity or for personal goals can trigger the stress response.

In the setting of acute and emergency medical care, however, this fight-or-flight response can no longer serve its purpose: When confronted with a severely injured child, there is no way one could "fight" physically with an adversary. Moreover, as healthcare providers have the obligation to care for their patients under all circumstances, flight is not an option, either. Critical situations in healthcare do not require the means the stress response provides – on the contrary, it can sometimes create more problems than it can solve.

9.2.2.1   Physiology of the Stress Response

Whenever people perceive that they are in a dangerous situation and that they are unable to cope with this situation, this awareness causes an activation of the limbic system and the hypothalamus. From there two different pathways are pursued: one leads from the anterior hypothalamus to an arousal of the sympathetic branch of the autonomous nervous system (ANS) and to a release of epinephrine from the inner part of the adrenal gland, the adrenal medulla, into the bloodstream. The second pathway emerges from the pituitary gland, which is located close to the hypothalamus in the brain: the adrenocorticotrophic hormone (ACTH) is released

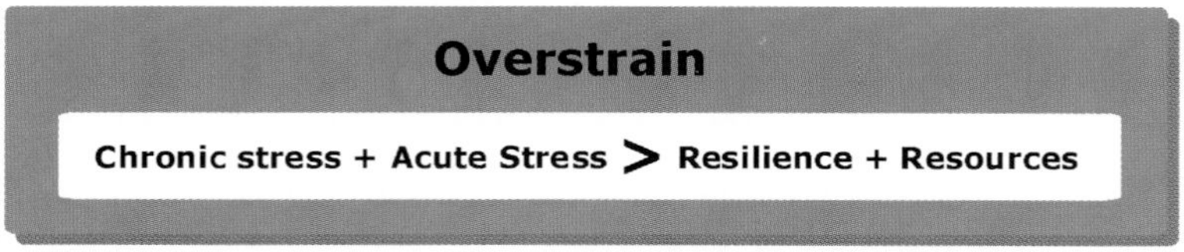

Overstrain

Chronic stress + Acute Stress > Resilience + Resources

◘ **Fig. 9.2** Factors that may cause excessive stress in an emergency situation. If and to what extent a person will be overstrained by a situation depends on the interplay of all four factors

into the blood, resulting in an activation of the outer part of the adrenal gland, the adrenal cortex. Consequently, the levels of cortisol and aldosterone increase, which in turn induce gluconeogenesis and inhibit regenerational processes. As a result of both processes the blood supply to those regions that govern motor functions and basic functions in the brain is increased as well as the oxygen delivery to skeletal muscles and to the heart. The stress response originated from evolutionary priority: to supply the organism with as much energy as possible so that it could deal effectively with threats (Semmer 1997). Cannon (1928) accordingly referred to the stress reaction as "physiological emergency reaction."

The stress reaction shows many unpleasant physiological symptoms which nevertheless are vital for survival. Among those symptoms are:

- Increase in heart rate
- Increased perspiration, cold skin
- Increased breathing frequency
- Increased strength of skeletal muscles
- Dry mouth
- Relaxation of bladder and intestine; urge to urinate and to empty bowels

Once the danger is over, the symptoms cease within the next 15 min; however, as the stress response is aimed at optimizing gross motor skills, the fine motor skills are affected considerably, resulting in tremor. This tremor can further increase problems in those stressful situations, where an unimpaired function of these fine motor skills would be more than necessary (e.g., difficult insertion of an i.v. line, emergency operation).

9.2.2.2 Alteration in Cognition and Emotion

If physiological changes, such as tremor, dry mouth, and increase in heart rate were the only noticeable effect of the stress response, people might still be able to successfully manage every emergency. Investing additional effort and concentrating on the task would help them to compensate for the physiological drawbacks. But the stress response also induces characteristic changes in the way people think and feel. Basically, the cognitive processes also organize around "fight or flight" – and this impairs our ability to recall data from memory, to analyze and reason, and to judge and make decisions. Fight and flight require first and foremost:

(a) focusing of attention; and (b) decreased resolution of the information processing.

If attention focuses on a single task, then people are able to concentrate on the essential. There will be an increased threshold for selecting another motive which basically helps people to become less distracted and to be able to stick to one task (▶ Chap. 4; Dörner 1999); however, there are several drawbacks to this cognitive change: If any other information is screened out, it becomes increasingly difficult to maintain situational awareness, because situational awareness depends on a situational image which is updated regularly. In other words: focusing competes with background control (▶ Chap. 8); we do not see or hear all the information that might be right in front of us. In hindsight people sometimes describe this experience as having had a "cognitive tunnel vision." In addition to a narrowed perception, focusing also implies a *narrowing of the very process of thinking*: because it is only the actual problem that counts the resulting behavior is guided by short-term goals. Complications, potential problems, and unexpected developments which may lie further along the road may not be considered when planning the next steps (Schaub 1997; Semmer 1997; Dörner and Schaub 1994; Dörner and Pfeiffer 1993). Stress makes it increasingly difficult for people to make choices from among alternatives. At the extent to which the information processing becomes coarse and superficial, simple explanations for a problem and quick and easy solutions are preferred. To make things even worse, the resulting behavior will not only be shortsighted but, in addition, strongly guided by emotions: A deeper reflection on, and analysis of, a situation is dispensed with and decisions are made inconsiderately. People under stress plan less and revert to automatisms and rules (▶ Chap. 2.2). As a result, only preexisting, well-practiced behavioral programs are activated, because only they allow fast action. This is true even in novel situations which actually would demand otherwise. Under stress, people tend to do what they *know* best rather than what would *be* best.

Stress-related alterations in thinking and feeling will increase the likelihood for errors in many ways. Once an error has occurred, the stress level may increase even further and as a result may promote even more errors. A poor judgment chain may be triggered (▶ Chap. 10).

9.2.2.3 Transfer of Stress into Other Situations

Once a person realizes that the threatening situation is over, the parasympathetic nervous system will help to restore the person to a state of equilibrium. Usually, this will take several minutes and has no residual effects on the individual. But the elimination of stress hormones takes longer than the actual situation so that there is a hangover of activation. Often also the mental preoccupation with an emergency will outlast the actual critical situation and consequently will lead to a prolonged elevated stress level. Stress can thus be carried from one situation to the next, and also from the working place into the private life, and vice versa. This way stress can accumulate (Semmer 1997).

9.2.3 Chronic Stress

If the triggering situation for the stress response remains active, the acute stress reaction ("alarm reaction") will be displaced by the General Adaptation Syndrome (Selye 1956). This "resistive reaction" enables the organism to adapt to prolonged stressful conditions. A state of apparent resistance against the stressors is achieved by increasing cortisol levels. This results in essential hypertension, an elevated heart rate, high blood sugar levels, and a weakened immune system. Regenerative processes are inhibited. If this arousal remains for weeks or months, resistance is no longer possible, exhaustion follows, and physical and mental health are in danger.

9.2.3.1 Results of Long-term Stress

Chronic stress can manifest in many ways: cardiovascular, psychosomatic, and psychiatric diseases (e.g., depression), cognitive and behavioral changes and dysfunctional interpersonal relationships may all indicate that a person's limit to stress had been exceeded long time ago. There is no such thing as *the* classical stress disease; in fact, every organism yields at its most vulnerable point. Stress also tempts people into unhealthy behavior such as smoking, alcohol, or drug abuse, and an unbalanced diet.

The psychic responses to long-term stress are:

- Problems with concentrating, poor attention, and forgetfulness

- Low productivity and poor time management
- Emotional disturbances such as anxiety, worry, and confusion
- Emotional instability, bad temper, and testiness
- Sleep disturbances/insomnia
- Addictive behavior (mostly alcohol and smoking)
- Behavioral abnormalities such as chewing fingernails, nervous tics, grinding one's teeth, etc.

The effects of chronic stress will add to acute stress and thus can have a negative impact on patient safety (Fig. 9.2). Although the knowledge about the relation between stress and personal performance should be familiar to every healthcare provider, an attitude of personal invulnerability seems to be a professional attribute especially among physicians: When compared with other professional groups, a higher percentage of physicians held unrealistic attitudes about their performance capabilities when faced with various kinds of stressors. Every second doctor endorsed the unrealistic attitude that his or her decision-making was the same in routine situations as well as in emergencies (Fig. 8.3) (Sexton et al. 2000; Flin et al. 2003).

9.2.3.2 From Long-term Stress to Burnout

When chronic work stress in a healthcare setting is maintained on a high level for a long period of time (e.g., long working hours, great amount of on-call duties, insufficient sleep, bureaucracy, unsympathetic superiors), it can develop into a maladaptive response pattern which has a far-reaching impact on a patient's emotional health and attitude towards life: the burnout syndrome. According to New York psychologist Herbert J. Freudenberger, who coined the term, "burnout" aimed at explaining the process of physical and mental deterioration in professionals working in areas such as healthcare, social work, or emergency legal services (Freudenberger 1974). Subsequently, burnout syndrome was defined as a sustained response to chronic work stress comprising three dimensions (Maslach and Jackson 1981):

- Emotional exhaustion: an increased feeling of emotional exhaustion. As emotional resources are depleted, workers feel they are no longer able to provide care for others. Emotional exhaustion is the hallmark of burnout.

- Depersonalization: negative feelings and cynical attitudes toward the recipients of care. A callous or even dehumanizing perception of others can lead staff to view their patients as somehow deserving their trouble.
- Lack of personal accomplishment: tendency to evaluate oneself negatively, particularly with regards to one's work with patients. General feelings of low accomplishment and of professional failure.

The classical burnout syndrome with its etiology as a response to occupational stress in human service professionals and its sequential order of development of the three dimensions of burnout syndrome comprise (Maslach 1982):

- Over-commitment: There is no healthy distance to work; people tend to "give everything."
- Beginning exhaustion: The onset is slow. The early symptoms include a feeling of emotional and physical exhaustion; a sense of alienation, cynicism, impatience, negativism and feelings of detachment to the point that the person begins to resent the work he or she is involved in and the people who are a part of that work. There is a constant feeling of tension and errors are committed with higher frequency
- Increased exhaustion: Healthcare providers start to develop hostile feelings and a negative attitude towards both, their own profession and their patients. The personal engagement at work is reduced and emotional reactions such as feelings of guilt, self-pity and helplessness, emerge.
- Feeling "burned out": If the stress level is kept high, a feeling of depleted energy and an inner distance from work will emerge. The ruling

feelings are shutdown numbness, mood swings, helplessness, and desperation. Individuals who once cared very deeply about fellow human beings will insulate themselves to the point that they no longer care at all. Psychosomatic disorders increase in frequency and can lead, as a worst-case scenario, to a nervous breakdown and to reactive depression.

9.2.4 Moderate Stress Is Good For You

Stress does not only have negative aspects. On the contrary, in order to be able to perform at all people need a certain level of stress. The cortico-cerebral activation which is part of the stress response makes us move and enables us to focus on the essential. Up to a certain level of stress this will result in an improved performance – if the person has enough resources to manage the situation or the task. If the level of stress is increased, which means that we have not got enough resources, performance will decline.

Under-challenge – a complete lack of stress – leads to worse performance. Additionally, under-challenge and boredom can be stressors themselves: We feel tense and even angry, which can lead to errors, too.

How much stress people need exactly for an ideal performance level depends highly on the task involved. Every task has its specific level of arousal with which it can be managed best. Too high and too low levels of stress will result in a suboptimal performance (Fig. 9.3).

Improved performance is one positive aspect of stress. A second equally important function of stress is the promotion of learning. Every stress-

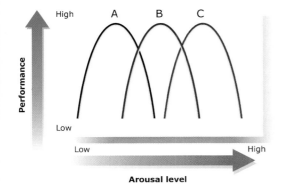

 Fig. 9.3 Relationship between activation and performance. An optimal performance in any given task depends on the degree of activation and the nature of the task. *A*, *B*, and *C* represent tasks with increasing difficulty. (After Yerkes and Dodson 1908)

ful situation carries an implicit message for the individual: you will either have to change the situation (e.g., by finding a solution) or modify your thinking and behavior. It is this kind of pressure that results in learning. Without the necessity for change people hardly ever will reconsider their cognitive models: We prefer to revert to the known and familiar rather than scrutinizing the obvious and finding new solutions.

9.3   Coping Mechanisms

The idea of "coping mechanisms" was first conceptualized by the working group of Lazarus and Folkman (Lazarus and Folkman 1984; Lazarus 1991) who defined coping as "those changing cognitive and behavioral efforts developed for managing the specific external and/or internal demands judged as exceeding or surpassing the individual's own resources." Coping strategies have customarily been classified according to the specific method (active/assertive vs passive/avoiding) by which a problem is addressed, thereby reflecting the "fight-or-flight response" on a cognitive level.

- Active-cognitive: The assessment and reevaluation of one's understanding of a stressful situation. Potentially stressful events as well as painful emotions can be reinterpreted and thereby loose their destructive impact.
- Active-behavioral: Observable efforts which are aimed at controlling and managing a stressful situation.
- Avoiding: The refusal to face a problematic or stressful situation and to act accordingly.

Other classifications emphasize the distinction between coping oriented to the problem and coping oriented to the emotion (Lazarus and Folkman 1984; Edwards 1988). Coping oriented to the problem would represent an attempt to respond directly to the stressful situation; coping oriented to the emotion would consist of attempts to moderate the emotional response to stressful events.

Various studies have related coping strategies with burnout and other consequences of occupational stress in a healthcare setting. As a general result, active and problem-oriented strategies are in the long run healthier for the individual and provide greater capacity for coping with difficult situations than coping strategies addressed to avoidance: these have been shown to be positively related to

the three components of burnout. Which strategy people finally choose will depend highly on the situation itself and on the preferred coping manner. This manner is largely determined by a person's personality and his or her previous learning experiences (Weber 2004); however, it is not confined to these but can also reflect the self-conception of a person's cultural surrounding: The overt expression of strong emotions (e.g., joy, anger, and infuriation) is natural in southern European countries. In such a cultural setting strong emotions are self-evident parts of interpersonal communication and by no means have to indicate exceptional personal involvement on behalf of the person speaking. In most parts of Asia, however, an untamed expression of feelings would create quite a different response: In this cultural context an expression of strong emotions outside the family might be considered to be inappropriate and impolite.

9.3.1   Emotion-Oriented Coping Mechanism: Yelling at People?

Acute stress is a trigger for strong emotions. In order to reduce the impact of these strong emotions on decision-making and action, it can become necessary to deal with one's own emotions first (e.g., by calming down) before addressing the actual problem. The unreflective way of letting off steam by yelling at team members may provide short-term relief from emotional pressure but will be counterproductive for any further effective teamwork. If emotions are not dealt with appropriately, their unfiltered expression can damage one's own and social acceptance and will destroy functional social relationships (Billings and Moos 1984). Nobody will be willing to support and cooperate with a person who just devalued them in public.

But an emotionally charged situation can be perpetuated by the opposite approach as well: an active-cognitive coping strategy which pays too close attention to the present emotional state may amplify negative emotions, i.e., a person most certainly will experience their own activation (e.g., "I'm really mad at this person"); a perception which will then be further integrated into the future situational assessment (Baumeister et al. 1994). Situational assessment, emotion, arousal, and again situational assessment can lead into a vicious circle. An appropriate way of dealing with any strong feeling would be to "filter" these emotions beforehand and then to bring them into the situation in a cooperative and not destructive way (e.g., by telling team members that you are angry and why, but without attacking them personally). However, there is one major drawback for this preprocessing of emotions: It only works if people have a minimum of self-control and if this self-control is not impaired by too much stress. This, unfortunately, will bring us right back to the point where we started.

9.3.2 Cognitive Coping Mechanism: Try to See Things Differently!

If task demands exceed available resources and the stress level rises, it seems like a legitimate strategy to consider the possibility of reducing the difficulty of a task. If things can be made easier for the healthcare provider by reinterpreting the facts, then he or she might have a realistic chance of success: the available resources might just be enough to manage the critical situation. If a goal is utterly unrealistic in the first place, it might be more than appropriate to strive for more realism. This approach has some charm when dealing with chronic stressors and certain personality traits (e.g., perfectionism). For healthcare providers, however, who are faced with a critical situation, this strategy will be of limited value: If a patient ought to survive a medical emergency, then certain goals cannot be abandoned lightly. Despite being tempted by a strong "flight response," it was no option for the emergency resident physician to stop in the middle of his resuscitation efforts and to say to himself: "Well, I always knew this case was too big for me; I'd better stop treating the infant now."

In an effort to reinterpret a situation the cognitive coping strategy can actually do more harm than help: people start losing confidence in their capabilities and in any realistic chance for success. As a result, pessimism will take over and people will no longer expect any improvement of a situation. Instead of trying to control a situation, they resign and withdraw from any constructive action. If healthcare professionals repeatedly experience such situations, they may start to develop the hazardous attitude of resignation (► Chap. 4).

Coping strategies do not only have short-term benefits or disadvantages; there is always a price that has to be paid in the long run if people opt for a certain coping mechanism. This is especially true

for inappropriate strategies that help to end the stress response for the moment: Yelling at co-workers reduces emotional pressure but is devastating with regard to functional and healthy relationships. To be less ambitious and to reduce personal goals to a minimum will greatly relieve a person from chronic stress but may actually hinder his or her medical training and any further professional development. To work harder under unsatisfying work conditions can lead to burnout. Smoking may help people to calm down but will eventually lead to serious health problems (Semmer 2003).

> Some different coping strategies are as follows:
> − Active/assertive vs passive/avoiding
> − Active-cognitive vs active-behavioral
> − Problem oriented vs emotion oriented

9.4 Overwhelmed by Stress

The previous passages gave a brief overview of the physiological and mental effects of everyday stressors, both acute and chronic. In an acute and emergency care setting, however, the level of stress can strain the healthcare provider beyond limits, which will result in a characteristic narrowing of thinking and behavior. These psychological alterations have been termed, with reference to the physiological reaction in stressful situations, "*cognitive emergency reaction*" (Dörner et al. 1983; Dörner 1996; "*intellectual emergency reaction*" in Reason 1990, p. 93).

9.4.1 The Cognitive Emergency Reaction

Whenever things go very wrong, and problems become uncontrollable and impossible to solve, people will feel that their feeling of competence (► Chap. 4) is seriously threatened. Because a minimum feeling of competence is necessary for humans to maintain their ability to act, it has to be defended at any cost. For this purpose the cognitive system is "shut off": More important than the *solution* of a problem, as vital as it may be, will be the *upkeep of the feeling* that the situation (or at least some relevant aspect of it) is under control. As a result people try to avoid any additional strain on this feeling of competence (e.g., doubts about the mental model or the adequacy of a plan). They will end up seeing only what they want to see (distortion of information; ▶ Chap. 6.3) and will use the resource "conscious thinking" (e.g., reflection, planning) as economically as possible (principle of economy; ▶ Chap. 6). The cognitive emergency reaction shows the symptoms given below.

9.4.1.1   Externalization of Behavior

- People focus less on internal cognitive processes (e.g., thinking, planning) than on overt behavior (▶ Chap. 4).
- The more the process of thinking and planning is reduced, the more behavior will be guided by external triggers and less by goals. This will result in erratic actions.

9.4.1.2   Quick Fixes

- People regress to familiar schemata of thinking and acting (methodism).
- Quick and simple solutions are preferred.

9.4.1.3   Inappropriate Reduction of Complexity

- Simple and reductionist mental models are formed.
- One's own (reductionist) situational model will be defended against any other point of view. This will result in dogmatism, bossiness, rejection of criticism or doubt, and the avoidance of the word "but …"
- New information will no longer be taken into account and analyzed; contradicting information will selectively be blinded out: at the end we will protect our mental model even against reality.
- Ignorance or the bad motives of other people will be made responsible for problems rather than the complexity of the situation or environment (personalization).

9.4.1.4   Dispensation with Self-reflection

- Self-reflection is markedly reduced. Subjects no longer pause to evaluate the progress of previous

actions. Instead, task performance is reduced to a series of disconnected actions.

Healthcare professionals are generally unaware of the way their decision-making and emergency management is affected by the cognitive emergency reaction.

9.4.2   Teams Under Pressure

Teams basically respond to stress in a way similar to the reaction of an individual: They try to guard their feeling of competence and not to be overwhelmed by destructive emotions. In addition to the above-mentioned reactions, team members show behavioral patterns (Badke-Schaub 2000) which can further compromise patient safety (▶ Chap. 11.2) in the following ways:
- Data collection is abandoned early
- No reflection on the problem
- No discussion about goals
- No search for alternative solutions
- Group pressure, suppression of disagreement
- Risk shift
- Diffusion of responsibility
- Lack of coordination
- Call for a strong leadership

When team leaders are stressed, team dynamics and team effectiveness will be impaired in two ways: On the one hand, leaders will feel compelled "to do something" in order to maintaining a sense of control and a feeling of competence. As a result, they will perform many tasks by themselves and will delegate less. On the other hand, their thinking and behavior will focus on their own person instead of on the entire team. There will be less communication about goals and plans, resulting in the "leader goes solo" (▶ Chap. 13).

9.5   Coping with Stress

9.5.1   Resilience: a Fourfold Strategy

There is no easy solution to the problem of how stress can be reduced in an emergency situation. A certain amount of stress will be the acute and emergency healthcare provider's lifelong companion (Jackson 1999); however, as over-strain in a critical situation results from several factors, four starting points can be identified which could help to reduce the occurrence and to mitigate the effect of the cognitive emergency reaction.

There are three basic strategies with which the problem of stress can be tackled (Weber 2002; Lehrer and Woolfolk 1993):

— Problem oriented (e.g., problem-solving strategies, resource allocation)
— Regenerative (e.g., relaxation, sports and other physical activities)
— Cognitive (e.g., change in attitude, "inner alertness," self-instruction)

For the four starting points in ◘ Fig. 9.4 we give some examples of how the implementation of these basic strategies might look in everyday life.

9.5.1.1 Reduction of Chronic Stress

Stress management can imply that people should do the following:

— Strive toward a relaxed and easygoing attitude toward life, thus minimizing private stress.
— Identify those factors which operate as personal stressors. In addition, they should become familiar with the way they react to these stressors and which options they have to influence them deliberately.
— Care about their life balance: Stressful times should always alternate with times of recreation.

9.5.1.2 Reduction of Acute Stress

There are some helpful rules which may help you to reduce stress in an acute emergency:

— Make it a habit to plan with foresight. Always try to stay ahead of the game. Use periods of low workload to prepare for possible upcoming events or necessary measures (e.g., by preparing i.v. drips, etc.).
— Try to stay in active control of your behavior. As soon as stress increases, this will be one of the first things you will abandon.
— Try to apply good strategies of action (► Chap. 10) whenever possible.
— Try to minimize the narrowing impact of the stress reaction: Step back and take a different perspective; scan your environment and ask yourself: What else could be important?
— Make sure that you pursue realistic goals. A realistic goal is a goal that you and your team can reach given the specific context of the critical situation.
— Try not to be emotionally overwhelmed by a problem. Of course, it is easier said than done: "don't panic!"
— If you have committed an active failure, try to see it as an isolated event and not as the confirmation of you being a faulty person or lacking the necessary capabilities.
— Sometimes it is helpful to apply a body-oriented strategy: step back, pay attention that you feel "firmly grounded" at the place you stand, and start to breathe consciously and in a controlled way.

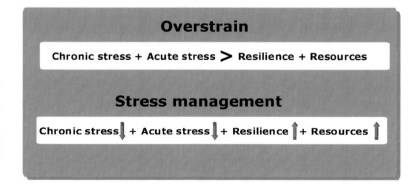

◘ **Fig. 9.4** Factors which lead to excessive stress in a critical situation and practical aspects of how the resistance to stress might be increased

9.5.1.3 Increase Your Personal Ability to Work Under Pressure

- Take a cautiously optimistic attitude towards life.
- Sports and other physical activities, as well as a balanced diet, are not only generally good for your health, they also help to build up physical resources, which you might need in stressful situations.

9.5.1.4 Increase Your Resources

- You can best practice the management of critical situations and team behavior in a realistic yet safe environment: Simulation-based training programs are available for a variety of acute medical care specialties (▶ Chap. 15).
- Knowledge and skills will help to reduce stress. That is why skills should be practiced regularly, knowledge should be acquired, and problem-solving strategies should be trained. To keep your medical knowledge up to date can further improve your capability for crisis management.
- Know your environment well. Do not depend on other people telling you where to find critical resources (e.g., difficult airway equipment, defibrillator).
- Once you are in a critical situation, you should call for help early, enlarge your team, and get sufficient resources.

9.5.2 Lead Teams Out of Stress

Your team is the most important resource in a critical situation: Be it the acquisition of knowledge, the development of situational models, the formation of goals, and the execution of tasks, in every single task team members can support each other. The necessary prerequisite is good communication and a good team climate. Leaders should distribute the "resource team" adequately among the different tasks and should try to maintain an overview of the situation. Furthermore, they should help their team to arrive at a shared mental model by naming the problem and by indicating the future direction of action. Team members under stress need clear commands as well as respectful communication (▶ Chaps. 12, 13).

9.6 The Role of Organizations in Reducing Stress

From the point of view of work psychology, the role of an organization in the development and prevention of stress is just as important as the behavior of individuals and their coping strategies. To change the stressful working conditions which have a long-term impact on employees is much more effective than investing great effort in trying to change individual behavior. In the acute and emergency healthcare setting many acute stressors are inevitable and part of the job – the sight of a severely injured person, the experience of suffering and death, personal tragedies, and in midst of it all the overwhelming feeling of helplessness. The same is true for some chronic stressors: night shifts and on-call duties most probably will remain an inevitable part of any healthcare system. Other stressors, however, to which health care providers might have gotten accustomed over the years, can and should be changed. Organizations can foster an effective stress management of their employees by doing the following:

- Creating a climate of support: In all sections of a healthcare organization it should be self-evident and natural that people can voice any concerns they have and call for help at any time. There is a clear structure as to where help can be found and who can be asked.
- Caring for the regeneration of the employees: Breaks and working schedules are maintained, there are appropriate on-call rooms or staff rooms, and the alimentation is good.
- Providing a constructive atmosphere for dealing with critical situations: debriefings.
- Fostering learning: The possibilities of continuous medical education, regular seminars, and morbidity and mortality conferences are provided.

9.7 "Stress": in a Nutshell

- The stress response is a stereotypical response of the human organism intended to secure the physical integrity and survival of the organism. It prepares the organism for a rapid and goal-directed action.
- Stress is not an external event that befalls people out of the blue sky. Instead, the stress response

results from a person's active perception of a novel situation and the ensuing subconscious and holistic assessment.

- Whether or not a situation will trigger the stress response depends largely upon the (subconscious) situational assessment ("Does this situation threaten my goals"? "Is it neutral or favorable?") and the resource assessment ("Will I be able to manage this critical situation?")
- The stress response prepares people physically and mentally to either fight a threat by means of a quick and goal-directed action (if the danger is perceived as weaker than one's one strength) or to fly from the danger (if an attack seems futile; fight-or-flight response). This is even true in settings such as acute and emergency healthcare, where neither fight nor flight are viable options.
- Stress does not only alter the physiological but also the psychological response patterns (e.g., thinking and feeling) of an individual; hence, it is one of the most important forces impacting human cognitive functions and the ability to make decisions based on analysis. The focus of attention is on the actual problem ("cognitive tunnel vision") and the degree of resolution in the information processing decreases.
- Stress hampers sound choices from among alternatives and leads to simple explanations and quick solutions to complex problems.
- The physical reactions of stress (e.g., tremor) can add additional stress to a critical situation.
- A moderate level of stress results in an improved performance; too much stress has the opposite effect.
- Chronic work stress in a healthcare setting can ultimately lead to a maladaptive response pattern with a strong impact on a person's emotional health and attitude toward life: the burnout syndrome.
- The three dimensions of burnout are: emotional exhaustion; depersonalization; and a feeling of professional failure.
- Mechanisms for coping with stress can be classified according to their mechanism into active-cognitive, active-behavioral and avoiding, and according to their object into problem-oriented and emotion-oriented.
- If healthcare providers are overwhelmed by a critical situation, a characteristic narrowing of thinking and behavior will follow. This cogni-

tive change is called the "cognitive emergency reaction."
- Teams respond to stress in a way similar to an individual. In addition, team members display other behavioral patterns which can further compromise patient safety.
- The role of organizations in the development and prevention of stress is just as important as individual behavior and related coping strategies.

References

Badke-Schaub P (2000) Wenn der Gruppe Flügel fehlen: Ungeeignete Informations- und Entscheidungsprozesse in Gruppen. [Dysfunctional processes of information management and decision-making in groups] In: Mey H, Lehmann H, Pollheimer D (eds) Absturz im freien Fall oder Anlauf zu neuen Höhenflügen. vdf, Zürich, pp 113–130

Baumeister RF, Heatherton TF, Tice DM (1994) Losing control: how and why people fail at self-regulation. Academic Press, San Diego

Billings AG, Moos RH (1984) Coping, stress, and social resources among adults with unipolar depression. J Person Soc Psychol 46:877–891

Cannon WB (1928) Bodily changes in pain, hunger, fear, and rage. Appleton–Century–Crofts, New York

Dörner D (1996) The logic of failure. Recognizing and avoiding error in complex situations. Metropolitan Books, New York

Dörner D (1999) Bauplan für eine Seele [Blueprint for a soul]. Rowohlt, Reinbek

Dörner D, Kreuzig HW, Reither F, Stäudel T (1983) Lohhausen: Vom Umgang mit Unbestimmtheit und Komplexität. [On Dealing with Uncertainty and Complexity]. Huber, Bern

Dörner D, Pfeiffer E (1993) Strategic thinking and stress. Ergonomics 36:1345–1360

Dörner D, Schaub H (1994) Errors in planning and decision-making and the nature of human information processing. Appl Psychol Int Rev 43:433–453

Edwards JR (1988) The determinants and consequences of coping with stress. In: Cooper CL, Payne R (eds) Causes, coping, and consequences of stress at work. Wiley, New York, pp 22–48

Flin R, Fletcher G, McGeorge P, Sutherland A, Patey R (2003) Anaesthetists' attitudes to teamwork and safety. Anaesthesia 58:233–243

Freudenberger HJ (1974) Staff burnout. J Soc Issues 30:159–165

Jackson SH (1999) The role of stress in anaesthetists' health and well-being. Acta Anaesthesiol Scand 43:583–602

Lazarus RS (1991) Emotion and adaption. Oxford University Press, Oxford

Lazarus, RS, Folkman S (1984) Stress, appraisal, and coping. Springer, Berlin Heidelberg New York

Lehrer PM, Woolfolk RL (1993) (eds) Principles and practice of stress management. The Guilford Press, New York

Maslach C (1982) Burnout. The cost of caring. Prentice-Hall, Englewood Cliffs, New Jersey

Maslach C, Jackson SE (1981) The measurement of experienced burnout. J Occup behav 2:99–113

Reason J (1990) Human error. Cambridge University Press, Cambridge UK

Schaub H (1997) Decision-making in complex situations: cognitive and motivational limitations. In: Flin R, Salas E, Strub ME, Martin L (eds) Decision-making under stress. Emerging themes and applications. Ashgate, Aldershot, pp 291–300

Selye H (1936) A syndrome produced by diverse nocuous agents. Nature 138:32

Selye H (1956) The stress of life. McGraw-Hill, New York

Semmer N (1997) Stress. In: Luczak H, Volper W (eds) Handbuch Arbeitswissenschaft [Handbook Work Science]. Schäffer-Pöschel, Stuttgart, pp 332–340

Semmer N (2003) Individual differences, stress, and health. In: Schabracq MJ, Winnubst JA, Cooper CL (eds) Handbook of work and health psychology, 2nd edn. Wiley, Chichester, pp 83–120

Semmer NK, McGrath JE, Beehr TA (2005) Conceptual issues in research on stress and health. In: Cooper CL (ed) Stress medicine and health. CRC Press, Boca Raton, Florida, pp 1–44

Sexton JB, Thomas EJ, Helmreich RL (2000) Error, stress, and teamwork in medicine and aviation: cross sectional surveys. Br Med J 320:745–749

Ulich E (2001) Arbeitspsychologie. 5.Auflage [Work psychology, 5th edn]. Vdf, Zürich; Schäffer-Pöschel, Stuttgart

Weber H (2002) Stress management programs. In: Smelser NJ, Baltes PB (eds) International encyclopedia of the social and behavioral science, vol 22. Elsevier, Amsterdam, pp 15.184–15.190

Weber H (2004) Explorations in the social construction of anger. Motiv Emotion 28:197–219

Yerkes RM, Dodson JD (1908) The Relation of strength of stimulus to rapidity of habit-formation. J Compar Neurol Psychol 18:459–482

10 Strategies for Action: Ways to Achieve Good Decisions

10.1 Case Study

On the pediatric cardiology ward the on-call pediatric resident was asked to evaluate a 6-year-old patient who was complaining of nausea and dizziness. The child was postoperative day 5 after cardiac surgery. His symptoms had started about 2 h earlier and worsened gradually. By the time the resident arrived at the bedside, the patient's clinical condition had deteriorated further and he was showing signs of impaired consciousness. The pediatrician transferred the child to the examination room and attached him to the monitors. The blood pressure was 60/40 mm Hg and the ECG showed sinus tachycardia with a heart rate of 130 bpm. The saturation was fluctuating between 88 and 92%. Knowing that the chest drain had been removed the day before, the physician listened to the lungs next. Auscultation revealed diminished breath sounds over the left lung and distant heart sounds. In addition, she noted the child's neck veins to be markedly distended. At this point the most likely diagnoses were considered to be tension pneumothorax following the removal of the chest drain and pericardial tamponade. Supplemental oxygen via facial mask and a volume load of 250 ml of crystalloid solution were administered, but the child's condition continued to remain unstable. The resident considered intubation, but cognizant of the detrimental effect that positive pressure ventilation might have on the hemodynamic parameters, she decided to first optimize the patient's status. An epinephrine infusion was started. As a result, the blood pressure improved, and the patient was stable enough to be transferred to the Pediatric Intensive Care Unit. There, transthoracic echography showed a large circumferential pericardial fluid collection and right ventricular diastolic collapse. With the diagnosis of pericardial tamponade, the patient was immediately taken to the operating room where exploratory thoracotomy was performed.

A pediatrician is confronted with an emergency in which the leading symptoms can result from a variety of causes. Just by means of clinical examination she can get no further clues as to which etiology might be responsible for the clinical deterioration. What makes the situation especially tricky is the fact that some possible therapeutic actions which could relieve the symptoms in one case (e.g., intubation, insertion of a chest tube) would actually worsen the patient's clinical condition in an-

other case. This means that if her initial diagnosis proves wrong, the physician may harm her young patient considerably. Although the patient's vital status is serious, it does not mandate any of these procedures as an immediate action. Instead of choosing one of the potentially harmful interventions, the physician takes additional measures to stabilize the patient's vital functions. The resulting clinical improvement buys her time for additional diagnosis. Once the cause of the clinical deterioration becomes evident, she can take specific therapeutic steps. Because the resident displays far-seeing and cautious behavior, she can prevent further harm to her patient which might have followed an unmindful action. With her example of deliberate judgment she demonstrates that the human factors are not only a source of many errors but also the important safety resource for good management of critical situations.

10.2 Strategies for Good Actions

10.2.1 "Good Decisions" in the High-Stakes Environment of Acute Medical Care

The pediatric resident's primary goal is to successfully treat a severely ill and vitally threatened child. But in order to be able to act successfully she has to make good decisions in a context where complexity and dynamic change make it a difficult task to achieve. What then are the characteristics of "good decisions" in a high-stakes environment?

A "good decision" in an emergency situation achieves the following:

— Supports an effective task management in terms of patient safety, efficiency of measures taken, and of the resources applied.

— Takes the present situation into account in which the healthcare provider finds himself or herself. Options of planning and acting are limited by the time available and the finite resources.

— Respects the "psychological condition" of human beings: The information processing capacity is limited, and motivation and emotion influence behavior. As there are limits to mental and physical workload and to the resistance to stress, good strategies will not overstrain a person.

— Results in a strategy of action which can actually be put into practice in a timely and feasible manner.

However, a good decision is not equivalent with:

- A good result: Decision-making is primarily concerned with the way how people come to certain conclusions. It is not uncommon that "shortcuts" and violations can result in good outcomes and thereby reinforce the same hazardous attitudes which lead to the decision in the first place. On the other hand, there will always remain an element of risk for patient safety despite good decisions: When debriefing an unsuccessful cardiopulmonary resuscitation the team members may nevertheless come to the conclusion that all decisions and actions were correct. Last but not least, people may find themselves in situations where they may say in hindsight: "It was pure luck that things turned out that way!"

- A good intention: Good intentions do not guarantee good outcomes. Any action planned has to be tested for inherent risks and for the probability of success. An immediate intubation of the child would have been done with good intentions; however, it might have caused more harm than it would have helped. In addition, an intention should match reality: If I intend to go for a specific treatment, it is only worth considering it if I'm actually capable and have the necessary resources of putting it into action. "Bearing good intentions is an extremely lowbrow mental activity" (Dörner 1996).

- The best possible decision: In hindsight to a critical situation people will often find even better solutions to their problem. As soon as the stress wears off and other team members share their thoughts on critical issues, some previously unconsidered options may arise. Unfortunately, in the time-critical situation itself, these pieces of information, ideas, and opinions were not available, and therefore "the best possible decision" could not be made. Healthcare providers should always bear this critical restriction in mind if they do not want to find themselves trapped in nagging thoughts of "I could have/should have done otherwise or better."

Critical situations differ with respect to situational demands: It can be that certain skills are needed, appropriate rules have to be applied, or a completely new solution has to be found (▶ Chap. 2). Whether or not a decision in the high-stakes environment of acute medical care can be called "good" will be characterized by its ability to meet the requirements of the emergency situation.

10.2.2 Maximum "Efficiency and Divergence"

The moment the resident has her first contact with her pediatric patient she only can assess the current clinical status of her patient. She can neither foresee spontaneous developmental tendencies nor can she tell how certain therapeutic actions will influence the situation. Both, success and failure of therapeutic measures, are within the realms of possibility, but it will only be in hindsight that the resident can know whether or not there would have been a better path to take. With this possibility in mind of choosing the wrong track and continuing until one finally finds oneself stuck at a dead end, it could be of vital importance to keep as many doors open as long as possible. Therefore, it will be part of a good strategy not to tie oneself down to a single treatment path too early. With the awareness of a possible detrimental effect of positive pressure ventilation on cardiac preload in patients with impaired ventricular filling, the resident decides against intubation and instead chooses to increase blood pressure by starting a continuous infusion of catecholamines. She manages to achieve a stable blood pressure and a tolerable arterial saturation which gives her the possibility to initiate further diagnostic procedures until the pathophysiological cause for the critical situation can be identified. Although this practice should be an integral part of patient care in a high-stakes environment, healthcare providers should nevertheless intentionally strive for such clinical conditions of "maximum efficiency divergence" (◻ Fig. 10.1; Oesterreich 1981). A situation characterized by high efficiency divergence offers many different possibilities (hence, "divergence") for actions that have a high probability of success ("efficiency"); thus, intermediate goals set according to this criterion target clinical conditions with many degrees of freedom from where one can move efficiently in many different directions.

10.2.3 Five Steps of a Good Strategy

The management of the critically ill child confronts the pediatrician with a novel situation to which she cannot simply respond by applying rules. The puzzling questions she is faced with are: "What is actually the problem?" and "What am I supposed to do about it?" Instead of simply activating behavioral

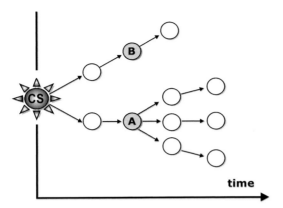

time

☑ **Fig. 10.1** "Maximum efficiency divergence" as a strategy for good action (Oesterreich 1981). Patient treatment is thought of as the sequence of different clinical situations (*circle*). In critical situation (*CS*) there are usually several options for action from which to choose. Some goals (*B*), however, have only one degree of freedom and therefore the development will go in one direction only. If a condition of maximum efficiency divergence is targeted (*A*), many different possibilities for actions are kept open

programs, she has to manage the critical task by applying problem-solving to the situation. Conscious thought, however, the very "tool" humans need to deal with unknown realities functions slowly and is not capable of processing many different pieces of information at the same time. As a result there is an ever present temptation for decision makers to abrogate problem-solving somewhere along the path and to switch to the application of rules simply in order to get rid of this tiresome business of thinking hard. This type of decisional situations, where both the causes of, and solutions to, a critical situation are unknown pose the biggest challenge for the healthcare provider in a high-stakes environment. Therefore, splitting this decisional process up into systematic steps can help to improve actions in the context of complexity and dynamics. There are several decisional aids in the literature on decision-making in critical situations (e.g., Runciman 1988; Gaba 1992; Risser et al. 1999; Small 1999; Murray and Foster 2000). All of them contain, in one way or another, the following five steps of a good strategy:

1. Preparedness
2. Analysis of the situation
   - Gathering of information
   - Building of mental models
3. Planning of actions
   - Formulation of goals
   - Risk assessment
   - Planning
   - Decision-making
4. Execution of action
5. Review of effects
   - Review of actions
   - Revision of strategy
   - Self-reflection

10.2.4 Decisional Aids

Experiences from other complex working environments have demonstrated that people can actually reduce their tendencies for hasty decisions by structuring and organizing their decision-making with the help of decisional aids (Benner 1975; Orasanu and Connolly 1992; Jensen 1995). This structured decision-making process has been shown to be an effective way to a safer operation in any high-risk environment. Decisional aids are often formulated as acronyms (i.e., pronounceable words formed from the initial letter of each of the constituent words) to facilitate memorization. Each time judgments or decisions have to be made under uncertainty, the systematic application of these aids can help to organize one's thoughts and to prevent impulsive action, shortcuts, and neglecting facts that may be important.

10.2.4.1 Decisional Aids for Time-Critical and Limited Problems

Two six-element decision-making models from nonmedical high-risk working domains have been adapted to acute medical care and have been proven to be helpful:

- DECIDE from the domain of firefighting (◘ Table 10.1; Benner 1975): The emphasis of this model lies on the safety aspect of a critical situation.
- FOR-DEC from the domain of civil aviation (◘ Table 10.2; Hoermann 1995): This model emphasizes the way to a risk-balanced decision.

Both decisional aids describe a "closed-loop" process: As soon as an action has been executed, thinking goes back to the beginning and the situation is reviewed anew: In both cases, if the situation has changed and if an action did not bring the intended result, decision makers return to the begin- ning of the loop. Because these acronyms describe decisional aids, they always presume that decision makers are clear about their goal. This explains why, in both models, the formulation of goals has not been implemented.

The important feature of these decisional aids is the fact that it enables all team members to share the same approach to decision-making and action. Once the decision-making process of FOR-DEC or DECIDE has become the implicit structure of problem-solving of all team members, the collection of facts, the generation of options, and the risk assessment will not be the solitary task of an individual but teamwork at its best.

10.2.4.2 Decisional Aids for Complex Problems with Moderate Time Pressure

Some of the problems healthcare providers are confronted with are characterized by a high complexity

◘ **Table 10.1** Decisional model "DECIDE". (After Benner 1975)

	Question/statement	Meaning
Detect	"Something has changed!"	The decision maker detects that a change has occurred which requires attention
Estimate	"Does this change have any significance for me?"	The perceived change is assessed for its significance for the patient and for the future course of events
Choose	"I will choose a safe action!"	The decision maker *explicitly* decides to choose the safest option possible
Identify	"Which reasonable treatment options do I have?"	The option with the fewest risks and the highest probability for success is chosen
		In addition, a "plan B" is mapped out in case the first choice should fail
Do	"I will act on the best options!"	The action is planned and executed
Evaluate	"Which effect did the action have?"	The effect of the action is evaluated
		The intended and factual course of action are compared
		Ask yourself: Has the situation changed in the meantime? Is this plan still appropriate?
		If necessary, return to "Detect" or "Identify"

▣ **Table 10.2** Decisional model "FOR-DEC". (After Hoermann 1995)

	Question/statement	Meaning
Facts	"What is the problem?!"	The need for a decision is detected
		The situation is analyzed and facts are collected
		The urgency is assessed: How much time do we have until a decision has to be made?
Options	"Which different options do we have?"	All team members contribute their point of view on available options
Risks/**B**enefits	"What are the pros and cons for every option?"	The benefits and the probability for success as well as the risk of each option mentioned are evaluated
		The degree of uncertainty is estimated
Decision	"That is what we will do!"	A decision is made by choosing the best option. The best option will be the one with the fewest risks and the highest probability for success
		At the same time, a "plan B" is formulated in case the first plan fails
		Before the plan is executed, the situation is rechecked: Is the initial analysis still appropriate?
Execution	"Who will do what and when?"	The decision is executed
Check	"Is the decision still correct?"	The action is checked
		A critical comparison of the factual and intended effect is made
		If necessary, the decisional process returns to "facts"

but fortunately only by moderate time pressure. Into this category many intensive care patients would fall whose clinical condition has been deteriorating over the past hours. In such cases the formulation of goals is of great importance. The model shown in ▣ Fig. 10.2 has been successfully implemented into the organization of behavior in other high-risk working domains (Dörner 1996; Dörner and Schaub 1994). The arrows indicate that the steps do not have to be processed in a sequential order: Depending on the problem, it might become necessary to spend considerable effort on the gathering of information before intermediate goals can be de-

fined; or it might become necessary to revise goals during the process of planning because certain planning prerequisites have changed. The model of action organization works more like a checklist and is intended to remind people to spend an adequate amount of time on every sequence of the organization of complex actions.

Goals, *plans*, *models*, and the handling of information are the topic of the Chaps. 6 and 7.

Review of effects is the control of the results of action, a central feature of any decisional aid. The review of effects can be made difficult by time delay and the overlay of the effects of many actions: This

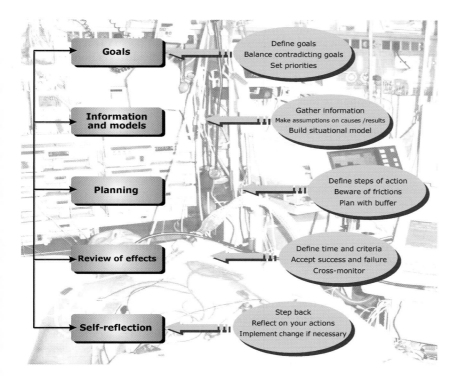

Fig. 10.2 Action organization: a decisional model for situations with moderate time-pressure and high complexity. (Modified after Dörner 1996)

way it becomes difficult to attribute clinical effects to the result of single actions. The review of effects is a way of information management and therefore all the restrictions to information management described in Chap. 6 apply. In addition, the avoidance or superficial performance of review of effects may help to protect the feeling of competence, especially if there is a substantial chance for failure.

Self-reflection describes the conscious analysis of one's own behavior (alone or as a team task). Self-reflective persons try to understand the reasons for success or failure and ask how the strategy for future action has to be adapted; however, self-reflection is uncomfortable and it is difficult to find an appropriate point of time for it: In a critical situation self-reflection it is only partially possible – if at all. After a critical situation, other problems may have arisen and often people are quite reluctant to return to the past. Nevertheless, self-reflection is essential for those working in complex domains: It enables us to learn consciously and to change our behavior.

10.3 Strategies for Coping with Error

10.3.1 Detect Errors Early

An error is an action which does not reach its intended goal. Errors and mistakes do not origin from pathological cognitive mechanisms but instead from useful psychological processes and from a limited cognitive capacity. This is the reason why it is impossible for humans not to make mistakes; however, in order to mitigate the effects on patient safety of those inevitably occurring mistakes, we need to detect them as early as possible and to correct them. But this is a difficult task to achieve for the person who committed the error. We are not prone to having a close look at things: We readily think that our mental model is correct even if there is only a loose match between data and our mental model. This tendency to see things the way we want to have them means that we easily overlook our own errors. But if we apply certain strategies to critical situations situation, we may detect errors more frequently.

The following suggestions are concerned mainly with the individual. Organizational error management will be a topic of Chap. 14.

10.3.1.1 Always Expect: "It Can Happen to Me!"

Because errors are committed all the time, it is necessary to expect them in the context of one's own behavior. A self-critical attitude and an awareness of the ever-present possibility of errors can help to suspect an error behind any deviation of the factual from the intended course of action.

10.3.1.2 Improve Your Perception: Look for Contradictions of Your Model

Any action which gives an immediate physical feedback can provide clear indicators for an error (e.g., accidental puncture of the carotid artery when trying to insert a central i.v. line). Much more difficult, however, is the detection of an error in clinical situations where no immediate feedback about success or failure is provided. In addition, confirmation bias becomes more marked with the experience of failure for the simple reason that it reduces insecurity and encourages the feeling that the critical situation is under control, despite the evidence. It is therefore crucial that the decision maker searches actively for information which could refute his or her situational model or which could indicate that plans do not go as intended. In order to be able to question one's assumptions in an emergency (where one is glad that one "knows" what to do), it has to become a habit in less critical situations to search for pieces of information which contradict or even disprove current assumptions about the situation.

10.3.1.3 Ask for Feedback of Team Members

Other team members are the most valuable resource for the detection of inadequate plans or erroneous actions; however, there is still reluctance among healthcare providers to accept the fact that two pairs of eyes can see more than one, and that this cross-monitoring is an effective means to enhance patient safety (Risser et al. 1999): Instead, it is not uncommon that the monitoring of one's own actions by a second person is regarded as a meddling with the individual's autonomy. This is especially true for physicians. Nevertheless, in addition to the detection of mistakes this dual control can promote a fresh understanding of the situation:

"Those who enter the situation afresh at some later point are not so theory-bound, at least initially. The nakedness of the emperor is readily seen by those who have not come to believe him clothed" (Reason 1990, p. 169).

10.3.2 Mitigate the Effects of Errors Committed

10.3.2.1 Break the "Poor Judgment Chain"

One single error does not cause a fatal outcome of a critical situation. It is only the sequence of poor decisions and the inability to recognize them early and to correct them which leads to accidents and patient harm.

Poor decisions can (a) reduce the safety margin for effective management, (b) undermine the personal feeling of competence, and (c) create feelings of shame and guilt and thereby increase the level of stress.

All these reasons taken together increase the probability that a single error will cause additional errors thereby resulting in a poor judgment chain (Jensen 1995). Once error has been added upon error and the situation threatens to become unmanageable, people will start to act in a "mindless" way. But we are no helpless victims to that mechanism: Critical self-assessment of the results of errors on one's own judgmental and decisional processes can be learned.

10.3.2.2 Use Your Team

The consequences of an error committed can strain any healthcare provider beyond his or her mental and physical limits. In that case it becomes virtually impossible for this person to correct the sequels all by himself or herself. Whenever a severe error is committed, other team members should join the case and give their support.

Coping with Errors Committed

In summary, to detect errors early, it is important to do the following:
- Always expect: "It can happen to me!"
- Improve your perception – look for contradictions in your model.
- Ask for feedback of team members.

To mitigate the effects of errors committed, the following two points are relevant:
- Break the "poor judgment chain."
- Use the team members' resources.

10.4 Tips for Clinical Practice

- Apply the above-listed decisional aids (DECIDE, FOR-DEC) when working in a team environment.
- If you want to be able to apply these decisional aids in critical situations, you should practice them regularly in advance. In a stressful situation you will withdraw to familiar patterns of thinking and behavior.
- "Only by doing nothing you can avoid doing something wrong." Sometimes you have to come to a decision and hazard the consequences that you decided wrong; however, this can never be a license for carelessness.
- Correct any mistake immediately – rectification outranks justification!
- Call for help early! Ask colleagues who are unburdened to join you in the critical situation. Again: ask, your only risk is pride!
- Make it your habit to thank team members for any input they may give on your performance or on suspected errors. Thank them even when you did nothing wrong. The long-term consequences will be that others know that you are a safe person to work with and that they can comment on your behavior without being asked. This input will become extremely helpful in the early detection of errors and mistakes.
- In turn, point out mistakes to other team members. The best way to do this is in the form of a question.

10.5 "Strategies for Action": in a Nutshell

- A good decision in the high-stakes environment of acute medical care is characterized by its ability to meet the requirements of the emergency situation.
- Part of a good strategy is not to tie oneself down to a single treatment path too early. Instead, one should always strive for clinical conditions with as many degrees of freedom as possible. From there on one can move efficiently in many different directions.
- A condition that offers several possibilities each having a high probability of success is called "maximum efficiency divergence."
- There are five steps of a good strategy: preparedness; analysis of the situation; goal setting and planning of actions; execution of action; and review of effects.
- The systematic application of decisional aids (DECIDE, FOR-DEC) can help decision makers to organize their thoughts and to prevent impulsive actions.
- The important feature of decisional aids is that they enable all team members to share the same approach to decision-making and action. Applying DECIDE or FOR-DEC to a critical situation is part of the teamwork, not the task of an individual only.
- It is impossible for healthcare providers not to make mistakes; however, if an error is committed, it is important that no "poor judgment chain" result.

References

Benner L (1975) D.E.C.I.D.E. in hazardous materials emergencies. Fire J 69:13–18
Dörner D (1996) The logic of failure. Recognizing and avoiding error in complex situations. Metropolitan Books, New York
Dörner D, Schaub H (1994) Errors in planning and decision-making and the nature of human information processing. Appl Psychol Int Rev 43:433–453
Gaba D (1992) Dynamic decision-making in anesthesiology: cognitive models and training approaches. In: Evans DA, Patel VL (eds) Advanced models of cognition for medical training and practice. Springer, Berlin Heidelberg New York, pp 123–148

Hoermann HJ (1995) FOR-DEC. A prescriptive model for aeronautical decision-making. In: Fuller R, Johnston N, McDonald N (eds) Human factors in aviation operations. Proc of the 21st Conference of the European Association for Aviation psychology (EAAP), vol 3, Avebury Aviation, Aldershot Hampshire, pp 17–23

Jensen RS (1995) Pilot judgement and crew resource management. Ashgate Publishing, Burlington, Vermont

Murray WB, Foster PA (2000) Crisis resource management among strangers: principles of organizing a multidisciplinary group for crisis resource management. J Clin Anesth 12: 633–638

Oesterreich R (1981) Handlungsregulation und Kontrolle [Action regulation and control]. Urban and Schwarzenberg, Munich

Orasanu J, Connolly T (1992) The reinvention of decision-making. In: Klein G, Orasanu J, Calderwood R, Zsamboka E (eds) Decision-making in action: models and methods. Ablex, Norwood, New Jersey, pp 3–20

Reason J (1990) Human error. Cambridge University Press, Cambridge UK

Risser DT, Rice MM, Salisbury ML, Simon R, Jay GD, Berns SD (1999) The potential for improved teamwork to reduce medical errors in the emergency department. The MedTeams Research Consortium. Ann Emerg Med 34:373–383

Runciman WB (1988) Crisis management. Anaesth Intensive Care 16:86–88

Small SD, Wuerz RC, Simon R, Shapiro N, Conn A, Setnik G (1999) Demonstration of high-fidelity simulation team training for emergency medicine. Acad Emerg Med 6:312–323

III   The Team

Part II dealt with the "psycho-logic" of cognition, emotion, and intention, and the different factors that influence a healthcare provider's behavior in a critical situation. Patient care, however, is seldom an individual's enterprise: There are always many different people from different professional groups and medical specialties involved. Teams are more than just the sum of individuals. Teams have their own strengths and weaknesses and can develop a specific dynamic. Part III will therefore deal with teamwork in a high-stakes environment from a human factors point of view.

The main questions are:

- Which requirements do teams in an acute care setting have to meet? Which are the typical team-related errors?
- Communication is the essential resource in teamwork. What are the characteristics of good communication in critical situations? What are typical communication problems?
- What role does leadership play in the successful management of emergency situations? What characterizes a good leader and which problems may arise with leadership?

Teamwork does not only depend on the people involved but also on the organization in which the team works. The organization sets the organizational frame for teamwork, allocates resources, and enables regular team meetings and team training. The implementation of teams into the greater concept of "an organization" is the subject matter of part IV.

11 The Key to Success: Teamwork

11.1   Case Study

A worker in a print shop attempted to remove a foreign object from moving print cylinders. During a brief moment of inattention, the cylinders caught the sleeves of his shirt and both of his arms were drawn into the machine. Despite an instantaneous shut down of the equipment by one of his colleagues, both arms were trapped up to the elbows. The EMS decided to send a physician to the scene along with the ambulance. When the emergency physician[1], who regularly works as a resident in internal medicine, arrived he found a patient with a reduced level of consciousness standing in front of the print cylinders. His colleagues were supporting him. The physician placed a large-bore peripheral i.v. line in a vein of the dorsal foot and started volume resuscitation. With repetitive small boluses of ketamine and midazolam the patient received adequate analgesia and sedation for the construction of a small temporary platform adjacent to the print cylinders. Initial assessment of the situation by the machine technician revealed a difficult and protracted disassembly. Since the print shop was not far from the local hospital, the emergency physician contacted the operating room and requested a surgeon and anesthetist to come to the scene of the accident. Because the patient was young and an amputation would impose severe risks, the emergency physician and the surgeon decided not to amputate the patient's extremities on site. Meanwhile, the fire department had arrived and, after the anesthetist had deepened the analgesia and sedation, helped the local technician with the difficult task of disassembling the press. Two hours later, both arms were free from the printing machine. Sudden pulsating bleeding was stopped by the inflation of upper extremity tourniquets, which had been placed on both arms before they were released from the machine. The patient was intubated on site and transferred to the operating room. Due to the rapid surgical intervention, both extremities were saved with a sufficient degree of functionality.

Both, the trauma mechanism as well as the pattern of injury of this occupational accident pose complex demands on the medical treatment of the entrapped patient. For a successful medical management of the patient, the Emergency Medical Team and the physician depend on the support of other professional groups, who, in turn, cannot simply go ahead with the technical rescue without having the medical team closely monitor and treat the vital status. The above example illustrates not only the dynamic and complex nature of the preclinical medical environment, but also the fact that teamwork is the ultimate prerequisite for a successful treatment in a high-stakes medical environment. The temporary team of physicians from different specialties, emergency medical technicians, fire rescue workers, and employees of the printing plant can successfully cope with the challenge because all necessary tasks are managed by the shared contribution of skills and experience of all team members. Successful teamwork, like in the case study, is often taken for granted. Usually, the question of how a heterogeneous group of people can actually work together effectively, and which factors account for the success, is not of interest – as long as the cooperation works well.

11.2   The Team

11.2.1   Why Teamwork Has Come into Focus Only Lately

Teamwork is the cooperative effort by members of a group or team to achieve a common goal. Wherever ill or injured people are cared for, healthcare providers will take care of their patients in groups of two or more people. Therefore, teamwork is an inherent feature of healthcare; there is virtually no healthcare possible without teamwork. Despite this fundamental feature of healthcare provision, the medical community has traditionally neglected to address this issue for many decades. The reasons for that are manifold:

Firstly, the widespread tendency of the healthcare community not to think in team concepts may reflect a *deep seated cultural issue*: Many team

---

1 Like in Chap. 4, this example is taken from a European emergency medical system, where a qualified physician (for reasons of simplicity called "emergency physician") joins the emergency medical team to treat a patient on the scene. Besides being on call for preclinical emergencies, the physicians regularly work as family practitioners or in hospitals and come from a variety of specialties (e.g., anesthesia, internal medicine, surgery).

members in Western societies are children of a culture which has come to cherish the individual human being in an unprecedented way. The pursuit of individual happiness and the fulfillment of personal agendas are unchallenged goals of our culture and have strongly impacted the way we perceive human relationships.

In addition, the foundations for a preference of individual achievements over social competence are laid early on: From birth through college, we nurture and praise the individual accomplishments of our children, as well as admire their cognitive faculties and the new skills they acquire, and thereby communicate the message that all that counts is what an individual can successfully accomplish single-handedly. Thus, contemporary Western culture has been unable to be a healthy corrective with respect to cooperation and teamwork for a medical community where medical quality and safety has historically been structured on the performance of expert, individual practitioners. The basic presumption that individual technical expertise will guarantee a desirable outcome has further found expression in the medical and nursing educational cultures: Healthcare providers have been taught intensively isolated technical tasks or clinical algorithms but have not been familiarized with basic concepts of communication and team performance; therefore, the presence of effective communication and teamwork has been assumed, but formal training of teamwork skills and assessments in these areas have been largely absent (Leonard et al. 2004). It is only with reluctance that wider parts of the healthcare community have come to accept the fact that healthcare provides no exception to the rule that a team of expert does not make an expert team.

In addition to the cultural assumptions about the value of individual expertise, another equally important reason has been identified for insufficient team performance and miscommunication: the *power relationships* that exist in healthcare. The existence of different groups of traditionally different status within organizations dominated by a strongly hierarchical structure has resulted in a concept of leadership that resembles the military model more than the mature interaction of adult healthcare providers (Firth-Cozens 2004). Considering the prevalence of this mindset, it is not astonishing that for decades the concept of teamwork has largely been reduced to a gathering of people who give and take orders. But even when a teamwork concept is basically embraced, physicians and nurses nevertheless have discrepant attitudes about the teamwork they experience with each other, including issues such as suboptimal conflict resolution and interpersonal communication skills (Makary et al. 2006; Thomas et al. 2003a; Undre et al. 2006).

11.2.2   Why Teamwork is Necessary

Fortunately, the past decade has witnessed an increasing concern among specialties involved in acute medical care about fundamental issues of successful teamwork. Stimulated by a large body of evidence from other high-stakes environments (e.g., civil aviation, military command operations, nuclear power plants, offshore oil platforms) healthcare providers have started to analyze the status quo of teamwork within their own fields of expertise and have tried to adopt and integrate team-training measures.

From a task perspective this approach to teamwork is long overdue: Many tasks impose mental and physical demands that are too strenuous even for the most experienced individual to perform in isolation. Furthermore, the task specifications very often demand that different groups of professionals cooperate if a problem is to be dealt with successfully. The case study at the beginning of this chapter represents such an interprofessional team approach.

The strongest support, however, for a cultural change and for a focus on teamwork in healthcare comes from the extensive body of research that has been directed at identifying the factors that contribute to an undesired patient care event. Unequivocally, working groups from different working environments have identified a close relationship between teamwork and performance in a high-stakes environment (e.g., Jain et al. 2006; Wheelan et al. 2003). The same is true for healthcare where effective communication and teamwork have repeatedly been shown to be essential for the delivery of high-quality, safe patient care. In turn, poor teamwork and communication between members of healthcare teams have emerged as key factors in poor care and for the occurrence of medical errors (Barrett et al. 2001; Morey et al. 2002). One of the consistently found reasons for poor team formation and teamwork is the lack of a shared understanding about necessity and forms of teamwork. As a result, emerging conflicts among team members and a breakdown in communication have impaired collaboration and resulted in an underutilization of available resources and the creation of new problems. In addition, team members failed to question actions of teammates, even when serious concerns about the adequacy of a diagnosis or a treatment existed (◘ Fig. 11.1; Risser et al. 2000).

Despite the delayed introduction of teamwork concepts in healthcare, there is a growing awareness of the significance of communication and team coordination for efficient task management in critical situations and the need to strive for cultural change. Interviews within all specialties of acute medical care have yielded comparable results: Healthcare providers in the operating room (e.g., Flin et al. 2003; Helmreich and Schaefer 1994; Schaefer et al. 1995; Sexton et al. 2006b), emergency departments (e.g., Barrett et al. 2001; Cole and Crichton 2006; Risser et al. 1999), adult intensive care units (e.g., Ohlinger et al. 2003; Reader et al. 2006; Sherwood et al. 2002; Thomas et al. 2004), pediatric intensive care units (Brown et al. 2003), labor and delivery units (Sexton et al. 2006a), and preclinical emergency medicine (Matera 2003) acknowledge the importance of human-factor issues and would like to engage in training measures that could improve their teamwork skills.

11.2.3 What is a Team?

Psychology knows many differing conceptual frameworks and theories concerning the nature of teams and team performance. Types of teams can be conceived to fall on a continuum, with highly structured, interdependent teams at one extreme and teams whose members interact minimally and perform greater parts of their tasks individually in a group context at the other extreme. Nevertheless, there are shared definitions of "team" which distinguish them from working groups or organizations (Kriz 2000; Katzenbach and Smith 1993; Risser et al. 2000; Salas et al. 1998).

A team in acute healthcare:

− Is defined as a distinguishable set of two or more people and is bound to the presence of these particular members. The team will change as soon as one of the team members drops out. In this respect teams differ from organizations or clubs, which exist independently of the people involved.

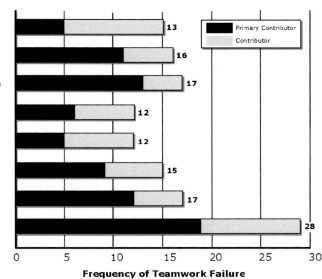

◘ **Fig. 11.1** The most frequent teamwork errors. Depicted is the data of 54 cases of a retrospective emergency department's closed-claims review where poor teamwork was judged to have contributed to clinical error. (From Risser et al. 2000)

— Has a task to fulfill.
— Consists of members with different roles and functions according to the professional group and the experience with the task assigned. Also knowledge relevant for the task is distributed among team members.
— Has a structured membership and decision-making process. The roles of the team leader and the followers are understood by every team member. Followers usually have an equal status (e.g., intensive care nurses, Emergency Medical Teams) and contribute a mix of skills to the successful task accomplishment. The decision structures can vary from distributed to centralized, depending on which levels of interaction and communication are needed to manage a task.
— Interacts dynamically and adaptively toward a common and valued goal, objective, or mission.
— Relies on a dynamic exchange of information and resources among team members for the coordination of task activities. Thus, a complementary relationship of interdependence exists. Member interdependency and the need for co-ordination are key elements which distinguish teams from a working group.
— Shares common explicit and implicit norms which allow decisions to be based on shared understanding.
— Has a limited lifespan in the present constellation: Teams are often confined to accomplishing a well-defined, time-bound task and will disperse eventually as a result of a task accomplished or a change in team composition.

11.3   Team Performance: Input Factors

Team performance research has been able to define major factors that affect the way a team will cope with a given task. Integrating these data into a conceptual framework, several theoretical models have been proposed (for an overview see Salas et al. 1998). Despite their diversity, they share an understanding which defines team performance as the result of how (process, throughput) a team utilizes its human and technical resources given a specific situational and task context (input factors). These results of the team performance (output) in healthcare are first of all safe patient care, but also error incidence, working climate, and team-member satisfaction (Salas et al. 1998; Mickan and Rod-

ger 2000; Paris et al. 2000). Knowledge of these factors is necessary for the advancement of teamwork in healthcare, but it is not a substitute for clinical skills, rules, or knowledge. Instead, it can help to sensitize healthcare professionals for team processes and it may serve as a guideline for strategies in team training (▶ Chap. 15). ◘ Figure 11.2 depicts a conceptual model of an integrated model of team performance in a medical high-stakes environment.

The input factors for team performance can be subdivided into:
— Individual characteristics
— Team characteristics
— Characteristics of the task ("emergency")
— Characteristics of the performance environment

11.3.1   Individual Characteristics

Every team member brings a set of individual characteristics (attitudes, motivation, personality), and individual skills (clinical experience, technical skills, and nontechnical skills) to the team. In addition to individual skills, every team member needs a defined set of team skills. Team skills are a set of nontechnical skills team members must develop before they can function effectively as a team: effective communication; adaptation to varying situational demands; compensatory behavior; mutual performance monitoring; as well as giving and receiving feedback (Burke et al. 2004). These team skills will ensure that the team members' abilities will be complementary, combining these resources to form relationships that enhance team performance; thus, somewhere "along the road" (and in acute medical care this should be very soon) teams must experience a merging of task-related skills and teamwork skills to perform a task successfully.

Integrating all factors, the individual's personal performance on the team can be understood as the product of three factors: individual characteristics; individual skills; and teamwork skills.

Another way to define this is: Personal performance on the team = Individual characteristics × individual skills × teamwork skills. Describing team performance as product shows that each factor is necessary: personality conflicts and varying levels of individual proficiencies can degrade team performance. In contrast, certain skills have been identified which make a person a successful team player.

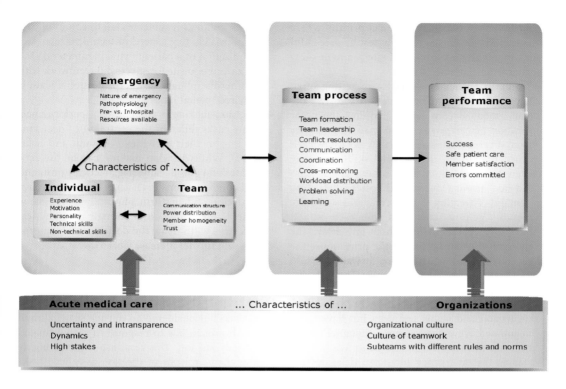

Fig. 11.2 Integrated model of team performance in a medical high-stakes environment. Successful teamwork is the result of an interaction of work and task characteristics, team characteristics (individual, team), and the team process over time. The organizational and situational characteristics influence input and process. The model is based on the theoretical framework of Salas et al. (1998)

A successful team player can:
- Listen and participate actively
- Ask the right questions
- Hold an opinion and then change their point of view
- Assess and value the qualities of other team members
- Assess what he or she can do best and where others have more experience
- Keep to an agreement and identify with a task
- Be self-critical
- Solve conflicts in a constructive way

11.3.2 Team Characteristics

General team characteristics define the team as an entity: team size (one of the main resources in critical situations); group cohesiveness; intra- and interteam cooperation; the power distribution within the team; communication patterns among team members; and the homogeneity and heterogeneity of the team members.

For these factors, desirable values have been described for teams in a high-stakes environment such as industrial or military teamwork. The research here is based mainly on established teams that have a lifespan of weeks or months in the identical formation. Acute medical specialties, however, such as aviation, work with "temporary" teams that are gathered in a random fashion ("ad-hoc teams"): The odds are low that the same group of Emergency Medical Technicians, physicians, and firefighters will ever again be dispatched for another medical emergency; therefore, members of ad-hoc teams need "portable" skills (Flin and Maran 2004) which are not dependent on the presence and combination of certain people but can instead be consistently applied in any given team situation. Rapid organization of such an ad-hoc team becomes a critical priority where patient safety is at stake. As a result, successful teams in a high-stakes medical environment show the following characteristics:

— Teams in an acute medical care setting often have to organize themselves "on the fly." The acute medical care setting requires the organization of caregivers – who may be strangers from diverse disciplines and may not know each other, their roles, their special skills, and may even be hazy about each other's goals – into "ad-hoc" teams (Murray and Foster 2000). Task demands ("treating the patient") and social demands ("getting acquainted with each other") have to go parallel and without any delay: The moment the team meets in the print house the severely injured patient is already waiting.

— The team is defined functionally. The task distribution during the parallel medical treatment and technical rescue operation is specified by profession and status and does not have to be negotiated. Nevertheless, some changes in function can be made during the treatment. For instance, the emergency physician delegates the induction and maintenance of anesthesia to the anesthetist and leaves the treatment of the extremity to the surgeon. The fact that role expectancies do not have to be negotiated anew in every single case is important for the stability of ad-hoc teams.

— Teams in an acute medical care setting are hierarchical. Hierarchy is necessary because in most medical emergencies eventually there has to be one responsible decision maker. Hierarchy supports the management of critical situations by clear paths of information flow and decision-making. Hierarchy can *hinder* problem-solving, on the other hand: Instead of actively participating in the acquisition of data and the contribution of options, team members leave everything to the team leader.

— The team often consists of subteams with specific rules and differing mental models. Multidisciplinary teamwork is a characteristic feature of acute medical care. Every medical specialty (emergency medicine, anesthesiology, surgery) or professional group (Emergency Medical Technicians, firefighters, and technicians) has a specific approach to an emergency situation and hence their own specific behavioral rules which are often unknown to others. This can re-

sult in conflicts if subteams fail to communicate appropriately (e.g., speed of technical rescue vs stabilization of a patient's vital parameters). The major prerequisite for successful teamwork with an interdisciplinary or interprofessional team is a shared mental model.

— Decision-making is embedded in performance. Team tasks differ in the centrality of decision-making in their activities (Orasanu and Salas 1993). While decision-making can be the central task for some teams (e.g., tactical command and control), teams in an acute care setting have to decide and perform physically at the same time. If attention focuses strongly on a physical task, this will impair the decision-making process and further increase workload.

11.3.3   Task Characteristics

A task can be considered an outside set of stimuli to which a team has to respond in a coordinated and timely fashion. This response depends highly on the characteristics of the task assigned: Tasks differ in their complexity (Xiao et al 1996), in task organization (i.e., the degree of interdependencies that exist between various subtasks of a team task), and task structure (i.e., the manner in which subtasks are assigned to, and shared by, various team members and different professional groups). These task characteristics have a strong impact on the communication structure of a team: If few interdependencies exist among subtasks (i.e., low task organization), team members are able to focus almost exclusively on performance of their assigned subtask. An example would be a domestic fire with the firefighters making their way through smoke-filled passages to rescue people who are trapped in the burning structure while the Emergency Medical Team is treating patients with smoke inhalation in the ambulance car; however, if subtasks of teams are highly interrelated (as in the case of the print-shop injury), the communication structure has to be quite elaborate in order to synchronize the different subteams, and team members must communicate frequently to coordinate the flow of individual work inputs and outputs.

Another aspect of the task are the resources at hand: External resources can limit or expand the possibilities for a successful team performance.

Equipment, staffing, and availability of special treatment options have an impact on whether or not a decision can actually be executed.

11.3.4 Characteristics of the Performance Environment

These task characteristics become especially demanding in the performance environment of high-stakes medical care. The foregoing case study calls attention to several characteristics of the environment healthcare providers frequently find themselves in:

- The task environment is characterized by complexity, uncertainty, coupling, and dynamics. There are several unique features that characterize decision-making and action in a medical high-stakes environment. They are explained in detail in Chap. 2.
- External circumstances hamper teamwork. Time and space matter in healthcare: Decisions have to be made under time pressure – the patient trapped in the press cannot wait for the team to organize. "Space" in acute medical incidents often means "no space" – the treatment of the patient on site or in an ambulance demands the ability to work in physical proximity and to coordinate actions. Especially in preclinical trauma patient care prehospital providers may have difficulty in accessing the victim. In the present case study the medical treatment of the patient cannot be performed in the familiarity of an ambulance but instead is, due to the entrapped arms, "bound" to the print roll. The problem of inaccessibility also applies in a moderate way to patients on ICUs who may be completely barricaded behind respirators, IABPs, hemofiltration devices, and dozens of tubes and i.v. lines.
- The task type can vary considerably, necessitating the availability of a broad spectrum of clinical skills, rules, and knowledge. In every medical specialty healthcare providers can be confronted with a great variety of medical or trauma emergencies. In addition, several specialties (e.g., anesthesia, emergency medicine) have to deal with a broad spectrum of patient characteristics (e.g., from neonatal to geriatric multimorbid patients) which demand a very specific set of clinical abilities.

11.4 Team Process

Team processes relate to the way team members communicate and coordinate their activities. Team processes have been an important focus for team research because they determine whether teams will be effective or ineffective. The individual characteristics that make a team member a good team player have already been listed; however, a successful outcome of teamwork requires adequate interaction of all team members involved. Several models (Fleishmann and Zaccaro 1992) have identified team-process factors which enable, support, and enhance team performance (◘ Table 11.1). These team processes are not a psychological end in itself but rather a management tool to expedite high-quality-care delivery to patients: They give caregivers increased control over their constantly changing environment and form a safety net which helps to protect patients as well as healthcare providers from the consequences of inevitably occurring errors (Sexton 2004). Teamwork will only function in critical situations if team processes have become habits and skills through daily practice – that is, we have to practice teamwork in everyday business so that in an emergency we can rely on it.

11.4.1 Team Formation and Positive Working Climate

Good teamwork provides the foundation for the daily operational task objectives, but it does not simply "happen": Teamwork grows in a trustful, cooperative climate which has to be nurtured, for example, by respectful communication. Team formation is a leadership task as well as the task of every single member. The cohesion within the team and good interpersonal relationships can both play a vital role in the successful management of a critical situation. When teams perform in any given climate, they perform better in a better climate.

11.4.2 Establish Team Leadership

The leadership role in an in-hospital emergency is usually assigned to a physician, whereas in the case of on-scene management the leadership role can vary between different people (e.g., emergency physician, EMS team leader, chief firefighter), de-

▢ Table 11.1 Characteristics of a good team process in a medical high-stakes environment. (After the MedTeams Project; Risser et al. 2002)

Team-process factor	Action
Team formation and positive team climate	Develop a "we" feeling
	Demonstrate mutual respect in all communications
Establish team leadership	Encourage leadership behavior in non-routine situations
	Establish a team leader
	Assign roles and responsibilities
Solve conflicts constructively	Try to see the positive aspects of a conflict
	Avoid struggle for power with team members
	"What is right" not "who is right" counts
Communicate and share your mental models	Create a "safe" environment for team members to speak up
	Offer and request information
	Develop and maintain a shared mental model
Coordinate task execution	Profit from implicit coordination and strive for explicit coordination
	Coordinate planned actions
Cross-monitor your teammates	Monitor your team-mates performance
	Address critical issues
	Anticipate possible evolutions
Share workloads and be true to your performance limits	Monitor the workload of team members
	Offer backup behavior
	Communicate clearly, when you have reached your performance limit
Apply problem-solving strategies	Use problem-solving strategies whenever appropriate
Improve team skills	Engage in informal and formal team training measures (personal feedback, team debriefing)

pending on which task is executed at the moment (e.g., medical treatment, technical rescue). In some emergencies (i.e., cardiac arrest in the general ward) the performance environment may be very noisy and chaotic, with many people involved but nobody in charge. In this case the person best capable of managing the crisis should actively take the role of the team leader. This is especially important for situations with an unrehearsed group, called together in an emergency from several different disciplines and professional groups (Murray and Foster 2000). This kind of leadership behavior should be encouraged in unstructured situations but not in routine tasks where roles and functions are clear. "Lead in a pinch, cede in a cinch."

Good leaders change their focus frequently between clinical task execution and team coordination issues, and seek to prevent overstrain of individual team members by distributing responsibility and task load in a well-balanced way.

11.4.3 Solve Conflicts in a Constructive Way

Conflicts are an integral part of team performance. Whenever different people assess the same situation, different points of view will emerge, as everybody has their own motivations, knowledge, and information about the situation. In this respect conflicts are necessary, helpful, and constructive: The contribution of diverse opinions can support a team to get a more comprehensive picture of the situation; however, if conflicts turn into power struggles they become destructive: "Who is right" instead of "what is right" is the kind of conflict that can severely impair team performance As a general rule, relational conflicts should not be addressed in an emergency situation but rather in the follow-up, when stress has eased and emotions have calmed down. In contrast, task-related conflicts (e.g., the choice of the right treatment) should always be resolved, even if it is cumbersome. There is always a chance that if a team member states his or her case they may actually promote an even better solution. Team members should learn conflict-resolution techniques which help to resolve disagreements in interpreting information or proposing courses of action. Open communication is the most important technique when dealing with conflicts.

11.4.4 Communicate and Share Your Mental Models

Only in a team environment that feels "safe" to team members will they speak up when they have safety concerns. Only the information team members actually share with their teammates will contribute to the overall situation and thus to the decision-making (Leonard et al. 2004). Good communication in critical situations is aimed at creating a shared mental model of patient-related and operational issues, thereby "getting everyone on the same page." Developing shared mental models for a problem will create a context within which decisions can be made and the cognitive resources of the entire team can be exploited (Stout et al. 1999). Such shared knowledge enables each person to carry out his or her role in a timely and coordinated fashion, helping the team to function as a single unit with little negotiation of what to do and when to do it. The greater the degree of accuracy and overlap among team-member mental models, the greater the likelihood that the team members will predict, adapt, and coordinate with one another successfully, even under stressful or novel conditions. Essential for the accuracy of the situational picture is a regular update of the members' shared mental models. This is achieved by team situation awareness (▶ Chap. 8): Team members regularly scan the environment for relevant cues and patterns, and then they communicate the information thus gained to the team and integrate it into existing knowledge structures.

11.4.5 Coordinate Task Execution

Coordination of actions is necessary because of time pressure, differing technical knowledge and roles, and parallel operations by team members. Shared mental models allow teams to anticipate, without much talking, each other's resource needs and actions (implicit coordination), especially when workload becomes high and the amount of communication decreases; however, if teams rely too heavily on implicit coordination, they may suddenly find themselves overwhelmed by a problem exactly because expectancies and previous experiences with comparable situations replaced task-oriented communication. A good team process will be characterized by team members defining the problem much more explicitly, volunteering relevant information, articulating plans and strategies, discussing contingencies, explaining the rationale for a decision to all teammates, and by allocating and coordinating responsibilities within the team (explicit coordination).

11.4.6   Cross-Monitor Your Teammates

Complexity, coupling, and opacity increase the likelihood of errors. In order to mitigate the effects of inevitably occurring errors on patient safety, healthcare providers should be encouraged to monitor their team members: Ask critical questions and voice concerns if you believe that an action may harm the patient ("four-eyes principle," cross-monitoring). If the clinical work environment can actively embrace the idea of mutual monitoring for errors by peers, cross-monitoring will help to reduce clinical errors considerably: One caregiver's error can often be prevented or corrected by another caregiver; however, cross-monitoring implies a working climate of open communication and a willingness to accept help from others, irrespective of their professional status. In a performance environment where this is not the case slips and lapses, as well as faulty plans, will go unnoticed or remain unchallenged. In a high-stakes performance environment where human fallibility is a constant threat, peer monitoring is beginning to be seen positively as a safety net that can protect both the patient and the caregiver.

11.4.7   Share Workloads and Be True to Your Performance Limit

Mutual monitoring is not confined to the detection of errors but also includes the workload status and the performance limits of each team member. High workload has been widely shown to degrade performance in individuals and to have a negative effect on team performance. In addition, workload increases the requirements for coordination in teams beyond that inherent in individual task demands (Urban et al. 1995). Critical situations can bring healthcare providers to a point where they will feel overwhelmed by the task load and by stress; therefore, team members should make it a habit to monitor the workload of other members and to offer help early and readily. On the other side, when team members feel that their personal limit is reached,

they should communicate this to the team ("Things are going too fast for me, please slow down" or "I'm not ready yet, please do not continue. I'll tell you when"). Do not hesitate to ask for help!

11.4.8   Apply Problem-Solving Strategies

The medical care of a patient with two entrapped arms is not an everyday problem. As a result, the practical approach to this problem cannot be deduced from a rule but instead needs problem-solving. Critical situations with moderate time pressure are best solved when a problem-solving strategy is applied. Chapter 10 deals with problem-solving in detail.

11.4.9   Improve Teamwork Skills

Teamwork skills are the cognitions, behaviors, and attitudes team members need to function effectively as part of an interdependent team. Research suggests that teamwork skills can be learned and systems can be designed to enhance team performance (Morey et al. 2002). The acquisition of new team behavior, however, requires a supportive organizational culture, sufficient time, and regular training. Team training measures can be both informal (e.g., situational learning, shift reviews of teamwork) and formal (e.g., educational forums). Feedback about team members' current team skills is vital for improvement. Feedback can take place as a personal conversation or as a team debriefing. If team members meet after an emergency or a difficult treatment and mutually debrief their experience, they can draw conclusions and identify consequences from their experience. This kind of learning demands fair and open communication; feedback guidelines should be learned and practiced (▶ Chap. 12).

11.5   The Result: Successful Team Performance

The combination of all the input factors (i.e., characteristics of the individual, team, performance environment, and available resources) with a good team process will result in a successful team performance and ultimately in low-error, high-quality patient care and high satisfaction of the healthcare providers. This will especially be true in a high-stakes environment or in critical situations where the patient's welfare is dependent on a team performing better than the sum of the individual's abilities.

11.6   Strengths of Teams

- Exceptional performance can be accomplished because of a sense of togetherness. In complex problems the team performance will exceed the expected sum of all single actions.
- Different talents and abilities can be used strategically as strengths and not as a factor of competition.
- Bigger cognitive capacity because of the many eyes, ears, and minds involved. More information can be gathered and processed. With this, more substantiated decisions are possible if communication works well.
- More standpoints and alternatives can be brought into a discussion. It is likely that a more comprehensive picture of the current situation will emerge. This in turn will help the team leader in the decision-making.
- Mutual monitoring can help to notice individual errors.
- Shared workload can help to prevent the overstrain of an individual and make sure that all tasks planned can be executed in a timely manner.
- Mutual support and encouragement can enable team members to master even the most difficult situations.

11.7   Why Teamwork Can Go Wrong

Given that teams represent increased cognitive resources compared with individuals, we might take it for granted that teams perform better than individuals: After all, they represent multiple ears, eyes, and brains which can contribute a substantial amount of information, situational models, and proposed courses of action. In addition, workload can be shouldered by all team members. Yet the presence of others can actually degrade the performance of an individual team member. If basic principles of a successful team process are neglected or if teams operate under stress, internal team dynamics may develop which will lead to a lower performance of the whole team than what would have been expected from the sum of its parts (Badke-Schaub 2000; Schulz and

Frey 1998; Orasanu and Salas 1993). What do we know about the underlying mechanisms?

11.7.1   Deficits of the Individual

Some teams will fail with their task assigned because individual team members lack the individual (professional) skills and team skills. Whereas in the first case the team members' contribution to the task accomplishment is minimal despite best efforts, a deficiency in team skills means that someone is unable to be a good team player despite his or her clinical experience. The reason can be either of the following:

- Individual characteristics such as personality structure or behavioral characteristics (e.g., self-centeredness, excessive perfectionism).
- The absence of skills that support the team process (e.g., communication skills). If it is the assigned team leader who lacks the necessary skills, teamwork will become virtually impossible: Instead of a team with a leader, there will only be several "supporting players" and one star.

Besides being unable to be a good team player, there is also the – admittedly rare – possibility that a team member is unwilling to work with other members of a team. This may be the case if team members:

- *Have* to work as part of a team, although they actually prefer to work alone
- Have to cooperate with people they dislike
- Try to solve an interpersonal conflict with other team members (often from other specialties of professional groups) by means of a patient case
- Seek to use a team for their own interests
- Use their role within a team to resolve power issues
- Do not work with full motivation but let others do the work and benefit from teammates efforts ("social loafing")

11.7.2   Team Deficiencies

11.7.2.1 Communication Deficit

Dynamic exchange of information and resources and coordination of actions are vital if a critical situation is to be managed successfully. Without communication, it is impossible to develop a shared understanding of the situation and problem and to act concertedly. If critical information is not shared, decisions have to be made on the basis of incomplete data. Misunderstanding can arise because there is no exchange of mental models. Lack of communication leads to a failure to announce tasks intended and a reluctance to challenge assumptions about the appropriateness of actions taken by other team members (Stout et al. 1999).

Due to the vital importance of communication regarding any team activity, Chap. 12 deals with the subject extensively.

11.7.2.2 Unclear Specification of Responsibility

If leadership is not clearly established in an unstructured situation, and if teams fail to agree on responsibilities in critical situations, we will regularly find a diffusion of responsibility (Darley and Latane 1968): Some tasks (e.g., the easiest) will be addressed by several team members, although one person would have been enough; other tasks remain undone, because everybody expects somebody else to take care of it. Time limits for critical tasks are exceeded because team members were unaware of being actually responsible for their execution. If several healthcare providers are in charge of an emergency without having appointed a team leader, then the tendency for risky decisions will increase because nobody will have to account for the outcome (risk shift; Kogan and Wallach 1969).

11.7.2.3 Shared Misconceptions

Teams easily develop a tendency to follow the majoritarian vote in their decision-making instead of rational arguments. Especially successful teams tend to succumb to the illusion of unanimity and invulnerability: "If every single team member agrees with a solution, it cannot be wrong." Because all team members are in agreement, they see no further need to discuss other possible options; thus, the search for solutions is abandoned early. Expert opinion from outside the team is not requested and the team suspends its rational judgment (*group think*; Janis 1972). Shared experience may also lead team members to assume shared understandings of words such as "risk," "threat," and "likely" when, in fact, everyone gives them a different meaning.

11.7.2.4 Development of Peer Pressure

If group cohesion is very important to the team, dissent and discussions are easily seen as a threat. Once the majority of the team members have formed an opinion they will stick to it even when faced with contradicting information which will prove the opinion as wrong and unrealistic. Criticism of dissenting members is suppressed, and disagreement is seen as disruption. Team members are voted down instead of convinced. Proposals from a leader unite the team, so they are not challenged. The danger of peer pressure lies in the fact that not all options are considered because only those pieces of information are used in the decision-making process which confirm a preexisting opinion. Once a treatment path has been chosen, there will be no further change, because nobody expresses doubt or asks critical questions.

11.7.2.5 "In-group" and "Out-group"

The feeling of togetherness can stimulate teams into an exceptional performance; however, if this feeling of togetherness is lived out excessively, teams tend to set boundaries between themselves and other teams. Whoever is not in the "in crowd" of a team will not find much appreciation and cooperativeness. This can also happen between subteams: "we" are right, "they" are wrong, "we" know best, "they" do not. Teamwork under these circumstances no longer encompasses all parties involved – group interests may outweigh the interest for the patient's health.

In addition to these deficiencies, which can become apparent in everyday situations, stress and the feeling of incompetence can further impair teamwork. Chapter 9 addresses the pathology of teamwork in emotionally straining situations.

11.7.3 The Organizational Context Hinders Teamwork

The organizational context or environment surrounding a team cannot be ignored. Much of what occurs in the environment may facilitate or hinder the team process and team performance. Although the emergency physician, the Emergency Medical Technicians, and the firefighters will be dispatched to many different sites and emergencies, they are nevertheless embedded in larger organizations (e.g., hospital, relief organization, fire department).

An organization can impact teams working in their sphere of influence via:

- Structure of leadership
- Working climate, corporate identity, culture
- Safety culture
- Resource allocation

If the culture within a hospital is defined by a disrespectful interaction among the different specialties, this will affect the cooperation in the emergency room, operating room, and intensive care unit. Healthcare providers then do not support each other more than necessary, and a real team spirit will not develop. On the other hand, if senior healthcare providers (e.g., physicians, nurses) ask their co-workers to monitor their actions and give feedback on possibly erroneous actions, then a top-down model encouraging safe behavior will develop.

However, organizational deficiencies do not always lead immediately to bad teamwork: Highly motivated teams can compensate for these problems for a long time, for instance by increasing personal commitment to patient care given a staff shortage on an intensive care unit. In the long run, however, this strategy will not pay off: Healthcare workers will become overstrained, and motivation and job satisfaction will decrease and possibly result in burnout (▶ Chap. 9). At the very least, at that point, organizational constraints will impact team work.

On the other hand, the organizational context can support and reinforce competent teamwork by creating a supportive safety culture and by providing sufficient resources in terms of staff and equipment. This will positively affect the stress level of team members and the quality of team performance. An elaborate information system, a functional educational system, and a reward system for safety-conscious performance can further propagate effective teamwork in a high-stakes environment. Chapter 15 covers this topic in greater detail.

11.8 Tips for Daily Practice

- If you want to profit from a good team process in a critical situation, you need to rehearse team skills on a daily basis. In an emergency situation, only habits and skills will be available (i.e., behavior that has been practiced time and again).
- Make heedful interacting a routine practice.
- Clarify roles and functions in an emergency. You cannot manage without them.
- You cannot expect people to read your mind. Therefore, state your opinions clearly!
- You will not succeed if you do not talk! Team members must develop and maintain a shared mental model. For juniors it is better to be blatant than to imply.
- If you want to reduce workload, the concept is simple: watch out whether your teammates need help and ask for help yourself.
- Teamwork and leadership are tightly connected: Many team problems are really problems of insufficient leadership, and vice versa.
- Everybody who is involved in the care of the patient belongs to the team.

11.9 "Teamwork": in a Nutshell

- Teamwork is the cooperative effort by members of a team to achieve a common goal.
- Teamwork is an inherent feature of healthcare: There is no high-quality, safe patient care without teamwork.
- Poor teamwork and a breakdown in communication between members of healthcare teams are among the key factors in poor patient outcome.
- Member interdependency and the need for coordination are key characteristics of a team.
- Superb individual clinical skills do not guarantee effective team performance in care delivery.
- A team of experts does not make an expert team: Communication is at the core of team performance. With it, teams will form more readily; without it, they may not function as a team at all.
- Team performance (output) is the result of how (process) a team utilizes its resources given a specific situational context (input factors). The results of good team performance are safe patient care, low error incidence, good working climate, and team-member satisfaction.
- Team tasks differ in their complexity, in task organization (i.e., the degree of interdependence that exist between various subtasks), and in task structure (i.e., the manner in which subtasks are assigned to, and shared by, various team members and different professional groups).

- There are several identifiable team-process factors which enable, support, and enhance team performance. These processes can be taught and learned.
- If people manage to work together as a team, then the performance in complex situations and under time pressure will become much more effective than the actions of an individual.
- Teams in an acute medical care setting show characteristic features and have specific problems.
- Teamwork can fail because team members lack individual skills and the generic and operational team skills.
- Individual skills and knowledge are not sufficient for successful team performance; individual resources must be appropriately utilized through interaction processes.
- Communication is used to build shared situational mental models when conditions demand nonhabitual responses. Once shared models have been created, they provide a context for interpreting information, making decisions, and planning actions. They also provide a basis for predicting behavior or needs of other team members.
- The presence of others can degrade the performance of an individual team member. The resulting behavior can actually threaten the successful treatment of patients.
- Teamwork behaviors and skills are teachable.
- Expert teams have been trained in both task work and teamwork skills.
- Organizations can reinforce competent task work by creating a supportive culture of safety and by providing sufficient resources in terms of staff and equipment.

References

Badke-Schaub P (2000) Wenn der Gruppe Flügel fehlen: Ungeeignete Informations- und Entscheidungsprozesse in Gruppen [Inadequate decision-making and infomation processing in groups]. In: Mey H, Lehmann Pollheimer D (eds) Absturz im freien Fall oder Anlauf zu neuen Höhenflügen. Vdf, Zürich, S 113–130

Barrett J, Gifford C, Morey J, Risser D, Salisbury M (2001) Enhancing patient safety through teamwork training. J Healthc Risk Manag 21:57–65

Brown MS, Ohlinger J, Rusk C, Delmore P, Ittmann P (2003) Implementing potentially better practices for multidisci-

plinary team building: creating a neonatal intensive care unit culture of collaboration. Pediatrics 111:482–488

Burke CS, Salas E, Wilson-Donnelly K, Priest H (2004) How to turn a team of experts into an expert medical team: guidance from the aviation and military communities. Qual Saf Health Care 13 (Suppl 1):i96–i194

Cole E, Crichton N (2006) The culture of a trauma team in relation to human factors. J Clin Nurs 15:1257–1266

Darley JM, Latane B (1968) Bystander intervention in emergencies: diffusion of responsibility. J Person Soc Psychol 8:377–383

Firth-Cozens J (2004) Why communication fails in the operating room. Qual Saf Health Care 13:327

Fleishmann E, Zaccaro S (1992) Toward a taxonomy of team performance functions. In: Swezey R, Salas E (eds) Teams: their training and performance. Ablex, Norwood, New Jersey, pp 31–56

Flin R, Fletcher G, McGeorge P, Sutherland A, Patey R (2003) Anaesthetists' attitudes to teamwork and safety. Anaesthesia 58:233–242

Flin R, Maran N (2004) Identifying and training non-technical skills for teams in acute medicine. Qual Saf Health Care 13 (Suppl):i80–i84

Helmreich R, Schaefer H (1994) Team performance in the operating room. In: Bogner M (ed) Human error in medicine. Erlbaum, Hillsdale, New Jersey, pp 225–253

Jain M, Miller L, Belt D, King D, Berwick DM (2006) Decline in ICU adverse events, nosocomial infections and cost through a quality improvement initiative focusing on teamwork and culture change. Qual Saf Health Care 15:235–239

Janis I (1972) Groupthink. Psychological studies of policy decisions and fiascos. Houghton–Mifflin, Boston

Katzenbach JR, Smith, DK (1993) Teams. Der Schlüssel zu Hochleistungsorganisationen [Teams. The key to high-performance organizations]. Redline Wirtschaft, Vienna, Austria

Kogan N, Wallach MA (1969) Risk taking. Holt, New York

Kriz WC (2000) Teamkompetenz. Konzepte, Trainingsmethoden, Praxis [Team competence. Concepts, training methods, practice]. Vandenhoeck and Ruprecht, Göttingen

Leonard M, Graham S, Bonacum D (2004) The human factor: the critical importance of effective teamwork and communication in providing safe care. Qual Saf Health Care 13 (Suppl 1):i85–i90

Makary MA, Sexton JB, Freischlag JA, Holzmueller CG, Millmann EA, Roven L, Provenost PJ (2006) Operating room teamwork among physicians and nurses: teamwork in the eye of the beholder. J Am Coll Surg 202:746–752

Matera P (2003) The power of teamwork. J Emerg Med Serv 28:26

Mickan S, Rodger S (2000) Characteristics of effective teams: a literature review. Aust Health Rev 23: 201–208

Morey JC, Simon R, Jay GD, Wears RL, Salisbury M, Dukes KA, Berns SD (2002) Error reduction and performance improvement in the emergency department through formal teamwork training: evaluation results of the MedTeams project. Health Serv Res 37:1553–1581

Murray WB, Foster PA (2000) Crisis resource management among strangers: principles of organizing a multidisciplinary group for crisis resource management. J Clin Anesth 12:633–638

Ohlinger J, Brown MS, Laudert S, Swanson S, Fofah O (2003) Development of potentially better practices for the neonatal intensive care unit as a culture of collaboration: communication, accountability, respect, and empowerment. Pediatrics 111:471–481

Orasanu J, Salas E (1993) Team decision-making in complex environments. In: Klein G, Orasanu J (eds) Decision-making in action: models and methods. Ashgate, New York, pp 327–345

Paris CR, Salas E, Cannon-Bowers JA (2000) Teamwork in multi-person systems: a review and analysis. Ergonomics 43:1052–1075

Reader T, Flin R, Lauche K, Cuthbertson BH (2006) Non-technical skills in the intensive care unit. Br J Anaesth 96:551–559

Risser DT, Rice MM, Salisbury ML, Simon R, Jay GD, Berns SD (1999) The potential for improved teamwork to reduce medical errors in the emergency department. The MedTeams Research Consortium. Ann Emerg Med 34:373–383

Risser DT, Simon R, Rice MM, Salisbury ML (2000) A structured teamwork system to reduce clinical errors. In: Spath PL (ed) Error reduction in health care. A system approach to improving patient safety. AHA Press, Chicago, pp 235–278

Salas E, Dickinson TL, Converse SA, Tannenbaum SI (1998) Toward an understanding of team performance and training. In: Swezey RW, Salas E (eds) Teams: their training and performance. Ablex, Norwood, New Jersey, pp 3–30

Schaefer HG, Helmreich RL, Scheidegger D (1995) Safety in the operating theatre, part 1: Interpersonal relationships and team performance. Curr Anaesth Crit Care 6:48–53

Schulz S, Frey D (1998) Wie der Hals in die Schlinge kommt: Fehlentscheidungen in Gruppen [Erroneous decision-making in groups]. In: Ardelt-Gattinger E, Lechner H, Schlögl W (Hrsg) Gruppendynamik. Anspruch und Wirklichkeit der Arbeit in Gruppen [group dynamics – ideal and reality of work oin groups]. Verlag für Angewandte Psychologie, Göttingen, S 139–158

Sexton JB (2004) The better the team, the safer the world: golden rules of group interaction in high risk environments: evidence based suggestions for improving performance. Published by Swiss Re Centre for Global Dialogue Rüschlikon, Switzerland, and the Gottlieb Daimler and Karl Benz Foundation, Ladenburg, Germany

Sexton JB, Holzmueller CG, Pronovost PJ, Thomas EJ, McFerran S, Nunes J, Thompson DA, Knight AP, Penning DH, Fox HE (2006a) Variation in caregiver perceptions of teamwork climate in labor and delivery units. J Perinatol 26:463–470

Sexton JB, Makary MA, Tersigni AR, Pryor D, Hendrich A, Thomas EJ, Holzmueller CG, Knight AP, Wu Y, Pronovost PJ (2006b) Teamwork in the operating room: Frontline perspectives among hospitals and operating room personnel. Anesthesiology 105:877–884

Sherwood G, Thomas E, Bennett DS, Lewis P (2002) A teamwork model to promote patient safety in critical care. Crit Care Nurs Clin North Am 14:333–340

Stout RJ, Cannon-Bowers JA, Salas E, Milanovich DM (1999) Planning, shared mental models, and coordinated performance: an empirical link is established. Hum Factors 41:61–71

Thomas EJ, Sexton JB, Helmreich RL (2003a) Discrepant attitudes about teamwork among critical care nurses and physicians. Crit Care Med 31: 956–959

Thomas EJ, Sherwood GD, Mulhollem JL, Sexton JB, Helmreich RL (2004) Working together in the neonatal intensive care unit: provider perspectives. J Perinatol 24:552–559

Undre SN, Sevdalis AN, Healey S, Darzi A, Vincent CA (2006) Teamwork in the operating theatre: Cohesion or confusion? J Eval Clin Pract 12:182–189

Urban J, Bowers C, Monday S, Morgan B (1995) Workload, team structure and communication in team performance. Milit Psychol 7:123–139

Wheelan SA, Burchill CN, Tilin F (2003) The link between teamwork and patients' outcomes in intensive care units. Am J Crit Care 12:527–534

Xiao Y, Hunter WA, Mackenzie CF, Jefferies NJ, Horst R (1996) Task complexity in emergency medical care and its implications for team coordination. Hum Factors 38:636–645

12 Speech is Golden: Communication

12.1   Case Study

On a late afternoon, the code team of an intensive care unit was called to a "code blue" on the general ward. Upon arrival, the patient was unconscious, two nurses were frantically performing CPR, and several other individuals were observing the events in disbelief. The first impression of the ICU physician was that the resuscitation was chaotic and uncoordinated. He took over the mask ventilation, announced in a loud voice that he would be running the code, and then allocated specific tasks to the medical staff in the room. Several minutes later, a surgery resident arrived and was immediately briefed by the intensivist. The initial diagnosis entertained by the two physicians was massive pulmonary embolism, but soon it was learned that the patient had just had an uneventful splenectomy. Suspecting hemorrhagic shock, the physician ordered aggressive fluid resuscitation. A large-bore Shaldon catheter was inserted into the right internal jugular vein, 2500 ml crystalloid solution was infused, and repeated boluses of epinephrine were given with subsequent improvement of the blood pressure. The OR desk was called to schedule an emergency exploratory laparotomy, and a request for emergency release of blood products was sent to the blood bank. A cell saver was also prepared in the OR. The patient was transported to the OR, where the intensive care physician gave a concise report to the receiving team and answered their questions. The hemoglobin concentration upon arrival was 3.8 g%. On abdominal exploration, a disengaged splenic ligature was identified, and the bleeding was controlled. Intraoperatively the patient was transfused with 9 units of PRBCs, 12 units of FFPs, and 2 units of platelets. The postoperative course was complicated by acute renal failure that resolved within the subsequent 3 weeks. The patient recovered completely and was discharged from the ICU without any neurological deficits.

A code team from intensive care is called to a cardiac arrest. Together with the staff from the general ward, the unrehearsed group of experienced and inexperienced nurses and physicians from different specialties have to manage the medical emergency. In his function as team leader the critical care physician has to cope with several parallel tasks: He has to assign tasks to the team members, coordinate the resuscitation efforts, and gather all available information which could explain the cardiac arrest. In addition, he has to initiate the preparations for an emergency operation while at the same time supervising the resuscitation efforts. A verbal handover of the patient to the OR team ensures that all relevant information is shared. The fact that the patient survives the cardiac arrest without any neurological impairment can largely be ascribed to the successful teamwork and the good communication during the emergency situation.

12.2   Organizing the Chaos: Functions of Communication

The most fundamental function of communication is to deliver a message from one individual to another. The case study, however, highlights a critical feature of good communication in critical situations: Communication is much more than just talking; it has to fulfill several important functions during a critical situation. The communication patterns necessary for this purpose may differ from those used in everyday conversations, as those might be inadequate during a critical situation. In the context of communication in a high-stakes medical environment, communication serves to promote the functions given below.

12.2.1   Build and Maintain Team Structure

In the case study the team is structured by the physician, who is authorized a priori by virtue of his profession. He can assign functions and roles to team members and can decide who is supposed to take responsibility for tasks such CPR, and who is supposed to take easier tasks such as running an errand. As in this case of cardiac arrest, every healthcare team needs structure in order to successfully manage its medical task. As life-saving critical care is performed by multiple caregivers from divergent professions and specialties ("ad-hoc teams"; ► Chap. 11) who may not know each other, their roles, their special skills, and each other's goals, task demands ("performing ACLS") and social demands ("getting acquainted with each other") have to run parallel (Murray and Foster 2000). Team formation has to make clear who will act in which role and whose instructions have to be followed. The team structure will be partly determined by professional roles and partly by explicitly allocating and coordinating responsibilities within the team, especially if "equal-rank" team members are present (e.g., nurses, physicians). It is crucial for a successful team performance to explicitly negotiate the leadership role and the allocation of responsibility and not to just assume it (explicit coordination). If a core team has already been formed (as in the case of a code team joining staff on ward), communication will help other staff members to find their role and will help to stabilize the team structure.

12.2.2   Coordinate the Team Process and Task Execution

From an operational perspective, communication serves as an enabling tool for achieving task objectives and for coordinating team efforts. The team leader in the case study coordinates work flow by assigning tasks in accordance with the team members' abilities. By concentrating all available resources on the management of the emergency and avoiding useless actions, the team leader can build a sense of confidence that the situation is manageable. This in turn reassures team members with little experience in emergency situations (e.g., inexperienced nurses from general ward) who gain confidence in their task execution. The less familiar a leader is with an emergency situation and with the team in its present constellation, the more effort he or she will have to invest in coordination; however, coordination is not confined to a top-down process by which a leader directs the activities of all team members. Coordination also implies that every team member is aware of the teammates' actions and the tasks accomplished.

12.2.3   Enable Information Exchange

Information exchange is the third function whereby communication contributes to the successful team performance on ward and to smooth cooperation with the OR team. An appropriate exchange of information is critical for an adequate situational assessment and a good strategy of action.

12.2.4   Facilitate Relationships

A cardinal principle of human communication is that it takes place in a social context; therefore, communication fulfills a fourth, ever-present function during the entire code: It facilitates and creates relationships among the team members. The way these relations are formed depends mainly on three factors:

- Which professional roles and necessary qualifications the participants embody
- Which behavior they display
- What they expect from each other and from their communication

The first three functions of communication (team structuring, coordination, information exchange) are unthinkable without this "being-in-relationship". It is impossible to exchange information with a mere matter-of-fact attitude without simultaneously establishing a relationship between the subjects who participate in this information exchange. This fact has direct consequences for a safe delivery of patient care: If a leader displays a calm and decisive attitude in an emergency situation, he or she will create a team climate characterized by confidence, reliability, trust, and the willingness to take responsibility for the situation. If a leader repeatedly behaves this way, the leader will soon have a reputation in the department or institution as a safe and competent person with whom to work. Team members will have positive expectations of their leader which, in turn, will characterize (and indeed facilitate) their next interaction. On the other hand, if a physician is reputed as being arrogant and bossy, team members will expect nothing but this attitude behind any of his or her utterances. If this particular physician gives brusque commands during a critical situation, team members will see their expectations confirmed – a vicious circle of expectations, perception, interpretation, and reaction arises. If the leader known as calm and decisive were to displace the same brusque behavior, the team might interpret these instructions differently: Since they know about the leader's affirmative personality, they would simply excuse these utterances as a slip; thus, questions of relationship and communication are inextricably bound together.

> **Basic Functions of Communication in an Acute Medical Care Setting**
> - Build and maintain team structure
> - Coordinate team process and task execution
> - Exchange information
> - Facilitate relationships

12.3 Understanding Communication

12.3.1 Basic Assumptions About Communication

There are many theoretical frameworks and definitions as to what actually constitutes communication (Griffin 1999; Miller 2005) and even more practical tips and suggestions on how to communicate well in everyday life (Knapp and Daly 2002; Hargie 2006). Throughout the book the following assumptions form the basis of our understanding of the term "communication":

— Communication is always intentional. A person wants to interact with another person. This interaction can happen verbally or nonverbally (e.g., head nods, smiling, frowns).

— Communication involves at least two people and implies that the thinking and behavior of one person is brought into relationship with the other person.

— Communication as a central form of human behavior depends on the situational context. Every time a person talks and behaves, this behavior can be perceived and interpreted by any other person. In addition to perceiving, the observer can relate this behavior to his person irrespectively of the intention of the sender: Some of the nurses standing by whom the critical care physician does not address explicitly could interpret his behavior as a indication that "the physician is ignoring us." This is a good example of one of the basic assumptions of communication theory, namely that communication has to be seen in a much broader context than mere verbal exchange: "We cannot *not* communicate" (Watzlawick et al. 1996).

— As we have no direct access to the mind of others, communication can never be a mere transfer of information from one person to another (Maturana and Varela 1992). Although the sender has many options to state his or her intention in a certain situation as clearly as possible, he or she has no influence on how the others understand this piece of information or respond to it. During the resuscitation in the case example, the critical care physician asks one of the nurses from general ward to go and fetch a Shaldon catheter from the crash cart. Because the nurse does not know this kind of catheter, his request "Could you please go and get me a Shal-don catheter from the crash cart?" has no informational value which could direct her behavior in accordance to the physician's intention; thus, the physician cannot achieve his goal with the nurse – he is unable to transfer information.

— We cannot determine how our counterpart will interpret words and behavior; therefore, "meaning" is not a settled variable which is transmitted along with the words spoken. As every message is subject to personal interpretation of the receiver, the result of this process will often differ considerably from the sender's initial intention.

— Cooperation within a team very often produces stable and relatively reproducible patters of team communication (Watzlawick et al. 1996). These communication patterns can be more or less appropriate for the demands of the actual situation: If a team is accustomed to discussing all pros and cons of a therapeutic measure in great detail, this can be helpful in providing optimum care for a critically ill patient; however, if the code team had applied the same communication pattern while performing CPR, this behavior would have been dysfunctional.

— A malfunctioning communication pattern is a pattern where all people involved have good intentions, but where the interaction nevertheless creates an unproductive and destructive system. A frequent example for such a cognitive and interpretative pattern is the widespread tendency of blaming other people for communication problems and the refusal to own a situation and take responsibility for it. The behavioral patterns of both communication partners form a system of circular cause-and-effect relationship. If two people cooperate (and communicate) ineffectively, the reason does not lie in problematic personalities (e.g., choleric surgeon, hysterical nurse) but in problematic communication patterns.

12.3.2 Sources and Squares: Theories of Communication

Several theoretical models have tried to conceptualize communication as the transmittal of signs and contents. In the context of team performance in a high-stakes environment two models are especially suited to explain the regular as well as the problematic aspects of human communication.

12.3.2.1 The Shannon–Weaver Transmission Model of Communication

In 1949 Claude Shannon and Warren Weaver, who were not psychologists but engineers working for Bell Telephone Labs in the United States, developed a technical model of communication which was intended to assist in developing a mathematical theory of communication. They proposed that all communication must include five components, if a message is to be transmitted successfully (◻ Fig. 12.1):

- Information source: It produces a message
- Transmitter: It encodes the message into signals
- Channel: Via a channel signals are adapted for transmission
- Receiver: It "decodes" (reconstructs) the message from the signal
- Destination: where the message arrives

A crucial prerequisite in this model is that transmitter and receiver share a common set of signs and common rules how to encode and decode the message. The quality of reception is determined by the kind of channel (which does not have to be speech), the channel capacity, and by perturbations (e.g., noise). The model "transmitter–channel–receiver" has been repeatedly applied to human communication, although it has too little components and is not complex enough to meet the requirements of the multilayered information processing of human communication. Apart from its obvious technological bias, this model nevertheless can emphasize certain interpersonal communication problems caused by the channel. Noise would be such a dysfunctional factor which causes channel interference. This interference with the message traveling along the channel may lead to a signal received being different from that sent or to a signal transmitted not being received at all. For example, if an emergency has to be managed in a loud and chaotic environment, a leader's instructions or a team member's feedback can easily be misunderstood or overheard. A second dysfunctional factor referring to the channel is that of channel overload. Channel overload is not due to any noise source but instead to the channel capacity being exceeded. In the context of high-stakes medical care this can happen all too easily if all team members talk at the same time: The channel "verbal communication" is overloaded by messages (and not by noise) and the receiving person has to filter "relevant information" from the incoming data (▶ Chap. 8). In this process important information can get lost. Another important aspect, which will be considered in greater detail in the second model, pertains to the message itself: Shannon's original paper, since it had all to do with information theory, discussed the transmission of information; however, as already stated, human communication is not merely about transferring information: Human beings do not process information but instead process meanings; thus, if this model is applied to human communication, problems arise with the assumption that meanings of a message can be encoded, transferred, and decoded. In addition, Shannon's model suffers from its obvious linearity: It looks at communication as a one-way process, although human communication relates to a verbal and nonverbal interaction of at least two subjects.

One last distinction, namely that of the physical context, is helpful when applying this model to the high-stakes medical environment (Kanki and Smith 1999). The location of a communication event may not affect the information content of the message, but it often affects the quality of transmission, impact, efficiency, and nature of the communication process. If sender and receiver are co-located, face-to-face communication can take advantage of the shared situation and can open the possibility of referring to nonverbal cues (e.g., facial expression, gestures; ▶ Chap. 12). In

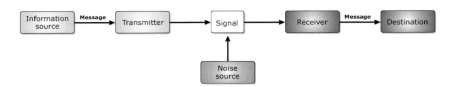

◻ **Fig. 12.1** Sender–channel–receiver. The Shannon–Weaver transmission model of communication. (From Shannon and Weaver 1949)

the absence of shared visual information (e.g., on the phone), many sources of information that can supplement communication are eliminated so that remote communication can only utilize verbal and paraverbal (e.g., intonation, phrasing) cues. If communicators are remotely located and speak via interphone (e.g., physicians from different departments) or via radio (e.g., EMTs and the dispatch center), it is crucial that information is transmitted reliably by closing the communication gap (read-back/hearback).

12.3.2.2 The Four Aspects of a Message

In contrast to technical models, psychological models of communication describe the interactions between subjects who communicate with each other. Psychological models distinguish between:
- The content of a message (content component)
- The relationship both subjects have with each other (relational component)
- The way a message can be interpreted (interpretational component)

Communication is not only a matter of sending and receiving but also of *what* is said, how it is said, and *how* the actors *understand* what has been said (Bühler 1934; Searle 1969). Psychological models emphasize the fact that we do not communicate merely on the grounds of factual information. Instead, "communication = content + relationship" (Griffin 1999). Moreover, apart from expressing the relation between the sender and receiver, every message contains also a (hidden) statement about the sender ("self-revelation"; Watzlawick et al. 1996).

The "square model" of communication based on work by Schultz von Thun (1981, English in Campbell and Bagshaw 2002) can help to explain and avoid misunderstandings in communication. In this model, every message has four aspects, such as the four dies of a square: content; self-revelation; the relationship between the actors; and appeal (◘ Fig. 12.2; ◘ Table 12.1).

Those four aspects of a message are equally relevant for the person talking and the person listening. You could say that we talk with four mouths and listen with four ears – and we can open them

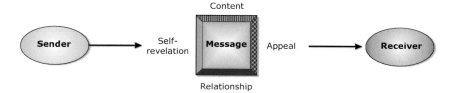

◘ **Fig. 12.2** The four aspects of a message. Schultz von Thun's psychological "square model" of interpersonal communication. (From Schultz von Thun 1981)

◘ **Table 12.1** The four aspects of a message: The "square model" of communication. (From Schulz von Thun 1981)

Content	Information about facts, objects, and events
Self-revelation	Information about the sender as person. This can either take the form of a voluntary self-presentation or an involuntary self-revelation
Relationship	Information about the relationship between sender and receiver. The sender reveals how he or she sees the receiver and their relationship is determined by the words chosen, by the intonation, and by nonverbal signals
Appeal	Information about an appeal to act. Every message tells the receiver what he or she is supposed to do or to leave. The sender prompts the receiver (not) to do something

more or less widely, according to our (not always conscious) intentions (▢ Fig. 12.3). Which of the four aspects the sender will emphasize (which mouth speaks most loudly) will be determined by his or her thoughts, intentions, and communication abilities. The receiver in turn has the possibility to react to each aspect of the message. Which of these aspects the receiver emphasizes (which ear listens intently) will be rooted in his or her present mental state, expectations, anxieties, and in previous interactions with the sender. The sender, however, has no means of influencing the listener's mind and therefore has difficulty in predicting the receiver's response to the message.

A clinical example might help to clarify this matter (▢ Fig. 12.4): After the patient has been weaned from cardiopulmonary bypass at the end of a coronary artery bypass operation the cardiac surgeon turns to the anesthetist and says: "The blood pressure is dropping! How high is your epinephrine running?" From the surgeon's point of view (he is the sender of the message) the content of the message refers to an observable change in hemodynamics and the resulting question about an appropriate catecholamine therapy. At the same time his question also has an appeal to the anesthetist. His request could be: "Have a look at your infusion pump and tell me the infusion rate." In addition, his question carries a self-revelation of his momentary mental state. One possibility could be that the question expresses his concern about the patient's current pathophysiological state and about the consequences if the hemodynamic situation is not improved quickly; however, it could

also be that the surgeon wants to clarify on the relational side the responsibility for all measures taken. He could reveal to the anesthetist by the choice of his wording, intonation, and mimic what he really thinks about his anesthesiological counterpart: "This is my patient, and I, as the responsible person, have no confidence in your capability to manage this situation. I have to tell you to increase the infusion rate and I think this case is too difficult for you."

The anesthetist (he is the receiver), however, will listen with his "four ears" to the different aspects of the message, opening one of them more widely than the others. If the content aspect is the most important one to him, he will respond to the question by stating the facts and telling the surgeon the infusion rate; however, if the receiver hears the self-revelation of concern about the patient's wellbeing in the question of the sender, then he might answer the question by mitigating the surgeon's concerns: "I'm taking care of the problem and have just increased the infusion rate of epinephrine. I'm confident that the blood pressure will soon return to normal values so you can actually continue to operate." Maybe the anesthetist has a very sensitive ear for the relational aspect of the message. In this case he will consider the question as a meddling with his area of responsibility and will hear disrespect for his capabilities. The answer then might be: "Mind your own business."

The reader might try to speak the sentences in the example with different intentions aloud – observe the tone of your voice, the emotions that go with it, and imagine the reaction of a counterpart.

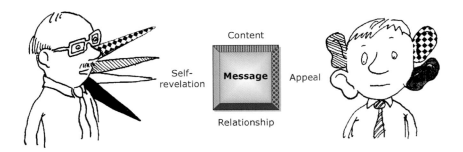

▢ **Fig. 12.3** The "four beaks" and "four ears" model. (From Schulz von Thun et al. 2000). Both, sender and receiver of a message, can emphasize one of the four aspects of a message. The sender has no means to predict the receiver's understanding of the message

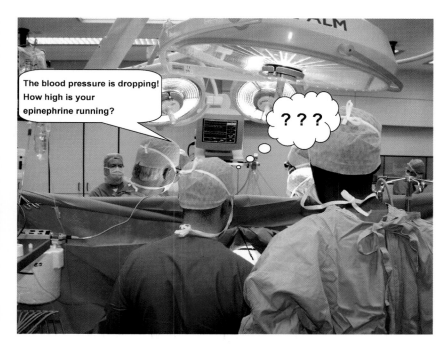

The blood pressure is dropping! How high is your epinephrine running?

? ? ?

◻ Fig. 12.4 Interpersonal communication during a critical situation while weaning from cardiopulmonary bypass. The anesthetist's reply to the cardiac surgeon's question will depend on which of the four aspects of the message (content, self-revelation, relationship, appeal) he will emphasize

12.3.3 It's Not What You Say, It's the Way You Say It: Nonverbal and Paraverbal Communication

Human communication uses different channels in a parallel way to transfer information. Besides the words we choose (verbal communication), we also transmit a messages through the tone, pitch, and pacing of our voices (paraverbal communication) and communicate through gesture, posture, facial expression, and eye contact (nonverbal communication). Communication can use many behavioral patterns; even silence can be "telling." People receiving a message will infer the information they believe relevant for joint action in the current situation from all three channels. Information conveyed by the nonverbal channel will "speak" to people much more directly than words and thus will have the greatest impact. Nonverbal and paraverbal information can help the receiver to understand the meaning of a message in its larger situational context. Nonverbal information is like a commentary or an instruction manual for the spoken sentences. The surgeons question "How high is your epinephrine running?" together with a frown on his face could be interpreted by the anesthetist as an expression of doubts about his competence. The same words spoken in a calm and friendly manner and with a knowing smile would signalize "I'm confident, you'll make it!" This interpretation takes place subconsciously: The nonverbal and paraverbal channel are much more colored by attitudes and emotions and are less under conscious control than the information processing of the verbal channel; however, if we feel that the verbal and nonverbal channel are at odds with each other because words convey one meaning and the nonverbal information indicates the opposite (incongruence), we will subconsciously place greater importance on the nonverbal and paraverbal cues: In case of doubt, we believe the tone, the mimic, gesture, and body language, rather than the spoken word.

If there are several possibilities of interpreting a message, we usually choose the one we expected or the one most probable in that situation. If incongruence leaves space for the receiver's interpretation, the result most probably will reflect the receiver's self-perception, anxieties, and expectations more than the sender's original intention; therefore, it is important to remember especially in critical situations that the messages sent via body language should conform to the spoken message (congruence).

12.4 General Disturbance of Communication

The case study describes a medical emergency situation during which communication is successfully used to structure and coordinate team activities. The outcome of this team process is rewarding: The patient survives his cardiac arrest and can be discharged from ICU without any neurological deficits; however, it is not uncommon that communication fails and compromises safe patient care. The disturbances can be rooted in any of the following:

- The characteristics of the message
- The process of receiving and interpreting the information
- The relationship of both dialogue partners

12.4.1 Misunderstanding

People communicate with the purpose of calling other people's attention to their intentions and goals of action. If the sender transmits information or instructions and a team member reacts in a way that is different to what the sender intended, a misunderstanding occurred. Under familiar and everyday conditions misunderstandings are seldom because both sender and receiver have similar mental models about the kind of behavior which would be best under these circumstances. Even if the message is transmitted incompletely (e.g., because of a noisy environment) and the receiver catches only half of the words, the situational context as well as his or her expectations nevertheless enable the receiver to guess the sender's appeal correctly; however, it is different in novel and ambiguous situations: In this case neither sender nor receiver can rely on familiar mental models. The situation has to be identified, assessed, and explained, and the future de-

velopment has to be predicted (▶ Chap. 6). Because this process depends highly on emotions, motives, available knowledge, and experience, there will be more or less overlap between the sender's and receiver's result. This gap in a shared mental model increases the likelihood for misunderstanding.

In casual conversation, small misinterpretations are tolerated – sometimes even intentional ones (e.g., jokes, ironic remarks). In a high-stakes environment, however, where complex tasks, ambiguity, and time pressure necessitate an effective team process, small misunderstandings and communication inefficiencies may have dire consequences.

12.4.1.1 Linguistic Ambiguity

Verbal messages can be misunderstood because phonation, grammar or dialect give an ambiguity to the sentences. The intended meaning must be derived from the situational context. If interference like noise, time pressure and distraction add to this process of understanding then the interpretation of ambiguous sentences can become faulty.

12.4.1.2 No "Square Clearness"

Successful communication is a "four-dimensional" affair, as every message contains four different aspects both for the sender as well as the receiver: Humans talk with "four mouths" and listen with "four ears" and thus will select one of the four aspects (◘ Fig. 12.3). Misunderstandings arise if the listener emphasizes a different aspect of the message than the one intended by the sender. This selection happens subconsciously and takes place even if the message was transmitted completely and without channel interference. If we want to avoid this kind of misunderstandings, we have to communicate in a congruent way: If, for example, somebody asks if you need help, do not say "I'm fine" with a desperate tone that could indicate your helplessness. Then it is not in your hands whether or not you get help.

12.4.1.3 Different Mental Models

Misunderstanding on a more complex level occurs if a team member's mental model and related plans for action differ from those of his or her teammates. This can easily happen if there is no explicit sharing of mental models. As a result, the team will be governed by the faulty assumption that all members have the same "Kopfkino" (i.e., "are sitting in the same movie") and are taking care of the same patient, whereas in reality each of them might be treating "a different problem." When mental models show little overlap, the likelihood that the team members will predict, adapt, and coordinate with one another successfully will be greatly reduced. The same is true for planning and the prediction of future developments: The more independent plans of action become from verbal feedback by other team members, the greater the danger of misunderstanding will be. If observations, assessments, and expectations concerning the future development are not shared, then team members will have no clue about the situational picture and the horizon of expectation of their teammates. As a result, a sender's information and instructions will increasingly be answered by a receiver's inappropriate actions; treatment plans of team members can develop in different directions.

12.4.2 Relational Problems

Most behavior in communication is strongly dependent on basic social and individual relationship patterns. It is crucial how the people concerned relate to each other. We speak of symmetric relationships if the persons involved are equal in position and the communication is "based on equal power," and of complementary relationships if one person is higher in the hierarchy and one is lower and communication is "based on differences in power" (Griffin 1999). Healthy relationships in the healthcare setting will have both types of power (Watzlawick et al. 1974).

Because communication is *the* way of relating to other human beings, a person's life-long interaction experiences will have led to personal assumptions and differentiated categories of how he or she thinks people behave and which personality traits they carry. Hence, if two people meet for the first time, they subconsciously will compare the perceived behavior of their counterpart with prestored categories. If this process happens too readily or rigidly, people will end up being pigeonholed from only a few moments of interaction. The next time these two people meet, they will have certain expectations about the behavior of their counterpart – expectations which are only reluctantly challenged. This is

the reason why the "first impression" (be it negative or positive) can have such a great impact on successful communication: The assumptions a person made about his or her counterpart will be a strong bias for every subsequent encounter. If the first impression is positive on both sides, this will foster a positive and constructive team climate; however, if the first impression is negative, a vicious circle can rapidly develop from the sequence of perception, assessment, categorization, and expectations. Expectations will rule perception and the message a person will receive from this encounter will in turn determine his or her reaction. Unfortunately, we are seldom aware of our bias towards other people and do not question the appropriateness of our expectations. Instead, we tend to ascribe the difficulties we have with certain people to their characteristics: We believe that it is not the problematic interaction (of which we are one part) but instead the problematic personality of the other which creates the problems. On the background of an expectation-driven interaction it can readily be understood why we find so many dysfunctional communication patterns at the work place. The most frequently encountered dysfunctional interactions are:

- Symmetric escalation
- Complementary escalation
- Reactance

12.4.2.1 "Tit for Tat": Symmetrical Escalation

Symmetrical communication describes a normal pattern of interaction which is based on the equivalence of both partners. Two people communicate symmetrically if the behavior of one person is mirrored by the behavior of the other; both partners strive for a reduction of differences (Griffin 1999). However, if the relationship between both communication partners is tense or if one has a competitive personality, the relational pattern will become dysfunctional. In this case symmetrical communication will escalate and individuals will compete for control: The result is symmetrical escalation with the motto "what you can do I can do as well!" A cardiac surgeon who had started training as anesthesiologist before changing specialties may try to compete with his anesthesiological counterpart in a symmetrical communication pattern. His statement "When I started my training we constantly had our finger on the pulse and could detect a low blood pressure without all this technical fancy" could be answered by "It's exactly this technical fancy which made it possible for you to perform this kind of operation on increasingly sicker patients." If both people continue this symmetrical pattern, they will continue arguing rather than solve the hemodynamic problem of the patient.

12.4.2.2 "What Goes Around Comes Around": Complementary Communication

Complementary communication patterns are differences of the communication partners that complement each other. The interaction stabilizes those differences. Moreover, one person's actions create the condition for the other person's actions, e.g., "order – execute," "ask – answer." Besides hierarchical structures or power gradients, the perception of an individual's behavior, too, can provoke a corresponding behavior in the other person: A dependent nurse will "force" her team leader to supervise her task execution closely and give very detailed instructions even if the senior nurse might actually dislike this kind of controlling behavior. The more controlling the leader will behave, the more dependently the nurse will confine herself to the mere task execution; thus, the unconscious subordination of the one person is a condition for the dominance of the other, which is a condition for the subordination. This dysfunctional communication pattern, too, can escalate: After a few "cycles" of such complementary communication, we have strong expectations about future behavior of the other person and it becomes increasingly more difficult to change such a pattern. It is possible that both partners actually are unhappy with this forced behavior because it contradicts their personal values, preferences, and the ideals of their professional roles. Other complementary interactions in healthcare include the physician–patient relationship and the teacher–student relationship.

12.4.2.3 "Don't You Tell Me What I'm Supposed to Do!": Reactance

Humans show a great interindividual variety in their ability to accept rules or regulations before they have the feeling that specific behavioral freedoms are threatened or eliminated. This feeling can arise in complementary relationships (e.g.,

when a person is heavily pressured to accept a certain view or attitude) as well as in symmetrical relationships (e.g., when the sender does not intend to manipulate but the receiver has a pronounced "ear" for the appeal of a message). In both cases people will show reactant behavior which is in direct contradiction to an appeal, rule, or regulation, and which has the purpose of communicating in round terms the message: "Don't you tell me what I'm supposed to do!" In more general terms, reactant behavior is a learned protective function resulting in mental and physical activation aimed at resisting other people's manipulative efforts and reconstituting a person's perceived behavioral freedom and freedom of choice (Brehm and Brehm 1981). Reactant behavior includes:

– Defiance
– Refusal
– Intentional failure
– Aggression
– Arrogance

Communication patterns governed by reactant behavior can play a major role when a healthcare provider receives instructions from a coprovider of another professional group (e.g., nurses from physicians), or when questions or instructions come from colleagues of other specialties (e.g., a cardiac surgeon asks an anesthetist "How high is your epinephrine running?"), would be an example of a question which could trigger reactant behavior in some anesthetists (if they listen with the "appeal ear" and hear "I'll tell you how to do it."). Reactant behavior would express itself in an emotional answer to the felt manipulation and the intonation of the answer: "I know how to treat my patient!"

12.5 Poor Communication in Critical Situations

Many problems in team performance can be traced to the abovementioned interpersonal communication difficulties that are found in routine situations and critical situations. As critical situations in the context of high-stakes medical care pose specific demands, there are specific opportunities for failure. Several communication patterns have been identified which can contribute to a faulty team performance in critical situations (Cushing 1994; Ungerer 2004; Hofinger 2005).

12.5.1 Unspecified Receiver

In critical situations, every message should be addressed to a specific person. If questions or instructions are simply put forward without naming the receiver, then nobody will feel concerned. Because nobody feels concerned, nobody will feel responsible either. The necessary process of closing the communication gap by ensuring that messages are correctly received and understood by the right person is often dispensed with when task load is high: Every team member is glad that he or she does not have to feel responsible for additional tasks when they have reached their personal limit with the current task. If none of the team members can tell to whom a certain instruction was addressed, then diffusion of responsibility will arise (▶ Chap. 11). Poor communication with an unspecified receiver can be seen in phrasings such as "could somebody ...", "does anybody ...", and "WE should do ..."

12.5.2 Problems with Speech: Articulation and Terms

Bad communication can result from bad articulation or mispronunciation. Talking in a low voice or too hastily, mumbling, talking in unfinished sentences, with a strong dialect, or with faulty grammar can contribute to misunderstanding.

Replacing medical terms by colloquial language and unofficial terms will create an "insider language," which may not be a problem as long as familiar team members cooperate; however, as soon as healthcare workers form other specialties are involved, the ambiguous and nontechnical terminology can lead to misunderstanding. In order to avoid misunderstanding, the healthcare provider would have to clarify the meaning of an expression by enquiring every single time he or she is confronted with an unofficial term. Such an enquiry takes time and can further increase time pressure in a critical situation.

12.5.3 Information Overload

There is an ever present danger in critical situations for a sender to overload a message with information. If this happens, the receiver has to separate the wheat from the chaff by deciding which part of the message is important. The criteria for this decision will then be guided by personal experience and expectations and often may not reflect the sender's primary intentions, again resulting in misunderstanding. The following signs may indicate an information overload (Ungerer 2004):

- Rapid sequence of instructions for actions which are unrelated
- Minimal pause between sentences (<2 s)
- More than one verb and object per sentence
- Long list with numbers or dosage instructions
- Aggressive and pressing intonation
- Long and detailed instructions
- Several questions within one question

12.5.4 Becoming Tight-Lipped

In critical situations the use of a precise and unambiguous language is necessary; however, if team members communicate hardly at all, this will threaten the team process and may even result in a complete breakdown of communication. Even worse, if team leaders become tight-lipped, the danger is great that the entire team will loose its shared mental model ("doc goes solo"). Among the typical indicators of an impoverished use of language are:

- Abandonment of explanations
- No reply to questions of team members
- No active communication of background information
- Closed questions
- Answers in monosyllables
- Long periods of silence

12.5.5 "Resolving" Conflicts by Passivity or Aggressiveness

Communication styles aimed at resolving a conflict can be arrayed on a continuum according to the degree to which they reflect a concern for one's own well-being at the possible expense of others, or vice versa (Jentsch and Smith-Jentsch 2001). The resulting behaviors on both ends of the continuum are:

- Passivity: Worded in the form of questions, passive responses often convey a watered-down expression of the sender's true intentions. Critique is "sugar-coated" and statements "beat around the b sh" instead of addressing the critical issue directly. As a result, valid and critical points do not carry the weight they should and therefore do not catch the attention of both, team members and the leader.

— Aggressiveness: Aggressive statements are direct and unambiguous and therefore leave no doubt about the sender's intentions. Unfortunately, as they generally take the form of accusatory, disrespectful, or even rude remarks and convey some form of hostility and defensiveness, team members will find it difficult to consider or even accept input or critique in this form, true as they might be. As a result, critical information or valuable suggestions will not be considered by the team or the leader because the form of the suggestions elicits a defensive reaction.

— Assertiveness: the divine "middle way" between these extremes of conflict resolution is discussed in greater detail in what follows.

12.5.6   Poor Listening

Communication is not a one-way street: Listening carefully and actively, actively inquiring through questions, and responding appropriately are just as important skills for effective communication as those needed to transmit information and instructions with the necessary clarity. Effective listening is a key communication skill but can be jeopardized in manifold ways. Indicators of bad listening are listed in the following summary (Jensen 1995; Transport Canada 1997):

— Interrupting: If someone constantly interrupts a conversation they are probably paying more attention to their own opinion and intentions than to what the other person is saying. They have preplanned their response and use short pauses to advance their own point of view.

— Diverting: People change the direction of the conversation by picking up irrelevant issues. Because they have not perceived the core problem, they pay undue attention to surface details rather than focusing on the substance of what is being said. Any key word may suffice to trigger the detour to other areas of interest.

— Debating: There is a fine line between challenging what someone said in order to obtain clarification, insight or more information, and arguing for the sake of arguing. People tend to

debate if they are more interested in winning an argument than in hearing the other person's position. In addition, some people want to play the devil's advocate and take the other side no matter what is said by team members.

— Quarrelling: If a conflict moves from the content level to the relational level, then personal differences will be carried out by verbally fighting the other person. A conversation can rapidly turn into a dispute and both partners may be more interested in offending the other than in solving the problem.

— Becoming reactant: In order to defend one's feeling of behavioral freedom an opinion is dismissed. Because people feel pressured by another person to accept his or her view, they reject both, the person and the corresponding opinion.

— Tuning out: When people think that their communication partner is not worth listening to, that they already know their counterpart's opinion, or when they are preoccupied with their own position, they will tune other people out instead of listening to their position.

12.5.7   Mingling of the Relational and Content Component

Sometimes team members allows relational and content components of a message to mingle. This happens if relational messages are hidden in a harmless phrase (yet clearly conveyed by tone or gestures) or if someone refuses a proposal simply because it comes from a person he or she dislikes. This mingling of messages will result in a breakdown in communication because the other team members will listen mainly to the relational message and react correspondingly. Reasons for this mingling are:

— Antipathy between team members
— A working climate of disrespect
— Enforcement of personal preferences and habits
— Intolerance of error
— Power struggle for social status

Subtle relationship messages can emerge like "pinpricks from below" (◘ Fig. 12.5) within a discourse which is apparently concerned with facts and goals. Messages in the form of "pinpricks" can be deliv-

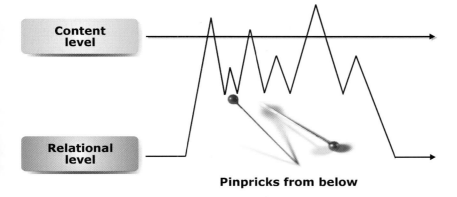

Pinpricks from below

▢ **Fig. 12.5** A discussion about facts can be disturbed by subtle devaluating messages on the relationship level ("pinpricks from below"). (From Schulz von Thun 1981)

ered by any team member, even those who allegedly have a lower social status.

Typical examples how the relational and the content component can be interwoven in a critical situation are:
- Decisions in a solo attempt: If someone acts in a critical situation without involving team members in the process of decision-making, he or she will signalize: I consider your contribution as unimportant. I can do without you!
- Enforcing decisions through loudness: If leaders treat their team members according to the maxim "the loudest argument wins," they will transmit the message: I disrespect you; the only thing that counts is me and my opinion.
- Appeal with a subtle dispraise: Antipathy can take the form of subtle relational messages: "Mr. Smith, you could go and fetch the bronchoscope so that for once you do something useful."
- Open insult: If stress and the experience of failure lead to a loss in self-control, rude or even hostile remarks can follow. Remarks of this kind indicate the lack of respect and esteem for others. The cost to repair a thus shattered relationship is immense.

12.5.8 Clarifying Relationships at the Wrong Time

Negative relationship messages have no place in critical situations; however, if they do occur, the relationship problem should be settled *after* the critical situation. This is not a defensive or conflict-avoiding approach; instead, a critical situation is a work phase which is absolutely inappropriate for the clarification of relationship issues. Even if communication style in a critical situation can become unpleasant from time to time (i.e., loud and harsh commands) and team relations might be strained, the rule is: First cope with the emergency situation and then discuss your personal feelings and the relational issues so that next time communication can be more effective.

12.6 Good Communication in Critical Situations

12.6.1 Give Luck a Bit of a Boost

Considering all the pitfalls in human communication, the fact that we all talk with "four mouths" and hear with "four ears" (▢ Fig. 12.4), and the way in which poor approaches to communication can exacerbate problems, it is surprising that we actually succeed in delivering a message from one person to another. From this perspective, constructive communication seems to be the lucky exception rather than the rule; however, there are some basic rules for good communication which can help to improve personal communication skills and communication in critical situations.

12.6.2 Communicate Congruently

Verbal, paraverbal, and nonverbal messages should correspond. If there is a gap between those clues, the receiver of a message can no longer be sure which message he or she should trust. Every speaker can provide a *congruent* communication by matching body language, nonverbal signals, and the words spoken.

12.6.3 Select the Same Aspects of a Message

Communication partners can try to select the same aspect of a message and make it their shared objective. It the content component is in the foreground, then both partners should use their "content mouth" and "content ears". If the self-revelatory aspect is especially important, then it is helpful if both partners join a level of personal statements.

12.6.4 Raise the Issue of Communication Failure

Communication partners should be able to talk about communication failure. Often communication fails because:

- A disturbance in the relationship has been transferred to the content level.
- The debate about the relationship is avoided by pretending that there is only communication about facts and goals.

If communication partners are able to talk (after the critical situation!) about the way they interact and how they interpret the words of their counterpart, precarious situations can be best avoided and a productive cooperation is (again) possible. Such communication about the situation in which communication takes place is called *metacommunication*.

Besides those general aspects, good communication style in critical situations is further characterized by the behaviors given below.

> Characteristics of good communication in critical situations are:
> - Communicate congruently

> - Select the same aspects of a message
> - Address communication issues at the right time
> - Speak unambiguously
> - Close the communication gap
> - Brief team members
> - Search actively for information
> - Advocate your position
> - Voice concerns
> - Listen actively

12.6.5 Speak Unambiguously, Avoid Ambiguity

Language is never completely devoid of ambiguity. For this reason a extreme clarity at the content level is a sign of good communication. A shared phraseology is helpful. Every speaker should explicitly identify the receiver of information best by making eye contact and using the name of the person addressed. Information should be forwarded concisely and with few items per sentence. Sentences should not consist of several verbs and objects. All difficulties, negative trends, and unexpected problems should be stated clearly (e.g., "I cannot find a vein which I can puncture").

12.6.6 Close the Communication Gap

"Things said are not things heard and things heard are not things understood." This places great importance on communication practices that limit the occurrence of errors due to problems in speech exchange. A safety process which ensures that messages are clearly "received" and understood requires "readback/hearback," as described in the following sequence (Brown 2004):

- The "sender" concisely states information to the "receiver."
- The receiver is then required to read back or say what she or he has just heard. By reading back an instruction the receiver implicitly asks: "Did I get the information right?" Readbacks allow the sender to verify whether or not the receiver understood what was said.
- The sender then provides a hearback, acknowledging that the readback was correct, or if necessary, makes a correction.

— The readback/hearback process continues until a shared understanding is mutually verified.
— The instruction is then carried out and the task execution is announced. This closes the communication gap.

Readback/hearback is an efficient way of helping teams to achieve a verified mutual understanding of the situation and of helping healthcare providers to avoid errors arising from informational gaps and misunderstandings. This is all the more important in a high-stakes medical environment where complexity, uncertainty, and time pressure increase the likelihood of errors occurring. Better to identify misunderstandings by closing the communication gap than by detecting them later on during task execution. Although this process may seem unfamiliar and cumbersome at first, it can become a fluid part of the fabric of messaging and decision-making in critical situations if it has been practiced repeatedly in everyday situations.

12.6.7 Brief Team Members

Briefings, although standard practice in many high-stakes environments (e.g., civil aviation, military command), have been uncommon in clinical medicine. Spending a few minutes at the beginning of a shift can get everyone at the same starting point, help to avoid surprises, and positively affect how the team works together (Leonard et al. 2004). Shared mental models are the basis for joint action (► Chap. 11). For this reason it is recommendable to brief the team in advance along general lines on the planned course of action. This is especially true for any critical action with several possible alternatives (e.g., difficult airway management, endotracheal tube exchange, coordination of medical management, and technical rescue). The common mental model enabled by a team briefing allows every team member to show initiative and think ahead. If a critical situation has a phase with low workload, the time should be used for a situational update and a forecast on the possible development of the situation. Briefings help to proactively focus individual plans and intentions on the "big picture" and to align mental models, thereby creating space for enquiry, concerns, and suggestions.

12.6.8 Search Actively for Information

Good decisions are based on good information, so seeking and gathering information are vital to safe patient care. Right at the beginning of critical situations healthcare providers will find themselves in the predicament that initial diagnosis or decisions most certainly will be based on incomplete information. In addition, the information available is filtered by the biased search for those pieces of information which fit into and confirm the current mental model of the situation (► Chap. 6). In light of these severe limitations it should become a habit to actively search for information which actually contradicts current assumptions. This is best done by asking questions and continuing to do so until one is sure that one has all the information needed.

Sometimes people are reluctant to ask questions because they feel it is a sign of weakness. The may feel that they should already know the information and, by asking for it, are letting everyone know their inadequacy. Especially entrants are faced with the dilemma that their questions could produce the impression that they are bothersome, incompetent, or overcautious if they keep on enquiring. They fear that the person questioned may start to send devaluating messages on the relational level. As a result, people tend to settle for limited information, to keep quiet for the sake of ongoing harmony, and to perform as best they can by themselves. This kind of poor communication can jeopardize patient safety, as necessary information is withheld, on the one hand, and an emotionally charged atmosphere can arise, on the other hand. The price for not having asked for relevant pieces of information, or for not having challenged a presumably faulty assumption or erroneous action even in the face of resistance, may be high for both, healthcare providers as well as patients. For safe patient care healthcare providers should continue to press for the information they need, no matter how awkward they may feel.

12.6.9 Be Assertive: Advocate Your Position

Most people are not assertive for fear of displeasing others and not being liked. Because people want to be thought of as "nice" or "easy to get along with," they often keep their opinions to themselves, especially if those opinions conflict with those of elder and more experienced colleagues; however, it is indispensable for effective teamwork that your position or viewpoint be understood by your teammates and that their intentions and actions be questioned, if necessary. This necessity expressly includes the opinion of senior healthcare providers as well as leaders. There should be no taboo concerning criticism with regard to *any* team member, whomever it might be (▶ Chap. 13). One's own position must be advocated actively, continually, and emphatically until it no longer seems an issue or until concerns about the adequacy of actions performed by team members can be dispelled. The goal of assertiveness is to prompt other team members to diligently reconsider their point of view before a decision is made (Lorr and More 1980; Jentsch and Smith-Jentsch 2001). In case of conflict, people want to be convinced by facts, and not by the authority of the other, that a planned procedure is appropriate.

Assertiveness is not aggressiveness; instead, it involves communicating one's feelings, concerns, ideas, and needs to others in a clear and direct manner, but without demeaning or infringing on the rights of others. As such, assertive statements suggest a sense of personal responsibility for one's own thoughts and feelings, as well as a sense of honesty and fairness.

Nevertheless, it will always be an awkward situation for team members if they have an opinion that conflicts with, or even is ignored by, someone in authority. Under the influence of issues such as promotion, approval, and appropriate respect for seniority, it is difficult to disagree with a superior about specifics. The following approach may help to broach the issue in a constructive way, thereby balancing the need to be both assertive as well as respectful (Jensen 1995; Transport Canada 1997):
— Opening: Use the other person's name.
— State your concern: Make the issue yours, and use the first-person singular form of expression. The opening phrase "I am concerned ..." or "I feel uncomfortable with ..." is more productive than "Sir, you are wrong!"
— State the problem: Define the problem as clearly and concisely as possible. Your counterpart should perceive the message that you are focusing on *what* is wrong and not on *who* is wrong.

— Offer a solution: If possible, suggest at least one solution to the problem.
— Obtain feedback: It is important to get acknowledgement that your concern has been heard and understood.

If team members advocate their point of view, this will often imply that they are taking a position of power. On the relationship level the message can be perceived as a "what you intend to do will fail! Fortunately, I know what to do next!" For this reason assertiveness should always be coupled with the capability to talk about facts, concerns, feelings, and proposals. When advocating a position it is crucial to avoid both getting into personal issues and setting up a power game. Last but not least, there is also a line that can be drawn between assertiveness and aggressiveness. Assertive people state their opinions, while still being respectful of others. Aggressive people attack or ignore others' opinions in favor of their own. If healthcare providers fail to advocate their position adequately, this can lead to reactant behavior from the person questioned, or to rejection and hostility. Senior team members and leaders should apply a different strategy for stating their case than junior team members or entrants: They can facilitate advocacy in critical situations by actively encouraging team members to share their thoughts and voice concerns during everyday situations.

Assertiveness is both, an attitude as well as a skill. Several dimensions of assertiveness have been identified (Lorr and More 1980; Jentsch and Smith-Jentsch 2001):

1. Personal Factors
— Independence: the ability and willingness to resist conformity. As a result of a high degree of personal autonomy, opinions are not easily changed by those of other team members.
— Assertiveness: the ability and willingness to initiate action and to take on responsibility. When confronted with an emergency situation, team members who display assertiveness get people organized and take charge of the situation. Other persons' irritating behavior is challenged and requested to change.
— Social assertiveness: the ability and willingness to express, initiate, and maintain interactions with nonintimate others.

— Defense of interests and rights: the ability and willingness to stand up for one's rights and refuse unreasonable requests. The ability to say "no" and to let others know when they have overstepped the mark and violated the rights of others.

Although assertiveness has an attitudinal component, a number of studies suggest that individuals turn assertiveness off and on from one situation to the next. An individual's assertive response may vary as a function of several contextual factors, which include:

2. Situational Factors
— Type of interpersonal relationship: An individual's tendency toward team performance-related assertiveness may vary in situations involving strangers or people with whom a personal relationship exists.
— Teammate gender: Individuals consider the gender of the receiver when determining whether (or to what degree) they are willing to assert an opinion.
— Status difference: The probability of nonassertive behavior increases as a function of difference in social status or occupational title (i.e., physician vs nurse; attending vs resident). The cognitive processes responsible for this behavior may best be explained by status theory (Torrance 1955; Milgram 1974): Salient status characteristics lead team members to form assumptions and expectations regarding the competence of their leader or teammates: The fact that someone has a higher social status "automatically" implies that she or he is more capable to cope with any difficult or critical situation that may arise. This expectation of competence is generalized to a broad range of situations and can result in a subordinate behavioral pattern: Team members will feel less responsible for their own actions and will view themselves as an "agent" of their leader, simply executing his or her wishes.
— Team climate: The cohesion within the team and good team climate can both play a vital role for the successful team process in a critical situation (► Chap. 11). In addition, team climate has the potential either to facilitate or inhibit the use of assertiveness among team members. By observing the consequences of assertive behavior within a team, an individual will draw consequences for accepted norms. Depending on the perceived climate within a team and the acceptability of assertiveness, an individual will adapt his or her behavior accordingly.

12.6.10 Listen Actively

A great deal of listening is a passive undertaking. Often people catch themselves paying only little attention to their conversation partner but instead thinking about other things while listening. In critical situations, however, this mind drift can be hazardous. An effective countermeasure is active and purposeful listening. *Active* listening is hard work and is more than just incessant attention: Active listening means that every team member takes responsibility for understanding the point of view of his or her teammates. "Nobody has to be a sponge" (Jensen 1995). By listening actively team members do not make assumptions about a teammate's intention or expect others to be good at conveying what they really mean; instead, they are proactive and take up the point until doubtful issues are resolved. As personal filters, assumptions, judgments, and beliefs can distort what we hear, our understanding of a team member's message can differ dramatically from what he or she actually intended to say; therefore, as active an listener we use feedback as a means to ensure mutual understanding by restating what we think we have heard and by asking "Did I understand you correctly?" Active listening is a communication skill that requires acceptance and active attention for the person speaking. Only if these prerequisites are met can people follow the speech of another person, can enquire with greater focus, and can influence the conversation by nonverbal signals. Active listening facilitates the exchange of information and increases the likelihood that the listener will understand what the other person means. The following habits and behaviors indicate an active listener (Transport Canada 1997):
— Be patient: Wait with your response until the other person has finished speaking and do not interrupt. While the other person is talking, try to hear what his or her position is.
— Ask questions: Once the other person has finished speaking, ask for clarifications, details, and explanations.

— Observe and hold eye contact: Observe body language and listen closely to other nonverbal and paraverbal signals. You can learn a lot about what the other person is really trying to communicate.

— Paraphrase and mirror: Repeat important details (doses, names, and times) literally; otherwise, repeat in your own words what you understood. This can help to clarify your own thoughts as well as let the sender know how well he or she has been understood.

— Be supportive: Encourage, show respect, and say "thank you": This will help to create a supportive team climate.

12.7   Communication After a Critical Situation

Giving and receiving feedback and trying to resolve interpersonal conflicts are integral components of good communication. Because both require a calm atmosphere and sufficient time to be successful, their place should be *after* a critical situation.

12.7.1   Giving Feedback

Feedback can be given on statements as well as on the behavior of a teammate or the team leader. Feedback is an ideal tool for clarifying a misunderstanding, which is always a good learning opportunity. In order to make feedback an essential part of team communication, team members have to feel safe and have to be sure that feedback is both wanted and used in a constructive way. Communication among coequal healthcare providers is mostly symmetrical, and the resulting feedback is generally rich in positive and negative aspects. Feedback toward people higher up in the hierarchy has an inbuilt amplifier for the selection of positive aspects, because the communication pattern is complementary: Subordinates tend to appreciate or even praise positive behavior but are reluctant to address problems. To avoid this pitfall, it is a good strategy for a leader to ask explicitly for feedback concerning his or her behavior and for constructive advice. The following guidelines may be helpful for constructive feedback:

Basic Guidelines for Constructive Feedback
— Show a respectful attitude – everybody can learn from feedback.

— Choose an appropriate opportunity and facilitating setting.
— Give feedback when the receiver is ready for it.
— Give positive feedback first. Any critical issues will be accepted more readily.
— Never embarrass anybody – try to criticize problematic behavior in private.
— Make your feedback as precise and objective as possible.
— Address observable behavior – not characteristics of a person.
— Use "I" statements whenever you communicate observations.
— If possible, suggest an alternative behavior.
— Set a good example: Take feedback willingly and show gratitude for it.

12.7.2   Address Conflicting Issues

As different people will experience the same situation in different ways, this may result in divergent opinions, plans, and intentions. If a personal intention can only be realized in opposition to intentions of another person, a conflict will result. Most conflicts can be resolved by trying to harmonize both points of view or by finding a compromise. Either the best point of view can be identified and pursued, or the conflicting intentions are prioritized, or both points of view are dismissed in favor of a third possibility. If a conflict is resolved in a constructive way, a more comprehensive picture of reality and better solutions may emerge. In critical situations and under time pressure rapid decision-making is mandatory. Under these circumstances it is not uncommon that the resolution of a conflict does not find the appropriate time. If harsh instructions add to this situation, team members can easily interpret the situation as repudiation of their person, as a disqualification of their competence, and as a depreciation of their commitment. To prevent a breakdown in relationship, a debriefing after the critical situation should include such unintended situations and the resulting emotions and any other possible cause of conflict.

12.7.3   Address Relational Conflicts

If a conflict refers to medical issues, they generally can be resolved by discussing data, opinions, or evidence; however, as there are always *persons* behind a conflict, and as we cannot communicate merely on the grounds of factual information, the resolution of a conflict will always demand more than just the settlement on the rational level. Especially conflicts with a good deal of involvement on the relationship level can be very difficult to resolve. If such a conflict emerges during critical situations, motives such as protection of the feeling of competence can quickly decide the behavior. *Who* is right will become more important than *what* is right. As emergency situations can be characterized by tough disagreements and resource conflicts, and can quickly turn into a climate with immovable positions on both sides, team members as well as leaders should try to work at the relationship level once the critical situation has passed. There are no easy rules of thumb about how to resolve differences, but the knowledge of some basic guidelines may improve the ability to resolve conflict.

Resolving Conflicts
— Listen well: Try to see a conflict as an un-requested opportunity to hear additional points of view.
— "The *problem* is the problem!" Instead of attacking your counterpart, you should tackle the problem.
— The *patient* should be the winner and not one of the healthcare providers involved in the conflict. Conflicts should be no power struggle with an adversary. The goal of any conflict should be a win-win situation for every person involved.
— Bring out the differences: It is helpful to clarify the areas of both agreement and disagreement. Often there will be less disagreement than initially expected.
— Acknowledge feelings: People often take strong positions because of feelings rather than logic.
— Respect every team member: If the leaders disagree with other team members and decide on a different course of action, they should nevertheless let everyone feel that they respect the personality of their team members and that they weighed their opinions fully.

12.8 Tips for Daily Practice

— Practice good communication and good listening, and let it become a habit in your daily life. You will profit from this habit in critical situations.
— Be aware of your appearance and bearing: The first impression you make on other people (be it negative or positive) can have a great impact on successful communication.
— You cannot expect people to read your mind, so state your opinions clearly and voice your concerns.
— Remember: Nothing is so simple that it cannot be misunderstood.
— Things said are not things heard and things heard are not things understood.
— If you are in doubt: Ask! Your only risk is pride.
— Good decisions are based on good information, so you have to actively seek and gather information if you want to ensure safe patient care.
— In an emergency, active listening is a critical skill.
— In critical situations the odds are high that the initial mental model is faulty and incomplete; therefore, you should always search actively for information which *contradicts* your current assumptions.

12.9 "Communication": in a Nutshell

— In the context of a high-stakes medical environment, communication has a fourfold function: It enables and maintains team structure, it coordinates the team process and task execution, it enables information exchange, and it facilitates relationships.
— Human communication takes place in a social context. For this reason it is impossible to exchange information in a mere matter-of-fact manner without simultaneously establishing a relationship between the persons who are participating in the information exchange.
— "Communication = content + relationship."
— Communication is not simply about transmitting but also receiving, including ensuring that the transmission was understood in the way intended.
— Communication is much more than mere verbal exchange. Every action can be interpreted by others and thus can transport a message, in-

tentionally or unintentionally: "One cannot *not* communicate."

— Human communication uses different channels in a parallel way. Verbal, paraverbal, and nonverbal cues are transmitted.

— If the verbal and nonverbal channel are incongruent because words convey one meaning and the nonverbal or paraverbal information indicates the opposite, the receiver will place greater importance on the nonverbal cues.

— Good communication uses verbal and nonverbal cues congruently. Every speaker can provide a congruent communication by matching body language, nonverbal signals, and the words spoken.

— The meaning of a message cannot be transmitted; instead, it is "reconstructed" by the receiver. If a message is transmitted incompletely, then the listener will tend to "complete" the message by reading something into the unclear aspects.

— Symmetrical relationships are those in which the persons involved are equal in position. Complementary relationships are based on differences in power, with one person being higher in hierarchy than the other.

— General disturbances of communication can be rooted in the characteristics of the message, the process of sending, of receiving, and interpreting, and in the relationship of the dialogue partners.

— Usually it is *patterns not partners* that make communication difficult.

— Communication becomes dysfunctional when the people involved have good intentions but the interaction creates an unproductive and destructive system.

— The most common dysfunctional communication patterns are: symmetrical escalation; complementary communication; and reactant behavior.

— A misunderstanding occurs if the receiver of a message reacts differently to information or instructions than the sender intended.

— Effective listening is a key communication skill but can be jeopardized in manifold ways.

— Active listening means to take responsibility for understanding the point of view of another person.

— A safety process which ensures that messages are clearly received and understood requires "readback" (i.e., the receiver says what she or he has heard) and "hearback" (i.e., the sender

acknowledges whether or not the readback was correct).

— Assertiveness means that the own position must be advocated emphatically until concerns about the adequacy of decisions or actions of other team members can be dispelled. The goal of assertiveness is to prompt other team members to diligently reconsider their point of view before a decision is made.

— Only if a communication pattern has been practiced repeatedly in everyday situations can it become a fluid part of the fabric of messaging and decision-making in critical situations.

References

Brehm S, Brehm JW (1981) Psychological reactance – a theory of freedom and control. Academic Press, New York

Brown JP (2004) Closing the communication loop: using readback/hearback to support patient safety J Comm J Qual Saf 30:460–464

Bühler K (1934) Sprachtheorie: Die Darstellungsform der Sprache [Speech theory]. Fischer, Jena, Germany

Campbell RD, Bagshaw M (2002) Human performance and limitations in aviation. Blackwell, New Jersey

Cushing S (1994) Fatal words. Communication clashes and aircraft crashes. University of Chicago Press, Chicago

Griffin E (1999) A first look at communication theory, 4th edn. McGraw-Hill, Boston

Hargie O (2006) Handbook of communication skills. Routledge, London

Hofinger G (2005) Kommunikation in kritischen Situationen [Communication in critical situations]. Verlag für Polizeiwissenschaft, Frankfurt/M

Jensen RS (1995) Pilot judgement and crew resource management. Ashgate, Aldershot

Jentsch F, Smith-Jentsch KA (2001) Assertiveness and team performance: more than "just say no." In: Salas E, Bowers CA, Edens E (eds) Improving teamwork in organisations. Applications of resource management training. Erlbaum, New Jersey, pp 73–94

Kanki B, Smith G (1999) Training aviation communication skills. In: Salas E, Bowers CA (eds) Improving teamwork in organisations. Erlbaum, New Jersey, pp 95–127

Knapp ML, Daly JA (2002) Handbook of interpersonal communication (abridged). Sage, London

Leonard M, Graham S, Bonacum D (2004) The human factor: the critical importance of effective teamwork and communication in providing safe care. Qual Saf Health Care 13 (Suppl 1): i85–i90

Lorr M, More W (1980) Four dimensions of assertiveness. Multivar Behav Res 14: 127–138

Maturana HR, Varela F (1992) Tree of knowledge. The biological roots of human understanding. Shambala, Boston

Milgram S (1974) Obedience to authority. Harper and Row, New York

Miller K (2005) Communication theories: perspectives, processes, and contexts, 2nd edn. McGraw-Hill, New York

Murray WB, Foster PA (2000) Crisis resource management among strangers: principles of organizing a multidisciplinary group for crisis resource management. J Clin Anesth 12:633–638

Schulz von Thun F (1981) Miteinander reden [Talk with each other]. Bd 1. Rowohlt, Reinbek bei Hamburg

Schulz von Thun F, Ruppel J, Stratmann R (2000) Miteinander reden. Psychologie für Führungskräfte [Talk with each other: psychology for leaders] Rowohlt, Reinbek bei Hamburg

Searle JR (1969) Speech acts. An essay in the philosophy of language. Cambridge University Press, Cambridge UK

Shannon CE, Weaver W (1949) The mathematical theory of communication. University of Illinois Press, Urbana

Torrance E (1955) Some consequences of power differences on decision-making in permanent and temporary three-man groups. In: Hare A, Borgotta E, Bales R (eds) Small groups. Knopf, New York, pp 482–492

Transport Canada (1997) Human factors for aviation: advanced handbook. Transport Canada Civil Aviation Resources, Ottawa

Ungerer D (2004) Simple speech: improving communication in disaster relief operations. In: Dietrichs R, Jochum K (eds) Teaming up: components of safety under high risk. Ashgate, Aldershot, pp 81–92

Watzlawick P, Weakland JH, Fisch R (1974) Changing a system. Norton, New York

Watzlawick P, Beavin J, Jackson D (1996) Pragmatics of human communication: study of interactional patterns, pathologies and paradoxes. Norton, New York

13 Leadership

13.1 Case Study

A 12-year-old boy sustained a bicycle accident resulting in an open fracture of the mandible. Because the patient had a full stomach and mouth opening was reduced due to pain, the anesthesia resident decided to perform a rapid sequence induction with thiopental and succinylcholine. The orotracheal intubation was uneventful and anesthesia was maintained as a total intravenous anesthesia (TIVA) with propofol and remifentanil. After 30 min of uneventful anesthesia, the saturation began to slowly drop and a sinus tachycardia developed. Under the assumption of insufficient anesthetic depth, the resident increased the concentration of propofol and remifentanil. This intervention, however, did not affect the tachycardia. The anesthesia resident checked the i.v. line to rule out soft tissue infiltration and auscultated both lungs. Breath sounds were equal bilaterally. The patient required 70% oxygen to maintain saturations above 95%. Because the resident was unable to find any apparent cause for the clinical deterioration and because of the danger of the situation, he called for help from his attending physician. When the attending physician entered the operating room a few minutes later, the patient was receiving a minute volume of 9.5 l/min to maintain the end-expiratory CO_2 at 45 mm Hg. Infrequent monomorphic premature ventricular contractions were noted on the ECG. The attending told the resident to insert an arterial pressure line into the radial artery and to obtain an arterial blood gas. The lab results showed a combined respiratory and metabolic acidosis with a mild alveolo-arterial difference in the partial pressure of oxygen and a potassium concentration of 5.6 mmol/l. Based on the induction of anesthesia with succinylcholine in conjunction with the current clinical picture and the lab findings, the attending physician decided to interpret the clinical deterioration as symptoms of malignant hyperthermia and to treat it accordingly. The body temperature was 37.2°C (99°F). He informed the maxillofacial surgeons about the seriousness of the condition and asked them to interrupt the operation. Dantrolene was dissolved in solution and administered to the patient. The arterial blood gas was monitored closely and the appropriate treatments for pH abnormalities, hyperkalemia, and renal protection were initiated. Cardiovascular stability was maintained by catecholamine support. Due to an increase in the

patient's temperature to 39.7°C (103.4°F) over 20 min, the attending anesthesiologist initiated external cooling procedures which were accomplished by the surgeons and OR technicians. Twenty minutes after the administration of dantrolene, the heart rate began to drop slowly and the acid–base status began to improve. Minute ventilation and F_iO_2 were gradually reduced. Once the treatment began to indicate a reassuring response by the patient, the attending physician contacted the pediatric intensive care unit (PICU) and requested a bed for his patient. He informed the pediatric intensivist about the clinical course, the measures taken, and current clinical status. An hour later, the patient had further stabilized and was transferred to the PICU. Over the course of the next day the patient developed a compartment syndrome of the left lower leg requiring reoperation. The anesthetic was trigger free for malignant hyperthermia and proceeded uneventfully. The patient was extubated postoperatively and was transferred from the PICU to the general ward on the following day. He was discharged from the hospital without any residual symptoms. The patient and his family were tested for their susceptibility to malignant hyperthermia and both the patient and his younger brother had positive results.

13.2 The Case for Leadership

Successful team performance in healthcare and good leadership are two sides of the same coin. Teamwork in teams that are organized hierarchically cannot function properly without a sound concept of leadership, and vice versa.

If the issue of leadership in a high-stakes medical environment is addressed, leadership in everyday life has to be differentiated from leadership in a critical situation. Both situational contexts require a different leadership approach. Nevertheless, although the situational demands for leadership in a critical situation differ from those in everyday life, both leadership approaches cannot be considered independently from each other. The same senior healthcare providers will be responsible as team leaders for their staff members in routine situations as well as in emergency situations. The question as to whether or not leadership in a medical emergency can succeed will depend to a great extent on the daily interactions of the leader with the team.

What then are the core functional competencies of a leader and which behavior is required to lead successfully? Which personal characteristics and abilities are required to bring out the best in teams? How can leaders attain above-average results while maintaining an environment of trust, motivation, and high job satisfaction? Of the extensive body of research on this topic (overview e.g., Bass and Stodgill 2007; Neuberger 2002), the results most important for acute healthcare are summarized in what follows.

13.2.1 Leadership in Everyday Life

Leadership in everyday life has a threefold purpose. Firstly, leadership is directed at the *activities* of staff members. This is done by:
- Assigning tasks
- Defining goals
- Monitoring the execution and the results
- Resolving team conflicts

Secondly, leadership in healthcare has a lot to do with a leader *assessing* clinical skills and the training status of staff members. Leadership comprises creating learning opportunities for each staff member and supporting their future career steps; therefore, a leadership position in healthcare should always comprise human resource development efforts. By assuming a leadership position, healthcare providers volunteer to motivate staff members, to value their individual personality, and to empower teammates to increasingly take responsibility for their working environment. Leaders inspire staff members by who they *are*, what they *know*, and what they *do*.

A third aspect to leadership specific for high-stakes environments has been proposed by the IOM report (Kohn et al. 1999) and many other publications: Leaders in healthcare should also be *role models* for a patient-safety-oriented approach to patient care. In order to mitigate the effect of inevitably occurring errors in patient safety, leaders should create a working environment where healthcare providers feel encouraged to be alert to threats to patient safety, to voice concerns if they believe that an action may harm the patient, and to monitor task performance and workload of their team members (cross-monitoring; ▶ Chap. 11).

Hierarchy of authority frequently inhibits people from expressing themselves. Effective leaders

◻ Table 13.1 The most important words a leader can speak (author unknown)

The six most important words: "I admit I made a mistake"
The five most important words: "You did a good job"
The four most important words: "What is your opinion?"
The three most important words: "If you please"
The two most important words: "Thank you"
The one most important word: "We"
The least important word: "I"

flatten the hierarchy, create familiarity, and manage to create an environment that feels "safe" to team members so they will speak up when they have information or safety concerns. By inviting team members to contribute their thoughts and ideas, a leader can facilitate a shared mental model of patient-related and operational issues (▶ Chap. 11). This is done by communicating (verbally and nonverbally) a message of support and empowerment and about the normality of errors in a medical high-stakes environment (◻ Table 13.1).

Some of the basic principles of leadership in everyday life are:
- Set the example: Be a good role model for your staff, set a high standard for personal conduct, and adhere to this standard in all situations. Sincerity, integrity, and ethical demeanor are trust-inspiring characteristics and communicate to the team that you are a safe person with whom to work. Team members not only want to hear what they are expected to be or to do, they want to see it lived out in *your* life as well.
- Be technically proficient: As a leader, you must know your job and have a solid familiarity with all task demands.
- Know your staff members by name and look out for their well-being.
- Be supportive, advocating, and empowering: Believe in people and communicate that belief.
- Think and behave in team concepts: communicate to your staff that it is *we*, not *me*, who do the job.
- Keep your staff informed: Practice good communication skills (▶ Chap. 12).

- Foster a sense of responsibility within your staff.
- Resolve conflicts within a team: recognize areas of tension between individuals and apply conflict-resolution techniques (► Chap. 12).

13.2.2 Leadership in a Critical Situation

The case study of a malignant hyperthermia (MH) is an example of a time-critical medical emergency which necessitates "leadership in a critical situation" for successful management. In contrast to leading people in everyday life, leadership behavior in a critical situation is much more centralized. The main leadership tasks are:
- Maintaining team structure
- Applying problem-solving strategies
- Coordinating task execution
- Monitoring workload
- Reevaluating the situation

These requirements for leadership in an emergency situation are described in greater detail in what follows. Whenever possible, the team leader should stand back, physically and mentally, and avoid direct involvement in tasks that would distract him or her from assessing the overall picture. The team members become the sensors and effectors for the leader who is the central control (Murray and Foster 2000).

13.3 Leadership Theories

13.3.1 Approaches to Leadership

There are many diverse definitions of leadership which focus either on the position of the leader (singular or collective) or the purpose, process, and hallmarks of leadership. Most of these definitions come from an industrial or management setting and cannot readily be applied to healthcare. Leadership in the context of acute medical care can be defined as the process whereby a person influences and directs the performance of other team members by utilization of all available resources toward the achievement of a defined goal. A leader can be defined as a team member whose influence on group attitudes, performance, or decision-making exceeds that of the average member

of the group. Research on the nature of leadership has proposed several theories which all emphasize certain aspects of leadership. The earliest theories emerged during the early part of the twentieth century and focused on the qualities that distinguished leaders from followers. Subsequent theories looked at other variables such as situational factors and skill level. For the context of healthcare in a high-stakes medical environment the following theories might be the most relevant ones (Bass and Stogdill 2007).

13.3.2 "Great Man" Theories

This theoretical approach may still be rarely encountered among male physicians as the delusive self-perception of a person with respect to his leadership abilities. This theory originally assumed that the capacity for leadership is inherent and that great leaders are born, not made. The historical roots to this theory are based on the results of early research on leadership where the leaders studied often came from the aristocracy which contributed to the notion that leadership had something to do with "breeding" and the right genes. The leadership style of people who have this "great man" self-assessment will reflect this notion of personal distinctiveness: As a result, teamwork with such a leader might prove to be challenging.

13.3.3 Trait Theories

Trait theories assume that people have certain qualities and traits that make them better suited for leadership. Several research groups claim to have identified lists of personality or behavioral characteristics which are found in successful leaders (e.g., dominance, self-reliance). This theory seems to be confirmed by personal experience: There are very obvious people who have the right and sufficient combination of traits and who seem to be made of "the right stuff" for a good leader. The problem with trait theories is that traits useful for leadership usually have a downside (such as suppressing others, overconfidence) – no theory has yet stated "how much" of these traits really makes a good leader. In addition, trait theories promote the idea that (adult) people are as they are which makes educational efforts (development of leadership skills) seem worthless from the start.

13.3.4   Behavioral Theories

Behavioral theories of leadership are based upon the belief that leaders can be *made* and are not "born" leaders. These theories focus on the definable and learnable skills and the behavior of leaders, not on mental qualities or internal states. Among the skills a leader must have are interpersonal skills, conceptual skills, and technical skills. Successful leadership can thus be defined in terms of describable actions. This theory opens broad possibilities for leadership development measures and training interventions, because good leaders will develop through a never-ending process of self-study, education, training, and experience. In addition, behavior can be identified which contributes to teamwork failure, thus adding a second layer of understanding. This approach, too, seems to confirm personal experience, as most healthcare professionals can compare their present performance to the time when they first started the job and will find that their leadership ability indeed has improved. But behavioral theories tend to "throw out the baby with the bathwater" when they completely ignore the influence of personality. Yet not every person will be able to learn and show appropriate leadership behavior. This makes staff recruitment and selection as important an issue for healthcare providers as human resource development.

13.3.5   Situational and Contingency Theories

Situational and contingency theories are very similar in their core beliefs. They state that different types of situations demand different leadership behavior. The effectiveness of a given pattern of leadership behavior is contingent upon the demands imposed by the situation. Both types of theories focus on particular variables related to the environment that might determine which particular style of leadership is best suited for the situation. Success is a function of various contingencies in the form of subordinate, task, and group variables, including the leadership style, qualities of the followers, and aspects of the situation. According to this theory, no leadership style is best in all situations because different styles of leadership may be more appropriate for certain types of decision-making.

13.4   A Conceptual Framework for Leadership

For a successful leadership process in a high-stakes medical environment a synthesis of these theories (e.g., the situational leadership model) might be helpful. In the frame model introduced here (Gebert and Rosenstiel 2002), three factors influence the success of this leadership process: The personality characteristics of the person who leads (leadership personality) the way the leading is done (leadership behavior) and the situation in which leadership has to be assumed (◘ Fig. 13.1).

13.4.1   Leadership Personality

Grounded in the traits theory there have been many different studies of leadership traits and skills. Unfortunately, research on leadership has not yielded consistent results with respect to the characteristics of a successful leadership personality. Skills that leaders need are technical skills, conceptual skills (analytic and decisional), and human relation skills. Among the traits and skills repeatedly identified are: self-confidence; decisiveness; high activity

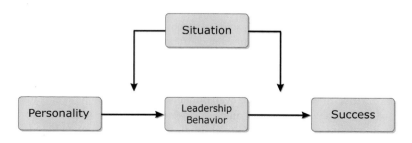

◘ **Fig. 13.1** Conceptual framework of leadership. (From Gebert and Rosenstiel 2002)

level (energetic); initiative; dominance; willingness to assume responsibility; intelligence; creativity; and being organized (Stogdill 1974).

13.4.2 Leadership Behavior

Leadership behavior equates to a great extent with communication. To lead basically means to communicate – with staff members and external resources (e.g., laboratory services, intensive care units from other departments, blood bank). Communication, however, is not an end in itself: Its purpose is to build a team out of individuals and to enable successful task performance. Leadership behavior can thus be described to fall on a grid, with relationship orientation (person preference) being one dimension and task orientation (performance preference) the other (Blanchard et al. 1985; Blake and Mouton 1961; Hersey and Blanchard 1977; Likert 1967). Research on styles began with Lewin et al. (1939) who described three basic styles:

The laissez-faire style (French: "just let things happen") is characterized by a low task focus and a low person focus: The leader has stepped back from the leadership role. The leader's involvement in decision-making is minimized, thus allowing people to make their own decisions and to do as they please. This leadership style is sometimes called a "delegation" or "free reign" style, although the "delegation" is often more the leaders' unwillingness to lead than a deliberate act of delegating responsibilities to staff members.

If a leader has a democratic leadership style, then his or her primary focus will be the well-being and the needs of the team members. The execution of task requirements is subordinated to the goal of team harmony and coherence. The democratic style is characterized by many discussions in which the tasks are democratically discussed and divided. The leader tries to listen to as many voices as possible and to compromise. Team members are involved in the decision-making even in situations where quick and unambiguous commands of the leader are necessary.

In clear contrast to this approach is the autocratic leadership style, which is defined by severe control, the focus on the execution of task demands, and efficacy, but with little concern for people. The leader uses pressure, threats, and other fear-based methods to achieve conformance. Lead-

ers are the only ones with solutions to problems, decisions are made without consultation, tasks are distributed with a detailed description of the procedure, and task execution is monitored closely. Communication is almost entirely top-down with a clear and strictly hierarchical decisional structure. There is a smooth transition from the authoritarian leadership style to arbitrariness and paternalism. An autocratic style would work in a performance environment where there is no need for input on the decision, where the decision would not change as a result of input, and where the motivation of people to carry out subsequent actions would not be affected whether they were or were not involved in the decision-making. This is clearly not the case in acute medical care. A modified autocratic style with its clear command structure is applied during cardiopulmonary resuscitation or during the management of natural or man-made disasters such as mass casualties. The modification would allow for a feedback and the volunteering of information. In the context of high-stakes healthcare, however, the autocratic leadership style causes the highest level of discontent among team members.

The integrative style combines a high focus on task execution with an equally high attention to the relation with and among team members. The concern of the leader is directed at the execution of tasks as well as the integration of all staff members. Leaders engage in discussion, convincing, and explanation to achieve a high degree of mutual agreement, shared mental models (▶ Chap. 11), and hence team task performance. Depending on the dynamics of a situation, the integrative style in a high-stakes medical environment can either be directive (authoritative) or cooperative (◘ Fig. 13.2). Other task-vs-person preferred models have been proposed. They share the believe that most effective leadership will load high on task and person orientation, and that successful leaders are able to switch between styles according to situational demands.

13.4.3 Leadership Situation

Healthcare providers in an acute medical care setting will find themselves confronted with different leadership situations: A surgical consultant may teach a young resident during an operation in the morning, be part of a trauma team at noon, and lead quality circles in the late afternoon. The range of leadership

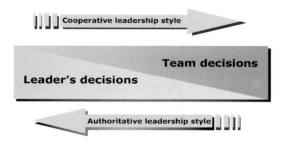

Fig. 13.2 Integrative leadership style in a high-stakes medical environment. Both, the cooperative as well as the directive leadership style are characterized by a balance between task orientation and relational orientation

situations may vary between leadership in everyday life and leadership in an emergency. Because these leadership situations differ from each other, different styles of leadership may be more appropriate for certain types of decision-making. Healthcare providers should be aware of the diversity of the demands and should adapt their behavior accordingly (McCormick and Wardrobe 2003).

13.4.4 Leadership Success

Leadership behavior will always have consequences, hopefully with overall success. Whether or not leadership in an emergency was successful has for a long time been dependent on the clinical course of events: The result in terms of survival and recovery was the touchstone. By which route this goal was reached was irrelevant, as long as the healthcare provider was able to improve patients' health status; however, the past decade has witnessed an increasing interest in the *process* of leadership. Successful leadership is no longer only a question of patient outcome, but in addition also that of a leader's interaction with the team members. Healthcare providers are adult and mature human beings and wish to be treated as such.

13.5 Leadership Tasks in a Critical Situation

The life-threatening situation from the case study necessitates "leadership in a critical situation" from the attending. His leadership behavior exemplifies the relevant tasks of a leader in a critical situation. (Note: The behaviors described here are good in critical situations – in routine situations they can be inappropriate or even wrong!)

13.5.1 Coordinate Tasks to Achieve a Particular Goal

The attending bears the responsibility that all team members direct their efforts to an effective treatment of the malignant hyperthermia. For this purpose he provides partial goals which he deduces from his medical knowledge, setting priorities according to the situational demands (▶ Chap. 7). The planned task execution is communicated to all team members in an appropriate way; individual tasks are distributed among the team according to skills and knowledge.

13.5.2 Centralize Communication and Flow of Information

All relevant information converges at the attending. This ensures that all relevant information concerning the patient's status can be integrated into the situational assessment. As every team member is aware of the fact that the attending is to be addressed with any information, the flow of information is formalized.

13.5.3 Generate a Comprehensive Mental Model of the Situation

One of the main factors for successful teamwork is a shared mental model (Stout et al. 1999). To have a shared mental model of the situation means a common understanding about the task or problem at hand, the resources, the team members' abilities and skills, and the situational context (▶ Chap. 11). The leader is responsible for the process of sharing mental models. In time-critical situations where there is no room for discussions, it is an important leadership task to define a model the group can share ("our problem is… the main risks are… the strategy is…").

13.5.4 Establish a Structure

If the teams perform repeatedly together in critical situations, a leadership structure will develop. Rules about how decisions are made and how communication is supposed to work will emerge and will be followed by all team members. As a result, the exchange of information, the planning of tasks, and the decision process will all run in an organized fashion (formalization of leadership). Because these rules have been fixed in advance, leadership in a critical situation will disengage from concrete persons and will become a function which can be fulfilled by different people. Which qualified person is called as attending to the critical situation of a malignant hyperthermia should be of no great importance for the majority of tasks involved. The team in the operating room expects from the person representing the function "attending" leadership behavior – irrespectively of the face which belongs to this function. The leadership behavior in the case study consists mainly of the delegation of tasks. Because the team in the case study has to deal with many concurrent problems under time pressure and limited staff resources, the team members are forced to repeatedly change their tasks. This change in task allocation is explicitly done by the anesthetist by ascribing new tasks to the resident and the nurses.

13.5.5 Stabilize Emotions

As a result of his leadership skills, the attending healthcare provider from the case study is sensitive to the impact of his own emotions and those of the team members on the ability to manage this critical situation. During the management of the malignant hyperthermia the resident is overstrained briefly with the situation because he blames himself for having chosen succinylcholine as a muscle relaxant for the induction of anesthesia. In this emotional turmoil he repeatedly makes frustrating attempts at inserting a central i.v. line into the internal jugular vein. As the negative emotions begin to spread across the team, the attending healthcare provider allocates the resident to a different task and has him supported by an emotionally stable team member.

13.5.6 Represent the Team

Because of the leadership function in this medical emergency, the attending healthcare provider represents the team externally. Outsiders can identify the team through the appearance and behavior of its representative. As the flow of information converges on him, he represents the team; however, team members also expect from their representative behavioral patterns such as integrity, adherence to moral standards, interpersonal skills, or certain political and religious beliefs. Although the extents to which these behavioral patterns are expressed in a leader do not directly impact task execution, they nevertheless play an important role in team cohesion.

> Leadership Tasks in a Critical Situation
> - Coordinate tasks to achieve a particular goal
> - Centralize communication and flow of information
> - Generate a comprehensive mental model of the situation
> - Establish a structure
> - Stabilize emotions
> - Represent the team

13.6 The Process of Leading

The purpose of leadership is to influence and direct the performance of team members toward the achievement of a defined goal (Murray and Foster 2000). Successful leadership requires that the leader be familiar with the five steps of a good strategy (▶ Chap. 10). This strategy has to be communicated to the team members step by step in a sensible way. The last critical step in a successful process of leading is monitoring whether information has been understood and tasks have been executed. This necessitates feedback by team members; thus, leadership is not a one-way street from the leader toward followers, but instead a constant interaction between both parties. To function effectively as part of an interdependent team, team members need the necessary cognitive, behavioral, and attitudinal teamwork skills (▶ Chap. 11); thus, successful leadership depends on both, the skills of the leader as well as the response pattern of the team members (Gebert and Rosenstiel 2002; Neuberger 2002).

13.7   Leadership Problems in Critical Situations

Leadership problems in acute care medicine can be traced to one core problem: A leader does not assume responsibility for the leadership position and does not act accordingly. The failure to take responsibility can show in various ways, as described below.

13.7.1   Without a Leader: When Nobody Shows the Way

If the leader does not fulfill the formal leadership function with the corresponding leadership behavior, the patient treatment in an emergency is jeopardized. Because decision-making in the high-stakes medical environment is based on an instructive leadership style, an indecisive leader will cause loss of coordination, failure to execute necessary tasks, and time delay. Recent work has demonstrated that despite having sufficient knowledge and training, teams managing a cardiac arrest were unable to follow guidelines successfully with the major obstacles being those of poor leadership and a lack of explicit task distribution (Marsch et al. 2004). This lack of leadership can partially be compensated if team members are familiar with each other because they have been working together for a while. In this case shared mental models allow each team member to anticipate each other's resource needs and actions (implicit coordination; ▶ Chap. 11)

13.7.2   Misled into Action

The main task of leadership in an emergency situation is to generate a comprehensive mental model of the situation, to define priorities and partial goals, and to coordinate the actions of all team members involved. This means that they have to refrain from operative actions. Unfortunately, leaders are not immune against a stress-related urge to

act ("do something now"). Once leaders have been misled into assuming tasks by themselves (e.g., inserting the central i.v. line, giving drugs, adjusting the ventilator settings), the danger is great that they will loose sight of "the big picture."; however, if it should become necessary that the leader, as the clinically most experienced person, perform a task (i.e., inserting the central i.v. line because the resident failed), this can only be a temporal exception which has to be followed by a "strategic" phase again.

13.7.3   Tasks Executed? Failure to Monitor

The leadership process is a goal-oriented, recurrent, closed-loop cycle of thinking and acting in order to execute a decision. Due to this circular structure, every leadership action is influenced by preceding actions. A crucial part of the process of leading lies in the monitoring whether or not an instruction has been correctly understood and executed, and if so, what the results are. If leaders fail to close the loop, consecutive decisions will be based on assumptions and expectations, but not on reality.

13.7.4   Strain: Leadership and Emotional Pressure

The anesthetist is confronted with a series of parallel task demands. He has to grapple with the medical problem (unclear diagnosis), has to assess the available resources, should satisfy the team members' need for adequate communication, and should regulate his own emotional reactions. Although the demands as a whole present an enormous challenge, leaders should be able to cope with them; however, if they are unable or not sufficiently able to do so, the danger is great that they may fall into the trap of the "cognitive emergency reaction" (▶ Chap. 9). Cognition and behavior will then no longer be directed at leading the team but instead at regaining the feeling of competence. Another frequently observable behavior is that the "leader goes solo": Under stress decision-makers tend to focus on their own thinking and acting. Team members can no longer participate in the leader's mental model of the situation; thus, they have no idea what the leader thinks, plans, or expects for support (Driskell and Salas 1991).

13.7.5 Change in Leadership – Change in Function

Healthcare providers in an acute medical care setting are sometimes forced to switch functions: Being a resident implies that the leadership role is up to him or her (e.g., in a case of malignant hyperthermia) until the attending arrives, a "code blue" is led by the physician on ward until the resuscitation team can take over the case. In both cases team members have to conform to the altered conditions and have to adapt their behavior. It is not uncommon in the healthcare setting that team members continue to assume a leadership role (e.g., by coordinating, defining structures) despite being assigned to a new task, subjective to directions.

13.7.6 "I'm in the Driver's Seat!" – Leadership and Power

Teams in an acute medical care setting are hierarchical. Hierarchy, however, always implies a power gradient. An autocratic leadership style can cause problems in teamwork. If a leader wields power insistently, he or she will give the impression of being master of the situation. An active participation of team members in the process of information gathering and situation assessment is seen as irrelevant and thus will be discarded. If the function of a team member is continuously abased to receiving orders, this can lead to hidden resistance, passivity, and wayward behavior. As teams in principle can refuse trustful cooperation with the leader, this can factually lead to a complete breakdown of teamwork. The other side to the coin is that a power gradient can be in the interest of the team: In critical situations humans tend to call for a strong leadership and dispense with responsibility. The consequences are the same. For this reason the participation and volunteering of information should be encouraged by the leader.

13.7.7 "There is Only Room for One of Us!" – Conflicts Among Coequals

When several leaders with a comparable position in hierarchy meet in an emergency (e.g., resuscitation on general ward, acute bleeding in the OR), the leadership position can become a matter of dispute. If there is no standing rule about the allocation of responsibility, it is helpful if the respective leaders agree explicitly on the most appropriate leadership model. This can either be the allocation of leadership to the most experienced person, or teamwork with equal partners; however, it is necessary that the leadership role and the allocation of responsibility be explicitly negotiated and not just assumed.

13.7.8 Handing Over Responsibility: the "Revolving-Door" Effect

During the management of the malignant hyperthermia the resident hands over the responsibility for all decisions to the attending physician. This handing over of responsibility generally corresponds with the necessary knowledge, expertise, and clinical skills of the leader and is done by sharing all relevant information and assumptions; however, sometimes leaders take over responsibility too abruptly: The resident could be sent away, ignored, or verbally be "pushed away." Because in this way the information the resident could share is lost, negative consequences for patient care a likely: Relevant information about the clinical development, important clues, procedures performed, and laboratory data requested will not be available for future treatment; instead, the leader arrives on scene, but team members leave and take crucial information with them (revolving-door effect). The advantage the new leader has with an unbiased approach to the situation is undone by the fact that team members stop participating in problem-solving as soon as they get the impression that their input is unwanted.

13.7.9 Invulnerable: Immunization Against Criticism

Leaders can make false diagnoses, can order controversial procedures, and can make mistakes. Because a leader's decision in everyday life often goes unchallenged, an immunization against criticism of team members can take place. Consequently, any decision a leader will make in a critical situation will underlie a taboo for criticism, too. Ideally, the interaction of team members with their leader should be characterized by a sound balance of respect and assertive behavior. The price for not having challenged a leaders' faulty decision can be high. Leaders can actively encourage team members to share their thoughts and to voice concerns if they manage to break open the "vacuum of criticism" concerning the position of leaders in healthcare.

> Leadership Problems
> — Leadership role is not assumed
> — Losing sight of the big picture
> — Failure to monitor
> — Overstrained with a situation (cognitive emergency reaction)
> — Assuming a leadership role despite being in a role which is subjective to directions
> — Exerting power with an autocratic leadership style
> — Conflicts among coequals
> — Assuming responsibility abruptly and thereby displacing team members with situational knowledge ("revolving-door" effect)
> — Immunization against criticism

13.8   Situational Leadership

Situational leadership is a term that can be applied generically to both, a recognized leadership model and a style of leadership. The model, created in the late 1960s, allows leaders to analyze the needs of the situation with which they are dealing, and then to adopt the most appropriate leadership style (Hersey and Blanchard 1977). The Situational Leadership theory is based on the amount of direction (task orientation) and amount of socio-emotional support (relationship orientation) a leader must provide given the situation and the level of maturity and commitment of the followers. Situational leadership is a holistic leadership concept which perceives and respects individual limits and tries to coach and motivate staff members as unique human beings. The four basic styles used for situational leadership are:
- Direct
- Coach
- Support
- Delegate

Leaders who apply situational leadership can always tell when they should use a certain style of leadership and whether they are able to keep it up: The interaction with an experienced and motivated nurse will be different from an interaction with a younger team member in training or with a colleague who displays a snappy and disrespectful attitude. Unfortunately, many leaders have great difficulty in adapting their leadership style to changing situational demands: Although an authoritative dictation of goals and task can be appropriate in a time-critical medical emergency, it will by unsuitable to carry on with this behavior when the situation has abated. A physician who tells a nurse in great detail how to plaster up an i.v. line would be another example of leadership behavior inappropriate to the situational context. Core functional competencies for situational leadership include:
- The ability to adapt the leadership style to the situational demands.
- The willingness to conceive the performance level and potential of a team member as a snapshot and not as his or her final and inalterable condition. This approach frees team leaders from the danger of jumping to conclusions about a team member too readily (▶ Chap. 12).

13.9   Tips for Daily Practice

- If you want to lead, you must like people. Leadership only works if leaders have a genuine interest in fellow human beings and if they show their appreciation. Make sure everybody counts and everybody knows they count. Without this core value of "liking people" nobody should strive for a leadership position.
- Leadership starts in everyday life. When confronted with a critical situation, leaders can only fall back on a behavior and team climate which has been established in the normal course of life.
- Leadership does not result automatically from a hierarchical position. Leadership is granted only if a person is qualified in terms of leadership *behavior*.

13.10   "Leadership": in a Nutshell

- Leadership in the context of acute medical care can be defined as the process whereby a person influences and directs the performance of other team members by utilization of all available resources toward the achievement of a defined goal.

- A leader can be defined as a team member whose influence on group attitudes, performance, or decision-making greatly exceeds that of the "average" members of the group.
- In the context of healthcare in a high-stakes medical environment four leadership theories are relevant: the "great man" theory; trait theories; behavioral theories; and situational and contingency theories.
- The success of the leadership process is determined by the person who leads (leadership personality), the way this leading is done (leadership behavior), and the situation in which the leadership role has to be assumed.
- Leadership behavior can be described as existing on a grid with relationship orientation and task orientation as both dimensions.
- Four leadership styles can be developed within this grid: the "laissez-faire" style; the democratic style; the authoritative style; and the integrative style.
- Leadership tasks in critical situations comprise task coordination, delegation, formalization of the flow of information, determination of structures, stabilization of emotions, and representation of the team.
- Successful leadership depends on the skills of the leader as well as the teamwork skills of each team member.
- A leader must have conceptual skills, technical skills, and interpersonal skills.
- Effective leaders delegate so that they can regulate: During high workload, the leading team member should manage the situation and team members should manage the technical tasks.
- Leadership problems in a high-stakes medical environment originate from the inability of a leader to assume responsibility of this leadership.
- No single leadership style is best in all situations. Different styles of leadership may be more appropriate for certain types of decision-making.

- Situational leadership is a holistic leadership concept which perceives, respects, informs, coaches, and motivates staff members as unique human beings.

References

Bass BM, Stogdill, RM (2007) Bass and Stogdill's handbook of leadership: theory, research, and managerial applications, 3rd edn. Free Press, New York and London

Blake RR, Mouton JS (1961) Group dynamics: key to decision-making. Gulf Publishing, Houston

Blanchard KH, Zigami P, Zigami D (1985) Leadership and the one minute manager: increasing effectiveness through situational leadership. William Morrow, New York

Driskell JE, Salas E (1991) Group decision-making under stress. J Appl Psychol 76:473–478

Gebert D, Rosenstiel L von (2002) Organisationspsychologie [Organizational psychology]. Kohlhammer, Stuttgart

Hersey P, Blanchard KH (1977) Management of organizational behaviour: utilizing human resources. Prentice-Hall, Englewood Cliffs, New Jersey

Kohn L, Corrigan J, Donaldson M (1999) To err is human: building a safer health system. Committee on Quality of Health Care in America, Institute of Medicine (IOM). National Academy Press, Washington DC

Lewin K, Lippitt R, White RK (1939) Patterns of aggressive behaviour in experimentally created "social climates". J Soc Psychol 10:271–299

Likert R (1967) The human organization: its management and value. McGraw-Hill, New York

Marsch SCU, Müller C, Marquardt K, Conrad G, Tschan F, Hunziker P (2004) Human factors affect the quality of cardiopulmonary resuscitation in simulated cardiac arrests. Resuscitation 60:51–56

McCormick S, Wardrobe J (2003) Major incidents, leadership, and series summary and review. Emerg Med J 20:70–74

Murray WB, Foster PA (2000) Crisis resource management among strangers: principles of organizing a multidisciplinary group for crisis resource management. J Clin Anesth 12:633–638

Neuberger O (2002) Führen und führen lassen: Ansätze, Ergebnisse und Kritik der Führungsforschung [leading and being lead – leadership research]. Lucius and Lucius, Stuttgart

Stout RJ, Cannon-Bowers JA, Salas E, Milanovich DM (1999) Planning, shared mental models, and coordinated performance: an empirical link is established. Hum Factors 41:61–71

Stogdill RM (1974) Handbook of leadership: a survey of the literature. Free Press, New York

IV The Organization

The fourth part of this book focuses on the influence of organizations on the performance of healthcare professionals in a high-stakes medical environment. At first sight many of these factors are beyond responsibility of healthcare providers: The organizational culture, basic concepts of patient safety, or principles of staff development seem to be set variables the individual has to take as they are; however, already the knowledge about the many ways an organization can impact patient safety can help healthcare professionals to understand basic mechanisms of accident evolution and may help to sharpen the focus for latent conditions in one's own work environment.

- Chapter 14 outlines a systemic view of organizations and discusses several influential organizational theories on error: Human Factors approach; Normal Accident Theory; and High Reliability Theory. We focus on key system issues for addressing error and safety in acute medical care and present several variables which seem to be especially relevant for the genesis of latent conditions.
- Chapter 15 deals with the possibilities in avoiding and managing clinical errors. Complex organizations such as hospitals, however, will not be changed by simple recipes and isolated measures. Instruments such as Incident-Reporting Systems, Continuous Quality Improvement efforts, simulation-based education, and regular team-training interventions should all become integral components of a comprehensive concept of organizational development. Given the current economical situation, it will become increasingly more important that every healthcare provider in hospital and prehospital medical care has patient safety on his or her personal agenda.

14 Organizations and Human Error

14.1   Case Study

A 32-year-old worker fell from the top of a 4-m scaffold and hit the ground on his right side. Emergency medical services (EMS) evaluated the patient, who was found to be alert and hemodynamically stable. He was transported to the Emergency Department of a nearby hospital for further evaluation. There, the emergency physician was extremely busy taking care of six emergencies while other patients were also waiting to be evaluated. On arrival, the blood pressure and heart rate were within normal limits and the lungs were clear to auscultation. The patient's chief complaint was localized pain on the right side of his chest that worsened with deep breathing and moving. The patient had a chest X-ray (CXR) done in the Radiology Department, but the radiology technician who had the habit of identifying patients based only on their last name erroneously distributed the wrong films. The patient received a set of normal CXR films that belonged to a different patient with the same last name. The patient returned to the Emergency Department accompanied by a student nurse who was asked to monitor the patient while the rest of the staff helped with another emergency. During the next half hour the patient became increasingly short of breath and anxious. The emergency physician was called by the nurse to assess the patient. He reviewed the CXR films, and after ruling out any chest and lung pathology, he prescribed boluses of morphine as needed for pain control. Shortly after morphine was administered, the patient became obtunded and the pulse oximeter which had just been brought in the room by the nurse recorded an oxygen saturation of 79%. Mask ventilation with an Ambubag was immediately initiated. After an uneventful intubation, the emergency physician noticed decreased breath sounds on the right side of the chest and subcutaneous emphysema. While he was preparing for chest tube insertion, the patient's oxygen saturation abruptly dropped to the 40s. The ECG monitor displayed ventricular fibrillation. A defibrillator was immediately brought at the bedside, but the shock was delayed because the operators were not familiar with the new version of the device. The resuscitation efforts were eventually successful and the patient regained spontaneous circulation. The CXR was examined again and the swap was discovered. The correct films were reviewed, and multiple rib fractures and a right-sided pneumothorax were identified.

A construction worker falls from the top of a scaffold and is transported by EMS to an Emergency Department. At the time of admission the Emergency Department is understaffed and many patients are waiting to be evaluated. Due to the hectic workflow, the only available physician performs only a very basic clinical check before heading for the next patient. Because the initial clinical findings suggest serial rib fractures, the physician orders a CXR. At the Radiology Department the CXRs are swapped and the patient returns to the Emergency Department with the wrong images. Because the patient carries the CXRs and because the family name on the film is identical to the patient's name, no suspicion arises that the films could be wrong. Neither first name nor date of birth are verified. The actual severity of his injuries is misjudged because an inexperienced student nurse accompanies the patient, and because vital monitoring (pulse oximeter) is not immediately available. When the patient's clinical status deteriorates, the physician cannot correlate the symptoms with the normal radiological findings. Because the CXRs shows no pathology, the resident neither crosschecks the radiological findings by repeating the clinical examination (e.g., chest auscultation) nor reexamines the CXR (e.g., verifying the patient's name); instead, he orders pain therapy with morphine which worsens the clinical situation. It is only after a successful intubation that new clues emerge (e.g., decreased breath sound, subcutaneous emphysema) which point to a pneumothorax. The situation is complicated by the fact that controlled ventilation precipitates a tension pneumothorax which rapidly develops into cardiac arrest. Moreover, the defibrillator that the code team carries is a new model with which nobody is really familiar. The delay of the first shock is caused by the conscious effort to identify the necessary steps for action.

Although the circumstances point at first sight to a concatenation of unfortunate circumstances, their occurrence is not accidental: This specific case can only occur in this specific hospital because it has been organized in a way that allows for such a concatenation of single factors and actions. What looks in the first instance like the faulty behavior of a few healthcare providers (e.g., radiology technician, student nurse, emergency physician) on closer inspection turns out to be based on flawed processes and structures in this hospital. Even if healthcare providers are unaware of the fact, organizational factors shape patient safety considerably (e.g., by setting a time budget for every patient, by providing training for medical equipment).

14.2 Organizations as Systems: Different Perspectives

Of all organizations in western culture healthcare delivery has certainly become one of the largest, most complex, and most costly of all. As public pressure increases to satisfy mutually contradictory criteria regarding improving efficiency and excellence, and at the same time cutting down on costs for healthcare, complexity of healthcare provision will most likely increase even more. Although healthcare delivery is usually not thought of as a system, being a *socio-technical* system is one of its most distinctive characteristic, defined as the way human behavior, an organization's complex infrastructures, and technology interact. The socio-technical system "healthcare" has many component subsystems: prehospital emergency medical service; hospitals (with their further subdivision into departments, wards, divisions, teams, programs); outpatient clinics; pharmacies; laboratories; manufacturers; government agencies; and patient organizations. Each of them represent a distinct culture with its own goals, values, beliefs, and norms of behavior, on one hand, and financial, technical, and personal resources on the other. Most of the problems within healthcare organizations do not exist in isolation; they interrelate with each other. In order to solve any specific problem within a subsystem, it is necessary to take a broader perspective, where local issues are seen as part of a coherent whole. *Systems thinking*, the "discipline for seeing wholes, recognizing patterns and interrelationships, and learning how to structure those interrelationships in more effective, efficient ways" (Senge 1990), has been applied to industrial and management issues for a long time; however, this conceptual framework has only recently been applied to addressing organizational issues in healthcare.

What, exactly, is an organization, though? Within social sciences many theoretical frameworks have been proposed for defining organizations: what organizations are, how they should work, and what can be done if they do not work. Several major schools of thought have evolved, each with its own perspective about characteristics of organizations, as described below:

— From a structural perspective organizations are created and exist primarily to accomplish specific goals. The organizational structure as well as processes and rules are determined mainly by the organization's goals, technology, and environment. Behavior in organizations is intentionally rational and governed by "norms of rationality"; organizations are "rational systems" (Gouldner 1959). System theorists would say that "a hospital *has* an organization." If the management of an organization takes a structural perspective, it will emphasize that goals, tasks, technologies, and structures are the primary determinants of organizational behavior; the needs, capacities, and self-interests of individuals or groups are less significant. The constant optimization and improvement of individual expertise and performance, and of cooperative processes, is best accomplished through the exercise of authority and rules, not by fostering creativity or participation. Organizational problems usually reflect inappropriate structure and can be resolved through redesign and reorganization.

— Whereas the structural perspective places rationality as its central motive, the human resource approach focuses on the relationship between organizations and people (e.g., Argyris 1957; Argyris and Schön 1996). In this framework, people are the most critical resource and organizations exist to serve human needs instead of humans existing to serve organizational needs. Topics central to self-concept of an organization include motivation, attitudes, participation, and teamwork. As a result, an organization is a permanent arrangement of social elements with a formal structure. The organizational members not only pursue factual goals but also personal interests (e.g., career, power, continuous education). If we say "the hospital *is* an organization," we emphasize the fact that people in organizations try to satisfy different needs and motives and are ready to align their behavior to shared values and norms. Such a hospital would place great value on the compliance with social rules. Organizational problems result from poor synchronization of human and organizational needs: The organization will become ineffective, people will feel exploited, or both. Remedial efforts would strive for a state where organizations can achieve their goals effectively while humans derive rewards and meaning from their work.

— The functional perspective on organizations centers on the process of organizing as *the* main leadership task (overview in Kieser 2002). This conceptual framework tries to identify and strengthen all processes whereby useful organizational structures, rules, and processes are created. If an organization takes this perspective, the core belief will be that an organization will never have reached its final structure; instead, constant reevaluation, reorganization, continuous improvement, and rationalization remain central tasks. Organizational problems may be rooted in an incomplete understanding of the way the organization functions under given circumstances.

Each of the drafted positions point to important phenomena in organizations and provide a valid and useful analytic framework of how structures, processes, people, and tasks interact. The outlined perspectives on organizations should be taken as complementary rather than mutually exclusive: Every organizational event can be interpreted in a number of ways, because organizations are "multiple realities" (Bolman and Deal 1984). Despite obvious differences, social scientists nevertheless agree that organizations generally develop as instruments for attaining specific goals: Organizations emerge in situations where people recognize a common or complementary advantage that can best be served through collective action; thus, by their very nature organizations imply an integrating and structuring of activities directed toward goal accomplishment. Organizations are consciously coordinated and deliberately structured social entities: a group of people intentionally organized to construct or compile a common tangible or intangible product or service (Alvesson 2002; Bedeian 1984; Black 2003; Bolman and Deal 1984). The goals an organization tries to achieve can either be deliberate and recognized (explicit; e.g., mission statement) or may operate unrecognized "behind the scenes" (implicit). Explicit goals of healthcare organizations can be safe patient care, medical excellence, or cost reduction, whereas implicit goals may comprise personal agendas of management, directors, or professional groups within the organization.

In order to balance contradicting goals and to accomplish specific goals, organizations have to coordinate recurrent tasks by setting up task plans. These task plans can be more or less complex and will comprise a multitude of single decisions that make it possible that people, material, and other resources are allocated in due time at the right place. At the early stages of organizational development, most of these task plans will emerge spontaneously, thereby reflecting a balance between effort and result. There will be a certain vitality and spontaneity to these task plans, like blood flowing through vessels providing an organism with new and fresh nutriments; however, when organizations exist for some time, experience with solutions to recurrent problems will be reflected in formalized structures, hierarchies, functions, and task descriptions. The constant flow of spontaneous and fresh ideas will gradually turn into an "accumulation of clotted decisions."

Finally, as human organizations have an essential social character, they are social systems with identifiable boundaries between members and nonmembers. By defining who belongs to the organization and who does not, organizations create an "inside" where people cooperate, share common rules, and agree upon the way power and responsibility are distributed, and an "outside" to which it can respond as a collective body.

14.3   Organizations, Human Error, and Reliability

14.3.1   Human Factors Engineering Approach

Human factors research has relentlessly pointed to the fact that active failures (► Chap. 3) rarely arise solely from negligence but are far more often the consequence of error-provoking circumstances (e.g., equipment design, software development, architecture of working place; Norman 1988; Vicente 2004). Errors are seen as "the downside of having a brain" (► Chap. 4; Helmreich 1998) rather than pathological cognitive processes that could be overcome by due effort or diligence. "Human error" is not mainly a property of humans – it is a property of systems that include humans. The contribution of the human factors approach to safe patient care and error reduction in a high-stakes medical environment has been mainly in three key areas (Moray 1994; Vicente 2004):
— Design of safe systems
— Ergonomics
— Importance of teamwork

Formal structures, hierarchies, functions, and task descriptions within an organization can be seen as "accumulation of clotted decisions." From this perspective latent conditions for errors (Reason 1990a, 1990b, 1997) are the "accumulation of clotted unsafe decisions": Decisions of people in no direct patient contact, such as systems engineers, managers, and others at the "blunt end" of an organization, who do not set safety as the top priority, or who, despite setting safety as the top priority, involuntarily create conditions that will weaken a system's protective barriers. Their decisions are permanently embedded in organizations and can have considerable side effects and long-range effects on patient safety. "Organizational accidents" result from the interaction of a long chain of latent failures, serious breaches in the defenses, and moments of inattention by the healthcare professional. Because almost all organizational accidents result from faulty systems that set people up to fail (Kohn et al. 1999), one of the main research areas of human factors engineers has been the analysis of *system design*.

The second main field of work within human factors research has been the application of scientific information concerning human limitations to the design of objects, systems, and environment for human use: the field of *ergonomics* (Carayon 2006). Often it is the design of medical equipment and the architectural layout of rooms that influence the likelihood of mistakes: Healthcare professionals are "forced" by inappropriate design of equipment and software to commit errors or are hindered by cable clutter, wires, hoses, and lines running across the floor to work properly and safely.

The information-processing capacity and decision-making capability of individual healthcare professionals have severe limitations within a high-stakes medical environment and under time pressure. In addition, poor *teamwork* and a breakdown in communication between members of healthcare teams can be the key factor in poor care and the occurrence of medical errors. As a result, Human Factors theory has emphasized the importance of group-level interactions and the use of multidisciplinary teams to detect, prevent, and manage error-associated incidents (e.g., Entin and Serfaty 1999; Burke et al. 2004).

Human factors engineering tries to optimize the relationship between humans and systems by designing systems and human–machine interfaces that are robust enough to reduce error rates and the effect of the inevitable error within the system.

14.3.2   Normal Accident Theory

In the aftermath of the accident at the Three Mile Island nuclear power plant in 1979, Yale University sociologist Charles Perrow introduced the idea that as soon as technological systems have become sufficiently complex, accidents will be inevitable or "normal." This conceptual framework has come to be known as Normal Accident Theory (NAT; Perrow 1999). Perrow explained his theory by introducing two related dimensions – interactive complexity and loose/tight coupling – which he claimed together determine a system's susceptibility to accidents.

Interactive Complexity and Coupling. The system dimension of interactive complexity is characterized by a multitude of positive and negative feedbacks between its components, most of them being either invisible or not immediately comprehensible. Unfamiliar or unexpected sequences of events can evolve in ways that cannot be predicted by the designers or the "user" of the system. As a result, apparently trivial incidents can cascade in unpredictable ways and with possibly severe consequences: The "harmless" habit of a radiology technician to call patients only by their family name can then contribute to a cardiac arrest in a young trauma patient.

The concept of coupling describes the proximity of connections or transitions between system components. Coupling can be either tight or loose. If a system is tightly coupled high interdependency exists: Each part of the system is tightly linked to other parts, and subcomponents of a tightly coupled system have prompt and major impacts on each other. In the absence of buffers, a change in one part of the system can rapidly affect the status of other parts. As a result, the quick response of system components to perturbations of another system may have disastrous consequences. The impairment of venous return by an increase in intrathoracic pressure, as in the case of a tension pneumothorax, would be a pathophysiological example of tight coupling. In addition, tight coupling and interactive complexity raise the odds that a healthcare provider's intervention will make things worse, since he or she might not understand the true nature of a problem: The true extent of the lung damage became evident only after the physician had intubated the patient, thereby precipitating the tension pneumothorax.

In contrast, if a loose coupling exists, then the part of the system either work relatively independently of each other or the system will have many buffers to absorb failures or unplanned behavior without destabilization. According to NAT, systems with interactive complexity and tight coupling will experience accidents that cannot be foreseen or prevented. The cascading of effects can quickly spiral out of control before healthcare professionals are able to understand the situation and perform appropriate corrective actions.

14.3.3   High Reliability Theory

Despite NAT's claim that accidents in complex systems are unavoidable, a set of organizations operate in a high-stakes environment and still manage to cause very little accidents (e.g., nuclear power plants, aircraft carriers; Roberts 1990; Weick and Sutcliffe 2001). These High Reliability organizations (HROs) achieve their high safety standard through mindful attention to ongoing operations. Although HROs resemble other organizations in their input processes, their adoption of precautionary beliefs and their susceptibility to surprises, they do differ in their commitment to *mindfulness* as a means of managing these challenges. The High Reliability Theory has a more optimistic approach and emphasizes that organizations can contribute significantly to the prevention of accidents through good organizational design and management. The High Reliability Theory identifies the important role played by the cultural features in an organization in promoting "error-free performance," while structural dynamics, such as in NAT, play a secondary role. The processes by which these reliable organizations mindfully pursue their goal are characterized by an "informed safety culture" (Reason 1997) and several other characteristics (Roberts 1990; Weick and Sutcliffe 2001). Of course, not all organizations in HRO domains work in that way, and not everyone in an HRO lives all these characteristics every day, but the research on HROs shows that it is possible for an organization to work safely even

under adverse conditions if the following ideas guide action:

— Preoccupation with failure: People in HROs are preoccupied with minor incidents and rare events rather than with accidents or complete failures. Because they view even the slightest incident as a signal of possible weakness in the system, they want to grasp every learning opportunity possible. This is evident in frequent incident reviews, the reporting of errors no matter how inconsequential they are, and employees' obsession with the liability of success. People in HROs are skeptical, wary, and suspicious of long and quiet periods of success, as they always anticipate the danger of complacency and inattention. Sensitive to the fact that any decision or action may be subject to faulty assumptions, they are "chronically worried about the unexpected." They hope for the best but anticipate the worst.

— Reluctance to simplify interpretations: HROs are just as preoccupied with complicating their simplifications as they are with probing their failures. The relentless attack on simplifications can be seen by the preference of differentiated and complex models about internal and external events. People in HROs know that simple mental models and expectations produce simple sensing and rash decisions. They know that it takes varied complex sensors to register the environmental complexities: "It takes variety to control variety."

— Sensitivity to operations: Normal work routines are constantly scrutinized for potential weaknesses of the system. The sensitivity is accomplished by building "a dense web of communication": Every staff member is provided with detailed real-time information on what is happening and what the ongoing operations require. Sensitivity to operations permits early identification of problems so that action can be taken before problems become too substantial.

Despite all efforts to anticipate and take preventive measures, critical events will occur. The mindset necessary to cope with these critical situations differs from the one needed to anticipate their occurrence. Once they are faced with critical situations, HROs will apply at least two processes that enable them to contain and bounce back from problems. These processes include:

— Commitment to resilience: To be resilient is to be mindful about errors that have already occurred and correct them before they worsen and cause more serious harm. Organizations which are committed to resilience always expect that they could be taken by surprise. To reduce the likelihood of such an occurrence they concentrate on developing general resources to cope and respond swiftly. The mindset of resilient people is cure rather than prevention; they think about mitigation rather than anticipation. They are attentive to knowledge and resources that relieve, lighten, moderate, reduce, and decrease surprises. They treat a problem before they have made a full diagnosis. Whereas anticipation encourages people to think and then act, resilience encourages people to act while thinking to implement the lessons learned from error (Hollnagel et al. 2006).

— Deference to expertise: In a typical closed hierarchical structure, important decisions are made by "important" high-ranking decision makers. Although hierarchical patterns of authority exist, in the case of HROs authority always shifts toward expertise wherever it lies, and not up or down the hierarchy toward seniority or rank. The designation of who is "important" in a certain critical situation keeps changing based on the decision maker's specialty and "migrates" to the person or team with expertise in that problem–decision combination.

Reliability-enhancing organizations encourage people to discuss the current state of the system, deviations, personal intentions, minimal events, and the occurrence of error. A climate of openness and a trustful relationship between employees and leadership are prerequisites. The constant reflection upon decisions made can prevent an effect of normalization when dealing with deviance. "Normalization of deviance" (Vaughan 1997) conceptualizes the gradual shift in what is regarded as normal after repeated exposures to "deviant behavior" (i.e., behavior straying from correct and safe operating procedures). Corners get cut, safety checks bypassed, and alarms ignored or turned off, and these behaviors become not just common but stripped of their significance as warnings of impending danger. Normalization of deviance is likely to occur within an organization if deviating events, deviating behavior, or violations of rules receive no immediate negative feedback. In the absence of a controlled punitive system safety hazards will slowly turn into an acceptable risk.

In summary, the three basic theories all address the issue of patient safety and human fallibility from a systemic perspective. All three theories provide helpful insight into the dynamics of error occurrence in a high-stakes medical environment. Each theoretical approach focuses on a different set of organizational dynamics (◘ Table 14.1); however, the assumption that by simply copying safety models from other high-stakes environments we will arrive at "model of success" in healthcare must be approached with skepticism (Thomas and Helmreich 2002).

14.4 Organizational Sources of Error

14.4.1 Key Systems Issues for Addressing Error and Safety in Acute Medical Care

Published almost a decade ago, the Institute of Medicine's (IOM) report "To Err Is Human: Building a Safer Healthcare System" (Kohn 1999) has triggered an unprecedented effort within the healthcare community to identify interventions that might decrease medical errors and enhance patient safety. A system-based approach to reducing error and the need for a strong patient-safety environment have begun to replace the focus on alleged incompetent or misguided individuals. Consequently, the medical community has directed empirical research to the linkages between organizational dynamics, medical error, and patient safety. A recent review of the clinical and health-service literature was able to identify the most discussed or analyzed organizational variables (Hoff et al. 2004). At present, however, there seems to be little scientific evidence for asserting the importance of one single individual, group, or structural variable in error prevention.

From among the analyzed variables the following seem especially relevant for the genesis of latent errors in a medical high-stakes environment (◘ Fig. 14.1; Cooper et al. 1978; Flin and Maran 2004; Morell and Eichhorn 1997; O'Connor et al. 2002):

— Structure and processes
— Equipment-related incidents
— Human resource management

▣ Table 14.1 Three theories addressing error and safety in terms of "system" issues. (From Hoff et al. 2004)

Theory	Key ideas around issue of errors	Key organizational factors implied by theory to reduce error	References
Human factors theory	"Latent" mistakes combine in a system to cause error	Decreased complexity; feedback loops; system redundancies; team cooperation; rapid response capability; operator communication; information systems; decentralized decision-making	Reason (1990a,b)
			Rasmussen (1982)
			Gaba (1989)
			Helmreich et al (1999)
Normal Accident Theory	Errors in complex systems are unavoidable; no design is foolproof; level of coupling between tasks and complexity of interactions determines error risk	Control over personnel; close proximity of elites to operating systems; no centralization; use of buffers between steps in process; information and feedback around critical phases and errors	Perrow (1984, 1994, 1999)
High Reliability Theory	Complex organizational processes can be designed for reliable performance	A "culture" of reliability and safety; system redundancies; training and education; decentralized decision-making; clear goals; measurement and feedback; use of routines	LaPorte (1982)
			Roberts (1990)
			Schulman (1993)
			Rochlin (1993)
			Weick and Sutcliffe (2001)

— Teamwork and leadership
— Communication
— Organizational culture

Here, we describe structure and processes, equipment problems, and human resource management. Teamwork, communication, and leadership are the topics of Chaps. 11–13. The significance of organizational culture is discussed in Chap. 15, where also formal teamwork-training interventions and simulation-based team training are discussed.

14.4.2 Structures and Processes

Medical and legal requirements are changing constantly. For this reason organizations have to adapt their structures and processes all the time. Historically grown structures underlie a certain inertia which causes a typical resistance to change within the organizations. As long as some people profit from the actual state, it will be difficult to change. Structures and processes in medical high-stakes environments which promote errors are:

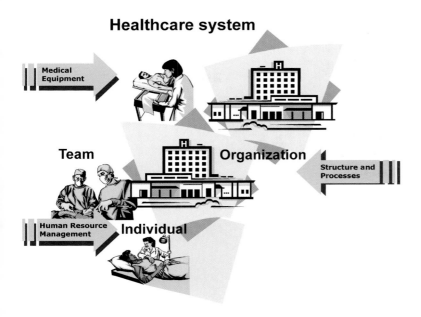

Healthcare system

Medical Equipment

Team

Organization

Structure and Processes

Human Resource Management

Individual

☐ **Fig. 14.1** Organizational sources of latent errors in a medical high-stakes environment

— Organizational culture: particular combination of safety, profit, and service
— Hierarchies, leadership principles
— Error concepts: person approach vs system approach
— Concepts of cooperation and teamwork
— Quality of information systems and flow of information
— Policies for shift work and hours of work

The Organizational Problem. The complete chain of patient care in a high-stakes medical environment involves different groups of staff across several organizations (e.g., ambulance crews, Emergency Department staff, diagnostic departments, labs, intensive care staff) that interact and constantly create vital patient-related information. Due to the many interfaces between the parties involved, important information can get lost. The fact that patient care is usually not organized as one complete process, but rather as the succession of many partial tasks executed by healthcare providers from different departments and specialties, is called the *organizational problem*: The shared goal of safe patient care can only be reached if several specialists are willing to work together and if their actions are coordinated. Because of that, the organizational problem is a problem of coordination and motivation (Jung 2001). So, dealing with motivation and cooperation at the interfaces within the organization is not a sign of faulty structures or processes but instead a normal feature of every organization.

The circumstances which lead to harm in the young trauma patient have their roots in such an organizational problem. An organizational problem is best addressed by creating structures and implementing strategies that improve the interaction and collaboration among healthcare professionals (☐ Fig. 14.2). In order to achieve this goal, an organization needs concepts for:
— Reliable communication at the numerous interfaces
— Interdisciplinary teamwork
— Efficient knowledge management
— Leadership performance

In addition to that inherent organizational problem, there may be goal conflicts: Despite the shared explicit goal of safe patient care, each department

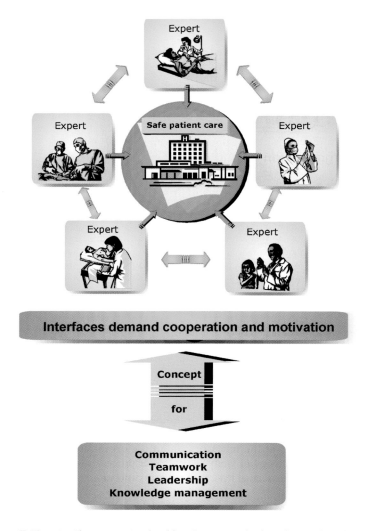

■ **Fig. 14.2** The organizational problem. Every expert has his or her own knowledge, experience, and motives, which are needed for constructive cooperation with experts from other specialties. The interfaces between professional groups demand cooperation and motivation as well as an institutional concept for communication, teamwork, leadership, and knowledge management

and specialty may pursue implicit goals which may serve self-interest more than patient well-being. Goal conflicts arise especially when resources are restricted. The understaffing of the Emergency Department in the case study may have been due to a conflict between "good medical treatment and "economic success," which was resolved in favor of short-time economic savings.

14.4.3 Medical Equipment-Related Incidents

Equipment-related incidents represent only a minority of incidents in a high-stakes medical environment (9–20% of all incidents; for anesthesia: Chopra et al. 1992; Cooper et al. 1978; Cooper at al. 1984; Currie 1989; Webb et al. 1993; for intensive care: Valentin et al. 2006). They nevertheless can have serious consequences if the equipment affected is highly invasive or life supporting, and if tight coupling exists between patient and device (e.g., infusion pump with vasoactive drug, ventilator, cardiopulmonary bypass pump). The problems and incidents reported can be divided into two groups: equipment malfunctions and user problems.

14.4.3.1 Equipment Malfunction

Equipment malfunction results from a technical problem that is not caused by the user. Instead device failures are caused by an inherent defect in the design, in faulty construction, or in poor manufacturing such as inadequate mechanical assembly. Equipment malfunction can be caused by software error or random failure of a component. In addition, many device components are not of adequate strength to survive reasonably anticipated conditions of use and break down after only a short service life. The majority of equipment failure can be detected by regular pre-use checks and service. Life of devices can be prolonged by regular equipment maintenance and servicing.

Given these reasons for malfunctioning, we usually find human error or organizational factors behind the "technical failure." Healthcare providers at the "sharp end" should especially acknowledge the importance of regular equipment checks and services.

14.4.3.2 User Error

More often than by a breakdown of faulty equipment, medical technology-related incidents are caused by the users themselves: User problems have been identified as the most frequent cause of medical equipment incidents; however, the term "user error" carries the problematic implication that the device malfunction was totally caused by, and therefore can be blamed on, the healthcare professional. The Human Factors Theory rejects this assessment of cause because bad design or a particular complex and tedious user interface and programming logic will "force" users to make predictable mistakes. In addition, the size, shape, and legibility of monitor displays, the position of controls, and the quality of alarms (to name only a few physical properties

of equipment) constrain the way in which a person can acquire and use information. In this perspective, bad designs have been considered "accidents waiting to happen" (Cooper and Newbower 1975). To the extent manual devices are giving way to computer-based systems, an adequate mental model of the programming logic and the different operational modes have become prerequisites for safe handling; otherwise, healthcare providers will have great difficulty in diagnosing difficult or unusual equipment problems (Woods et al. 1989).

As with "human error," "user error" also is not mainly a characteristic of the healthcare professional – it is a property of medical technology that includes the user. The likelihood for user errors is greatly increased in the presence of faulty engineering and in critical situations.

The following common user (and technology) errors have been identified (e.g., Hymann 1994; Weinger 1999):

- Ineffective user interface: Tools are too complicated for the operator to understand. Knobs are replaced by soft keys where the same physical button has different functions depending on the place in the software menu.
- Implementation of useless applications: Manufactures design complex medical equipment which offers much more capability than is usual or necessary in the application.
- Use of equipment under inappropriate circumstances, e.g., use of integrated ICU monitors for anesthesia resulting in displays with overly compressed information; use of critical care equipment in home care with unanticipated errors by users unfamiliar with complex electronic devices.
- Over-reliance on monitoring: Over-reliance on monitoring is most likely to occur during a clinical crisis in which the healthcare provider may avoid verifying any monitor value by clinical diagnostic.
- Insufficient setup and default modes: disabled alarms, inappropriate alarm thresholds.
- Inadequate feedback to device status: Especially elder generations of medical devices tended to surprise users by error messages such as "Error 22AE17." In addition, often information about fundamental device status (e.g., "on/off/standby") was missing.
- Inadequate task-specific training: Insufficient knowledge of the healthcare professional is

caused by a lack of standardized training. This can inadvertently lead to the nonappliance of the manufacturer's operating standards.

— Documentation is ineffective or incomplete.

14.4.3.3 Medical Device Clutter

A third category of equipment-related incidents is neither caused by faulty construction nor the user but instead by the simultaneous use of multiple devices from varying manufacturers for one patient. Because medical devices are often complex, durable equipment with a considerable lifespan, different technology generations with a different user philosophy may coexist in the same high-stakes medical environment (e.g., emergency room, operating room, intensive care unit). This results in physical and visual clutter common in many intensive care units and operating rooms. Clutter carries the risk of the healthcare provider confusing various lines, leads, and in tracking monitor alarms.

The regular less-than-optimum placement of monitoring equipment behind the anesthesia-provider equipment in the anesthesia environment is another example of workplace architecture which does not meet ergonomic criteria.

14.4.4 Human Resource Management

Accessible healthcare requires well-trained and well-motivated physician and nurse workforces of an adequate size that are able to deliver safe, high-quality medical services. Over the past decades, however, healthcare services have been losing their competitiveness as employers as moderate revenues concurrent with increasing workload and unsatisfactory career perspective have contributed to an increasing reluctance to enter healthcare. As a result, healthcare organizations have increased their efforts in developing human resource concepts contingent on organizational needs as well as economic and political circumstances. The theoretical underpinnings as well as practical techniques of managing a workforce are provided by Human Resource Management (HRM). In today's healthcare systems HRM tries to cover the gap between economic interests in healthcare and the individual employee's needs and objectives. The HRM takes a positive view of healthcare professionals, assuming that virtually all wish to contrib-

ute to safe patient care. Given the importance of skilled and motivated healthcare professionals for an efficient and safe delivery of patient care, and for the avoidance of errors, HRM has to serve six key functions:

— Determination of staff requirement: Long-term organizational goals determine the quantity of trained healthcare professionals needed; however, whether or not the planning can be put into practice is highly dependent on the way the organization solves the short-term conflict of available financial resources and staff requirement. A suboptimal solution of the dueling priorities leads to staff shortage, long working hours, and a decline in morale.

— Staff recruitment and selection: A thorough job analysis is required to determine the level of technical skills, competencies, and necessary flexibility of a potential employee. Despite the availability of adequate diagnostic tools for staff selection, current practice still seems to be that employees are hired according to personal "diagnostic standards" of chairmen and other responsible persons. As a result, certain personality traits may accumulate systematically within an organization: If the head of a department has a conflict-avoiding personality, he or she will prefer conflict-avoiding staff members. This tendency in turn may create a certain team climate where members are reluctant to advocate their position or voice concerns.

— Clinical job assignment: Staff assignment is responsible for task allocation "on site." Problematic aspects in staff assignment are constantly changing schedules for operations with surgeons operating or anesthetists anesthetizing patients of whose medical history they are unaware. Even worse, healthcare providers are assigned tasks which exceed their knowledge and experience, such as emergency physicians with limited experience with pediatric patients being responsible for any patient presenting at the Emergency Department.

— Evaluation of clinical performance: The HRM strategies include the design of compliant, consistent, and effective competency-assessment programs.

— Promotions and remuneration: In the face of a tightening market for qualified healthcare professionals, healthcare employers will have to compete for employees by offering financial rewards and fulfilling job opportunities.

- Human resource development: "Producing" better-trained healthcare professionals with relevant qualifications and higher clinical proficiency. This is best done by applying principles of knowledge management (▶ Chap. 15) and by integrating formal teamwork-training interventions (▶ Chap. 15) into quality-improvement efforts.

Human resource management affects patient safety directly, despite the fact that decision makers have no direct patient contact. This is quite obvious in the case study: The concatenation of unfortunate circumstances might not have occurred if the Emergency Department had been adequately staffed with physicians and qualified nurses; however, the strategic decision to provide a department or ward with enough qualified staff will only be made if patient safety is an organization's top priority.

In addition to the human resource issues, this century has seen another vital challenge emerge for the provision of acute medical care: On a national scale issues such as hospital emergency planning and disaster preparedness have come into focus. The constant threat of mass casualties caused by terrorist bombings and bioterrorism pose a completely new challenge for the provision of emergency medical care.

14.5 "Organizations and Human Error": in a Nutshell

- Although healthcare delivery is usually not thought of as a system, its most distinctive characteristic is its uniqueness as a socio-technical system, defined as the way human behavior and an organization's complex infrastructures interact.
- Organizational theory has different perspectives on organizations: the structural perspective; the human resource approach; and the functional perspective.
- Organizations develop as instruments for attaining specific goals: They emerge in situations where people recognize a common or complementary advantage that can best be served through collective action.
- The Human Factors approach studies human abilities and characteristics as they affect the design and smooth operation of equipment, systems, and jobs. From a human factors perspec-

tive "human error" is not mainly a property of humans – it is a property of systems that *include* humans.
- The Normal Accident Theory states the idea that as soon as technological systems have become sufficiently complex, accidents will be inevitable and therefore "normal."
- The High Reliability Theory emphasizes that organizations can contribute significantly to the prevention of accidents through good organizational design and management and mindful attention to ongoing operations.
- Key system issues for addressing error and safety in acute medical care include structure and processes, equipment-related incidents, HRM, teamwork and leadership, good communication, and organizational culture.

References

Alvesson M (2002) Understanding organizational culture. Sage Publications, London

Argyris C (1957) Personality and organization. Harper and Row, New York

Argyris C, Schön DA (1996) Organizational learning II: theory, method and practice. Addison–Wesley, Reading, Massachusetts

Bedeian AG (1984) Organizations. Theories and analysis. Saunders College Publishing, New York

Black RJ (2003) Organisational culture: creating the influence needed for strategic success. Dissertation.com, London

Bolman LG, Deal TE (1984) Modern approaches to understanding and managing organizations. Jossey–Bass, London

Burke CS, Salas E, Wilson-Donnelly K, Priest H (2004) How to turn a team of experts into an expert medical team: guidance from the aviation and military communities. Qual Saf Health Care 13 (Suppl 1):i96–i194

Carayon P (ed) (2006) Handbook of human factors and ergonomics in health care and patient safety (Human Factors and Ergonomics Series). Erlbaum, Mahwah

Chopra V, Bovill JG, Spierdijk J, Koornneef F (1992) Reported significant observations during anaesthesia: a prospective analysis over an 18-month period. Br J Anaesth 68:13–18

Cooper JB, Newbower RS (1975) The anesthesia machine: an accident waiting to happen. In: Picket RM, Triggs TJ (eds) Human factors in healh care. Lexington Books, Lexington, Massachusetts, pp 345–358

Cooper JB, Newbower RS, Long CD, McPeek B (1978) Preventable anesthesia mishaps: a study of human factors. Anesthesiology 49:399–406

Cooper JB, Newbower RS, Kitz RJ (1984) An analysis of major errors and equipment failures in anesthesia management: considerations for prevention and detection. Anesthesiology 60:34–42

Currie M (1989) A prospective survey of anaesthetic critical events in a teaching hospital. Anaesth Intensive Care 17:403–411

Entin EE, Serfaty D (1999) Adaptive team coordination. Hum Factors 41:312–325

Flin R, Maran N (2004) Identifying and training non-technical skills for teams in acute medicine. Qual Saf Health Care 13(Suppl):i80–i84

Gaba DM (1989) Human error in anesthetic mishaps. Int Anesth Clin 27:137–147

Gouldner AW (1959) Organizational analysis. In: Merton RK, Broom L, Cottrell LS (eds) Sociology today. Basic Books, New York

Helmreich RL (1998) The downside of having a brain: reflections on human error and CRM. University of Texas Aerospace Crew Research Project Technical Report 98-04

Helmreich RL, Merritt AC, Wilhelm JA (1999) The evolution of crew resource management in commercial aviation. Int J Aviat Psychol 9:19–32

Hoff T, Jameson L, Hannan E, Flink E (2004) A review of the literature examining linkages between organizational factors, medical errors, and patient safety. Med Care Res Rev 6:3–37

Hollagel E, Woods DD, Leveson N (eds) (2006) Resilience engineering. Concepts and precepts. Ashgate, Aldershot

Hymann WA (1994) Errors in the use of medical equipment. In: Bogner MS (ed) Human error in medicine. Erlbaum, Hillsdale, pp 327–347

Jung H (2001) Personalwirtschaft [Human resource management]. Oldenbourg, München

Kieser A (2002) Organisationtheorien [Organizational theories]. Kohlhammer, Stuttgart

Kohn L, Corrigan J, Donaldson M (eds) (1999) To err is human: building a safer health system. Committee on Quality of Health Care in America, Institute of Medicine (IOM). National Academy Press, Washington DC

LaPorte TR (1982) On the design and management of nearly error-free organizational control systems. In: Sills DL, Wolf CP, Shelanski VB (eds) Accident at Three-Mile Island: the human dimensions. Westview, Boulder, Colorado, pp 185–200

Moray N (1994) Error reduction as a systems problem. In: Bogner MS (ed) Human error in medicine. Erlbaum, Hillsdale, pp 67–91

Morell RC, Eichhorn JH (eds) (1997) Patient safety in anesthetic practice. Churchill Livingstone, New York

Norman DA (1988) The psychology of everyday things. Basic Books, New York

O'Connor RE, Slovis CM, Hunt RC, Pirrallo RG, Sayre MR (2002) Eliminating errors in emergency medical services: realities and recommendations. Prehosp Emerg Care 6:107–113

Perrow C (1984) Normal accidents: living with high-risk technologies. Basic Books, New York

Perrow C (1994) Accidents in high-risk systems. Technol Stud 1:1–38

Perrow C (1999) Normal accidents. Living with high-risk technologies. Princeton University Press, Princeton

Rasmussen J (1982) Human errors: a taxonomy for describing human malfunction in industrial installations. J Occup Accid 4:311–335

Reason J (1990a) Human error. Cambridge University Press, Cambridge

Reason J (1990b) The contribution of latent human failures to the breakdown of complex systems. Phil Trans R Soc Lond 327:475–484

Reason J (1997) Managing the risks of organizational accident. Ashgate, Aldershot.

Roberts KH (1990) Managing high reliability organizations. Calif Manage Rev 32:101–113

Rochlin GI (1993) Defining "high reliability" organizations in practice: a taxonomic prologue. In: Roberts KH (ed) New challenges to understanding organizations. Macmillan, New York, pp 11–32

Schulman PR (1993) The analysis of high reliability organizations: a comparative framework. In: Roberts KH (ed) New challenges to understanding organizations. Macmillan, New York, pp 33–54

Senge P (1990) The fifth discipline: The art and practice of the learning organization. Doubleday, New York

Thomas EJ, Helmreich RL (2002) Will airline safety models work in medicine? In: Rosenthal MM, Sutcliffe KM (eds) Medical error: What do we know? What do we do? Jossey–Bass, San Francisco, pp 217–234

Valentin A, Capuzzo M, Guidet B, Moreno RP, Dolanski L, Bauer P, Metnitz PG (2006) Patient safety in intensive care: results from the multinational Sentinel Events Evaluation (SEE) study. Intensive Care Med 32:1591–1598

Vaughan D (1997) The Challenger launch decision: risky technology, culture, and deviance at NASA. University of Chicago Press, Chicago, Illinois

Vicente KJ (2004) The human factor. Revolutionizing the way people live with technology. Routledge, New York

Webb RK, Russell WJ, Klepper I, Runciman WB (1993) The Australian Incident Monitoring Study. Equipment failure: an analysis of 2000 incident reports. Anaesth Intensive Care 21:673–677

Weick KE, Sutcliffe KM (2001) Managing the unexpected: assuring high performance in an age of complexity. Jossey–Bass, San Francisco

Weinger MB (1999) Anesthesia equipment and human error. J Clin Monit 15:319–323

Woods D, Cook R, Sarter N, McDonald J (1989) Mental models of anesthesia equipment operation: implications for patient safety. Anesthesiology 71:A983

15   Reliable Acute Care Medicine

15.1   Case Study

A patient was prepared to undergo major abdominal surgery and received a thoracic epidural catheter prior to the induction of anesthesia. At the end of the operation, a local anesthetic was given and a PCEA pump was connected in the recovery room. Following an uneventful postoperative course in the postoperative care unit (PACU), the patient was transferred to a general ward. He was awake and had stable vital signs. At 2:00 a.m. the anesthesia resident was paged by the night nurse and told that "either the catheter has become displaced or something's wrong with the pump." Further inquiry revealed that the patient complained about increasing pain that could not be relieved by boluses of local anesthetic. Upon arrival, the resident observed a patient who was fully oriented, had noninvasive blood pressure values of 100/50 mmHg, a heart rate of 45 bpm and a saturation of 94%. The anesthetist inspected the insertion site and catheter and realized that the PCEA line was not connected to the filter but instead to the central intravenous line. Because it was difficult to determine when the improper connection occurred, the exact amount of local anesthetic that was injected intravenously was impossible to calculate. The patient was transferred to the intensive care unit. Without any additional therapeutic measures, the blood pressure and heart rate returned to normal and the patient was transferred back to the general ward during the afternoon of the same day. The resident physician decided to enter the case into the hospital electronic critical-incident reporting system. While doing so, she realized that this was the third case in 1 year in which a PCEA pump had been inadvertently connected to a central i.v. line. These incidents were presented at the Anesthesia Department's next quality-control conference. A root cause analysis prior to the presentation indicated that the contributing factors were high staff turnover on the wards and a lack of familiarity with the technique and equipment. Furthermore, many of the new nurses did not know the difference between patient-controlled intravenous (PCIA) and epidural (PCEA) analgesia. In addition, the intravenous and epidural lines were similar in appearance and could be easily confused. The members of the quality-control conference suggested several solutions to the problem. Firstly, standard operating procedures were to be

developed allowing only nurses who had appropriate training in the particular technique to operate the pump. Secondly, the staff of the pain clinic was to devise a plan to have all the ward nurses trained on the use of the pump within the next few months. Thirdly, a label "for epidural use only" was to be attached to the epidural line as a reminder to the operator. The incident was presented at the next morbidity and mortality conference and was welcomed by the hospital simulation center as a new teaching case for resident physicians.

A patient receives a thoracic epidural catheter for postoperative pain relief. On arrival at the PACU the epidural catheter is connected to a delivery pump containing a dilute mixture of local anesthetic and opioid (PCEA pump; *Patient-Controlled Epidural Analgesia*). Satisfactory epidural blockage is established. Several hours after the operation, the patient is transferred to a general ward with stable vital signs and with efficient pain control. In the course of the next hours the line from the PCEA pump is disconnected from the epidural catheter for reasons unknown and improperly connected to the central i.v. line. This error is facilitated by the nurse's lack of familiarity with the different techniques of pain relief and the fact that both lines are from the same manufacturer and are similar in appearance. As a result of the misconnection, the pump infuses the local anesthetic and the opioid intravenously. Due to insufficient pain reduction, the patient requests PCEA boli more frequently; however, instead of relieving the pain, the requested boli now lead to short periods of dizziness. The incident is detected before toxic plasma levels of the local anesthetic are reached and thus has no long-term consequences for the patient. Because the hospital has established an Incident-Reporting System (IRS), the reporting physician is able to notice that two similar incidents had occurred within the past months. Because all three incidents reveal a similar pattern, a systemic problem seems much more likely than an isolated personal failure. The physician directs the hospital's risk management appointee's attention to these incidents. The root cause analysis results in several practical steps to solve the problem. The knowledge gained from these incidents is fed back into the system by creating guidelines and additional teaching opportunities (e.g., morbidity and mortality conference, simulation-based training).

15.2 Business Objective: Patient Safety

Despite all preventive efforts, critical incidents occur in high-stakes medical environment on a daily basis and in manifold ways. More often than not, faulty individual actions are identified as the last step in a chain of errors. It only takes a moment of inattention to improperly connect a plastic line, turning an efficient drug-delivery system into a vital threat to a patient. Fortunately, the majority of these incidents are detected and "defused" before a patient is harmed, but there is no guarantee that healthcare providers can correct every single error in due time: Several other healthcare providers had taken care of the patient prior to the anesthetist's intervention – without anyone noticing the improper connection and the associated hazard. Therefore, patient safety should never depend on specific individuals being at the right time at the right place and taking care of a problem they notice by chance. If patient safety is to become the main business objective in healthcare, the development of an efficient *safety culture* is a main task. The concept of a safety culture implies that all organizational structures and processes, all working places and equipment, the qualification standards of all staff members, and the relationship among the staff are shaped in a way that enables safe behavior at any time and at any given working place. Reliable patient care and maximum patient safety will only become reality if every single healthcare puts patient safety first on his or her personal agenda. It may seem a contradiction to say that safety must not depend on individuals, and at the same time that safety culture depends on every single person in the organization, but an individual's errors can only be reliably detected if structures and processes are organized in a way that others are willing and able to detect them. Only if the safety culture is supported by all staff will this work.

Unfortunately, the achievement of safety is no once-and-for-all event. Instead, safety is a "dynamic *nonevent*" (Reason 1997); "nonevent" because it cannot be described as the "presence of something" but rather as the continuous absence of accidents, the nonrealization of unwanted incidents. The fact that safe medical care can never be an everlasting condition makes it a "dynamic" task: We will have to strive relentlessly to maintain patient safety. Because complacency and inattention constantly threaten patient safety, every healthcare professional will be well advised to heed James Reason's warning: "Don't forget to be afraid" (◘ Fig. 15.1; Reason 1997).

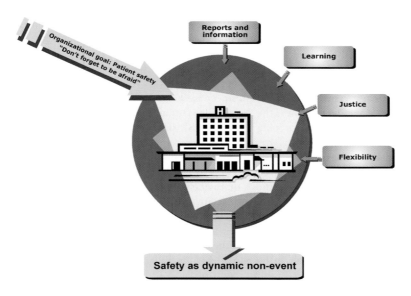

◘ **Fig. 15.1** Elements of a safety culture. Safety is not a static feature of a system but rather the dynamic absence of critical events for which a person or team has to continuously strive

In order to strengthen patient safety, it has to become the central management task for healthcare institutions: Hospitals will have to turn into High Reliability Organizations (HROs). Safety and reliability will then no longer be delegated to single officials such as health service managers, patient safety and quality officers, or risk management coordinators; instead, they will be the responsibility of every single member within an organization. Healthcare professionals on every level of the hospital, from management down to the actual providers of medical care, will cooperate to make patient safety *the* most important business objective.

15.2.1 Safety Culture Means Organizational Culture

"Organizational culture" defines the shared values, norms, and expectations that govern the way people approach their work and interact with each other. It is an amalgam of the values and beliefs of the people in an organization (Bedeian 1984), the silent governor of behavior, the way "how we really behave here." The culture of an organization is positioned at the heart of a system's vulnerability to error because of its role in framing organizational blindness to risk. The very nature of culture enforces conformity of organizational members and resists cultural change. Because cultural norms typically supported past success, it can be difficult to embed new norms that run counter to prevailing cultural values; however, if organizational culture is intentionally shaped around patient safety, and if safe patient care it is anchored as a central management task in the minds of all staff members, then the odds are high that patient safety indeed will become the defining characteristic of an organization.

Every healthcare organization has its own unique culture, even if there have been no conscious efforts to create it. In most organizations the prevailing culture has been created unconsciously, based on the values the founders and the variations of values that managers and clinical directors add. But it is also shaped by the staff's beliefs and attitudes. Organizational culture can be seen from the implicit rules and expectations with respect to an individual's behavior. The organizational culture is characterized by:

— The organization's mission statement
— Values, beliefs, norms, and maxims

— Traditional behavioral patterns ("the way we do it!")
— The character of interpersonal relationships (e.g., the way physicians of different specialties interact or physicians and nurses cooperate)
— The learning culture

A strong corporate identity with which all professional groups can identify ("we from the hospital X," "we from the intensive care unit Y," EMS from city Z") is a very powerful tool to embed patient safety in an organizational culture. During and after critical incidents, the quality of an organizational culture becomes most evident: The way patients are treated, how problems are solved, whether or not effective teams are formed across all boundaries of profession and specialty, and the way difficult situations are debriefed have a lot to tell about the organizational culture.

15.2.2 The Contribution of Organizational Theories on Error

Chapter 14 introduced three influential conceptual frameworks that address the issue of patient safety and human fallibility from a systemic perspective. Each theoretical approach focuses on a different set of organizational dynamics and provides a complementary insight in the dynamics of error occurrence for the development of a safety culture within an organization: The Human Factors approach emphasizes the limitations normal cognitive processes impose on decision-making, and that the systems of which humans are a part call forth errors from humans, not the other way around. "Human error" is not mainly a property of humans – it is a property of systems that *include* humans. Human factors engineering tries to optimize the relationship between humans and systems by designing systems and human–machine interfaces that are robust enough to reduce error rates. Furthermore, it encourages organizations to counterbalance the limitation of individual decision-making and performance by implementing formal teamwork-training interventions.

Normal Accident Theory (NAT) alludes to the structural factors (i.e., interactive complexity and loose/tight coupling) that shape the probability for the occurrence of incidents and accidents within an organizational system. According to NAT, no complex system with tight coupling of processes can be rendered foolproof; therefore, it is only a matter of time until the next accident occurs within an organization.

In contrast to NAT, which claims that it is impossible to prevent severe accidents in sufficiently complex system, the High Reliability Theory has a more optimistic approach and emphasizes that organizations can contribute significantly to the prevention of accidents. Organizational design and management, not structural dynamics, play an important role in promoting "error-free performance." Redundancies, simulations, decentralized decision-making, learning from mistakes, mindfulness, good training, and experienced personnel are seen as important requisites for a "culture of reliability." Some of these features are described below.

15.2.3 Safety Through Shared Information

Values and beliefs, relationships, learning, and other aspects of organizational safety culture are all about sharing and processing information. So, "safety culture" can be equated with "informed culture" (Reason 1997). An informed culture deals with the potential accidents and errors in an organization. This is done mainly by analyzing latent errors (▶ Chaps. 3, 14) and less by trying to detect single errors in hindsight. In order to establish an informed culture, organizations should strive for the following aspects (Weick and Sutcliffe 2001):

— Reports and information: If organizations want to learn most from the "lessons for free" that incidents provide, information about events, errors, and deviations is crucial. If members of an organization are expected to share information about situations where they made mistakes, the culture in an organization needs to be free of blame and open for communication. The management has to decide which kind of information about errors is seen as trustworthy (e.g., written or verbal information, information upon request or spontaneously delivered, anonymous, etc.). Incident Reporting Systems are an important part of this gathering of information.
— Justice: If a serious accident occurs, the focus will not be on blaming individuals; instead, great care is taken to analyze the event for latent errors. Nevertheless, personal responsibility

remains intact: There is no general amnesty for errors. Every member within an organization is aware of error-provoking actions that will not be accepted (e.g., disrespect for standard operating procedures, violations of safety rules, alcohol ingestion during work, etc.) and will have disciplinary consequences. So, the message is "we will not blame you for errors that occur if you work in a responsible way". Information about the line between forgivingness and sanctions are important for members' feeling of being treated justly.
— Flexibility: During emergency situations, decisions will be made by local experts at the "sharp end." The advantage of this procedure is that decisions can be made without having to wait for confirmation from higher levels of hierarchy. Every member knows which decision competence is expected and he or she will act accordingly. Leaders within the organization encourage other members to display flexibility during their decisions in critical situations. Information about competencies and ways of decision-making is part of this approach to safety!
— Learning processes: Learning, too, is an integral part of an informed culture. Every member, including management, is eager and capable to learn from incidents and change behavior.

15.3 Avoidance of Error

High reliability organizations strive to avoid errors; however, as they know that incidents and accidents will occur from the rare combination of latent and active failures (▶ Chap. 3) no matter how hard you try, they do not expect a faultless performance of the people within their organization; instead, they put great effort into the development of resilience in order to contain errors as far as possible. Concrete measures to avoid the errors discussed in this chapter are, on a superordinate level, the following:
— Imagination against accidents
— Improved qualification of healthcare professionals
— General measures of quality improvement

At the "sharp end" the measures are:
— Standards
— Checklists

15.3.1 Using Imagination to Avoid Incidents

A powerful tool to anticipate incidents and avoid errors is readily available: People can use their imagination to create "worst-case scenarios" and see whether they themselves, their team, or the entire organization would be prepared to cope with the situation. This approach is especially helpful with rare problems and events. Similar to planning (▶ Chap. 7) people can think through the implications of a certain situation or reflect on consequences of their potential actions. The mental simulation of hazardous situations has the big advantage that it is not real. Change can be initiated without a single patient having been harmed. From real events an organization can only learn once they happened. This would mean in the healthcare setting that learning opportunities arise only from patients being harmed. The disadvantage of using imagination could be overconfidence in one's own preparedness: Despite all creative imagination, there might still be some details missing: In "reality" some minor detail may jeopardize even the best plan.

Because accidents occur as a rare constellation of predisposing conditions and active failures it is very unlikely that the same combination of factors will ever again cause an identical event. Again, imagination will be helpful to get the most out of the actual incident or accident. Simply by asking: "What else could have happened? Are there any safety measures we could have taken in advance? How could a similar "trajectory" (▶ Chap. 3; Reason 1990) through all safety barriers look?" alternate scenarios can be created and analyzed.

In contrast to the anticipation of rare events, imagination is not as vital when dealing with routine actions: In this case the predisposing factors and conditions under which errors can occur are well known. These conditions can be systematically changed with the intention of completely avoiding errors.

15.3.2 Qualification

Skills and knowledge of healthcare professionals are the decisive human resource for an efficient and safe delivery of patient care and the avoidance of errors. The systematic enhancement of staff qualification by providing knowledge and training opportunities can be a major investment in patient safety. In recent years the healthcare community has started to incorporate nontechnical skills into the training of teams in acute care settings (e.g., Fletcher et al. 2002; Flin and Maran 2004; Reader et al. 2006; Yule et al. 2006): Structured teamwork of caregivers can considerably be enhanced by learning how to define, execute, and monitor the delivery of care in a coordinated fashion. Multidisciplinary simulation-based healthcare education and problem-based learning are two approaches to foster.

Leaders in the healthcare setting should embody this approach and should be role models as clinical teachers by providing clinical and educational supervision and by mentoring the trainee (e.g., bedside teaching; Kumar and Dodds 2003).

An organization which decides on integrating these approaches into their system, however, should maintain a realistic time frame and a reasonable conception about what is possible and what not: Civil aviation has been struggling for over three decades to create a culture supportive of human error-related issues, and to foster skills and attitudes of error avoidance and high-stakes team performance.

15.3.2.1 Simulation-Based Education and Crisis Resource Management

Simulation for medical and healthcare applications has revolutionized the way healthcare is taught. The number of centers with simulation labs has increased considerably over the past decade, from a mere handful at the end of the past century to alone over 500 in 2007 in the United States. Depending on the aspect of the environment which is replicated by a simulator, the devices can be classified as part-task trainer, low-fidelity screen-based simulators, intermediate-fidelity simulators, high-fidelity mannequin-based simulators, virtual reality, and, in its early stages, immersive virtual environments (◘ Figs. 15.2, 15.3; Cooper and Taqueti 2004; Gaba 1996; Glavin and Maran 2003; Mantovani et al. 2003; Reznek et al. 2002; Rosenberg 2000).

A special case of simulation is the use of standardized patients, actors who are trained to behave like patients with real diseases. Standardized patients are used mostly in the education of medical students where access to real patients with a

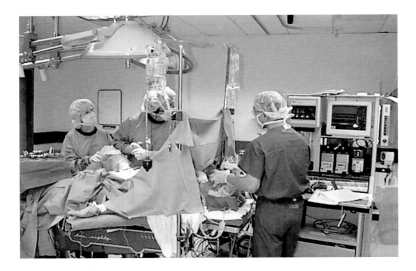

◻ Fig. 15.2 Simulation-based training of medical emergencies. (Courtesy of Center for Medical Simulation in Boston)

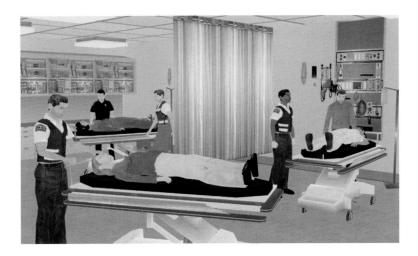

◻ Fig. 15.3 Virtual team training environment. The simulation is Web based and trainees are represented by avatars which participate with first responders and clinical staff (Courtesy of Forterra Systems Inc., U.S. Army TATRC, and the SUMMIT group at the Stanford University School of Medicine, Stanford, Calif.)

specific pathophysiology may prove difficult. Simulation covers almost all aspects of technical and nontechnical learning by providing tools to train skills, rules, and knowledge. In the context of training healthcare professionals to perform in a high-stakes medical environment, full-scale simulators, sophisticated human-like mannequins driven by physiological and pharmacological software models, are routinely used to substitute for an actual patient encounter. There are several advantages of simulation-based training over bedside teaching. The main benefits of high-fidelity simulation are (Glavin and Maran 2003; Jha et al. 2001):

– Any skill, procedure, or management of a critical situation can be practiced as often as required without any risk to the patient.

- Trainees can try to fend for themselves when faced with a critical incident. Because there is no need to hand the case over to a more experienced clinician, beginners can see the result of decisions and actions in their ultimate consequences.
- Errors are allowed to occur and reach their conclusion. Trainees are allowed to commit errors and will learn from these errors.
- The same scenario can be presented to learners many times and alternative strategies can be tried.
- Uncommon but critical events in which a rapid response is needed can be rehearsed, and a systematic approach to medical emergencies can be trained.
- Interpersonal skills can be explored; communication, teamwork, and leadership can be trained with staff members.

The most important development fueled by the availability of full-scale simulators was the possibility to train entire teams in a real-life setting by adopting the aviation concept of Crew Resource Management (CRM) for the purposes of acute medical care. Crew Resource Management, a safety training developed in the late 1970s by aviation psychologists, emphasizes the role of human factors in high-stakes environments (e.g., Helmreich et al. 1999). The CRM teaches crew members to use all available resources (information, equipment, and other team members) to achieve safe and efficient flight operations. Over three decades ago, anesthesia departments started to apply this training concept for the management of intraoperative complications (Runciman 1988). In the subsequent years basic components of CRM were tailored to the needs of clinicians and introduced as Anesthesia Crisis Resource Management (ACRM; Howard et al. 1992; for an overview see: Pizzi et al. 2001). Today, ACRM-like team trainings have been introduced in every acute medical care specialty (intensive care medicine: e.g., Kim et al. 2006, pediatric intensive care: e.g., Weinstock et al. 2005; delivery room: e.g., Halamek et al. 2000, emergency department: e.g., Reznek et al. 2003, Small et al. 1999; prehospital emergency care: e.g., Miller et al. 2001). Despite their diversity, all training interventions consist of similar modules:

- Information related to the Human Factors Theory

- Simulated critical incidents ("scenarios")
- Video-assisted debriefing
- Promoting of transfer

In addition to individual and team learning, the conceptual framework of CRM and related training concepts may stimulate healthcare professionals to engage in patient safety issues, the redesign of the working culture, and the error management strategies of their organization. High-fidelity simulation has recently been used to enhancing learning at a morbidity and mortality conference by recreating the actual patient encounter (Vozenilek et al. 2006).

Despite its great popularity, the true impact of CRM training in aviation and other complex working domains has yet to be determined. A review of 28 published accounts of CRM training in complex environments (e.g., aviation, medicine, offshore oil production, shipping/maritime, nuclear power domains; Salas et al. 2006) suggests mixed results of the impact of training on learning and behavioral changes. Findings indicate that CRM training generally produced positive reactions from trainees, but the transfer of the learned behaviors from the simulated environment to the job were not consistent. In cases where transfer was observed, it was based on the trainee's experience of a particular simulated scenario; thus, the powerful tool of simulation training needs to be explored further in order to yield optimal results.

15.3.2.2 Formal Teamwork-Training Interventions

Successful team performance is a significant tool for promoting patient safety and managing the change toward a fair and just organizational culture (Barrett and Gifford 2001; Firth-Cozens 2001; Frankel et al 2006; Powell 2006). Parallel to simulation-based training efforts, formal teamwork-training interventions have been introduced into many areas of high-stakes medical care (e.g., Morey et al. 2002; Thomas et al. 2006). Although the importance of teamwork is generally accepted in healthcare, the reality does not reflect this conviction: Most professionals work more in a parallel "play" understanding than in a real team concept. Teamwork-training interventions could cross divisions between professional groups and specialties within an organization, thus creating and maintaining true interdisciplinary teams;

however, these training interventions require unrestricted commitment and support by management and clinical directors: The culture in healthcare and lifelong habits will not be changed by an intervention lasting a day or two. In addition, as even the best results of team-training are simply diluted by time and inertia, the decision to provide team-training will require a long-term commitment to a training plan. If healthcare organizations decide on implementing team-training interventions, this will amount to an integrated and recurrent component of their healthcare provider's professional development, rather than being a one-time immunization.

Despite the many proven benefits for an organization, team-training interventions have not advanced significantly in medicine. The reasons may be either of the following:

- Most organizations in healthcare operate in a profit-motivated environment where decisions are often being made in antithesis to the principles of human factors and team-training. In contrast to many other decisions, financial investments in safety-relevant training efforts do not pay off immediately.
- Training in an interdisciplinary team is a personal challenge for every healthcare professional involved. Traditional boundaries between specialties and professions have to be overcome if all members want to function as a team. Long-held beliefs about own strengths make it difficult for individual healthcare providers to capitalize on the capabilities of the other professions and recognize their own limits.

15.3.3 Quality Assurance and Continuous Quality Improvement

The term "quality assurance" was initially introduced by business and industry and conceptualizes "all planned or systematic actions necessary to provide adequate confidence that a product or service will fulfill the requirements for quality as expected by the customer" (Bedeian 1984). In the context of healthcare, however, the "product" and "service" of interest are the patient's health and the quality of medical care. Quality assurance appointees systematically evaluate the quality of patient care as well as the design and establishment of mechanisms for improvement. The focus is on the structure (e.g., resources, personnel, facilities, equipment) and the process involved (e.g., the actual activities of

patient care, information management, teamwork, and leadership) as well as on the resultant outcome (e.g., wellness, length of stay, morbidity, mortality; see Eichhorn 1995). Continuous Quality Improvement (CQI) activities aim at delivery of the highest quality care. By focusing on latent errors and poor system design, CQI tries to eliminate preventable morbidity and mortality as much as possible.

15.3.3.1 Clinical Audits

A clinical audit is a systematic and objective evaluation of an organization (e.g., department, hospital, relief organization) that aims to improve patient care. Aspects of patient care – including structure, processes, and outcomes – are selected and evaluated against explicit criteria and, where necessary, changes are implemented at an individual, team, or service level (NHS 1996). Audit procedures include collecting, analyzing, interpreting, and documenting information by the auditors. These are either external auditors (independent staff assigned by an auditing firm) or internal auditors (healthcare providers from within the organization hired to assess and evaluate its system). Clinical audits are initiated and supported by the Board of Directors or top management. A clinical audit can be described as a cycle or spiral of several stages that follow the systematic process of:

- Problem identification
- Definition of criteria and standards
- Data collection
- Comparison of performance with criteria and standards
- Implementation of change
- Reaudit: sustaining change

Clinical audits in a medical high-stakes environment should focus on those structures and processes which are most likely influenced by latent errors: medical equipment (including maintenance); the preparation of planned procedures; patient positioning; drug administration errors; and the application of protocols and standard operating procedures (SOPs; Eichhorn 1995; O'Connor et al. 2002).

15.3.3.2 Quality Circles

A quality circle (QC) is a small volunteer group of healthcare professionals who meet at regular intervals to identify, analyze, and resolve workplace and patient-care-related issues (e.g., Robson 1989). Ideas and suggestions about how to improve the quality of healthcare processes and patient safety issues are presented to management. The QCs are usually led by a supervisor or a senior healthcare professional who acts as a moderator. The QCs can neither decide on changes nor put improvements into practice. Instead, they are based on two ideas: that employees can often make better suggestions for improving work processes than management and that employees are motivated by their participation in making such improvements. The acceptance of the instrument "quality circle" is highly dependent on the extent to which the management acts on suggestions from the QC. The working pattern of QCs should be systematized so that ideas for improvement are grouped according to central weaknesses of an organization (e.g., equipment, staff qualification, culture of leadership, communication, and cooperation).

15.3.4 Standards

Standardization, the deliberate strategy to maintain a high similarity in task performance, is aimed at guaranteeing the highest possible quality patient care in routine tasks. Standardization, however, can have a double-edged effect: On the one hand, healthcare professionals are provided with standards for professional conduct and instantly available sources of medical and procedural knowledge. This may help to prevent untoward outcomes or help to manage critical situations. On the other hand, many healthcare providers still perceive standardization as unnecessary bureaucratic drudgery and an unwanted restriction of the freedom they have in exercising their medical profession. Although the term "standard" is loosely applied to many elements of policy and procedure, the term "standard of care" carries significant medico-legal overtones: Once promulgated, a standard of care dictates mandatory practice. As an alternative, many departments have labeled their procedures as "guidelines," which serve to identify a responsible option and to guide task performance rather than dictating an approach. Standards can be agreed on within a group or department at a hospital (e.g., standards for patient hand-over) as well as on a superordinate level (e.g., local or state department, professional societies, accrediting body).

Apart from medical procedures, teamwork and communication can be the subject of standards: Standards in teamwork could apply to terminology, routine tasks, and emergency procedures (Buerschaper and St. Pierre 2003).

15.3.4.1 Standardization of Communication

Experience from other high-stakes environments (foremost civil and military aviation) has provided ample evidence that a standardization of communication technique can help to reduce misunderstanding in noisy and stressful situations (Conell 1996). Standard terminology (comparable to that of civil aviation) and the resulting avoidance of misunderstanding can help to reduce errors. Standards for communication processes ensure that messages are clearly "received" and understood. Those standards are termed *call-outs*, *readback*, and *hearback*. A call-out is a concise statement in a defined terminology (e.g., "Please step back, I will defibrillate"). Readback and hearback are a redundant procedure aimed at verifying that both, sender and receiver, understood what the communication partner said (▶ Chap. 12). The readback/hearback process continues until a shared understanding is mutually verified and the task has been executed. Due to a lack of familiarity with this technique, healthcare professionals tend to dismiss communication standards as unnecessary. Nevertheless, if healthcare professionals in a high-stakes medical environment want to reduce misunderstanding, the establishment of communication standards would be a promising way to go. These standards would have to become a habit in daily practice; only then would healthcare professionals be able to use them effectively in critical situations.

15.3.4.2 Standard Operating Procedure

A standard operating procedure, commonly abbreviated as SOP, is a detailed, written instruction to achieve uniformity of the performance of a specific function. Standard operating procedures exist for routine operations as well as for emergency situations. The SOPs for emergency situations should enable a structured approach to a critical situation and, at the same time, be flexible enough to meet situational demands. They emphasize the medical and technical steps and are complemented by general steps of organization of action (Cooper et al.

1993). The advantage is that SOPs describe successful guidelines for coping with an emergency situation. As a result, the individual has less to figure out, which is a relief in time-critical situations. Teams profit from SOPs because they offer a shared mental model of all steps and procedures involved. This facilitates coordination of joint actions. The availability of written checklists may help to unburden memory.

15.3.5 The Use of Checklists

15.3.5.1 Purpose of Checklists

Healthcare has relied heavily on clinicians' ability to recall critical information during a medical emergency. During stressful situations, however, memory is likely to be error-prone, resulting in a variety of planning and execution failures (► Chap. 3). Many inherently risky industries, such as commercial aviation and nuclear power, have tried to overcome this limitation by mandating the use and adherence to checklists and protocols. Critical situations in medicine, however, follow a much more unpredictable and disorganized pattern; therefore, a simple checklist may not be adequate to cover the complexity of acute medical care. Nevertheless, checklists could provide a cognitive aid for many unusual but acute conditions in medicine, which compensates for the limitations of human memory by providing additional therapeutic and diagnostic guidance to healthcare professionals (Harrison et al. 2006). Checklists can help to ensure consistency and completeness in carrying out all necessary procedures for a given task. In a medical high-stakes environment formal checklists can unburden memory and support individuals and teams in the following ways:

- Preparation and execution of routine tasks (e.g., preuse checkout of medical equipment, preparing for anesthesia induction)
- Anticipation of untoward events (e.g., preparations for weaning from cardiopulmonary bypass in cardiac anesthesia; preparing for a difficult-airway situation)
- Structured approach to problem-solving (e.g., troubleshooting malfunction of critical devices, ventilatory or hemodynamic problems in critically ill patients)
- Structuring of teamwork (e.g., team briefing, shared understanding of roles and responsibilities; see Buerschaper and St. Pierre 2003)

Checklists for routine tasks in complex systems contribute to a correct and complete execution of safety-relevant tasks. All steps involved are explicitly listed and have to be checked out in given order. An electronic checklist has been introduced that can give voice prompts and highlight errors to assist the healthcare provider in checking the preparations for general anesthesia (Hart and Owen 2005).

Checklists for unexpected problems can support the structured approach to diagnose a problem or find the cause of an event. If, for example, medical equipment fails, a checklist may help to localize the problem and find the most plausible cause in a meaningful order. Intraoperative problems may best be addressed by situational adapted checklists or by an electronic decision support system such as dynamically configured checklists (Sawa and Ohno-Machado 2001) which help to detect and manage problems in a timely manner by providing "intelligent alarms" for the most frequent intraoperative complications.

In contrast to routine tasks and problems accessible for a structured problem-solving (e.g., problems with technical equipment) checklists for emergency situations cannot cover in detail all steps involved, because every situation is a unique constellation of problems. Instead, they are directed at helping healthcare providers to consider possible causes and pay due attention to the necessary steps involved in sound decision-making (e.g., goal formation, risk assessment, effect control, ► Chap. 10). Checklists in an emergency situation are more a decisional aid than a check-off list. Due to these inherent limitations, healthcare professionals have generally preferred the use of algorithms over extensive checklists when faced with an emergency situation. Precompiled algorithms which can be applied quickly and effectively can facilitate a systematic and effective response to the wide range of potentially lethal problems. Intensive efforts over a period of more than 15 years have led to the development and testing of an algorithm for the management of any crisis under anesthesia (Runciman and Merry 2005).

15.3.5.2 Checklists: Necessary? Cumbersome?

Research on the use of checklists has provided clear evidence that problems with medical equipment as well as the likelihood of drug errors can be dramatically reduced when checklists are applied (e.g.,

Arbous et al. 2005; Kumar et al. 1988). Despite these and other examples, there still seem to be reservations among healthcare providers against introducing and using them. Not too long ago the Anesthesia Apparatus Checkout Recommendations (checklist) recommended by the United States Food and Drug Administration (FDA) was only reluctantly accepted and used in clinical practice (Klopfenstein et al. 1998; Laboutique and Benhamou 1997; March and Crowley 1991). Although there seems to have been a significant increase in the past decade in the proportion of anesthesia providers undertaking machine checks, machine checking guidelines are still poorly followed (Langford et al. 2007).

If an organization intends to introduce checklists, the following questions should be answered in advance:

— For which routine tasks do checklists make sense? Which safety-relevant procedures are difficult to standardize and should be addressed by a variable, open list?
— If a critical situation arises, when should a checklist be used? As soon as the development is noticed or only after a conventional rule-based approach fails? Which team member is responsible for working through the checklist?
— Which mode of presentation is most suited for the healthcare setting? A paper-based list, a handbook, software for the PDA, or an implementation into the monitoring system?

> Instruments to achieve error reduction are:
> — Using imagination to avoid incidents
> — Qualification
> — Quality assurance and continuous quality improvement
> — Standards
> — Checklists

15.4 Error Management

Accidents usually result from the often unforeseeable combination of human and organizational failures in the presence of some weakness or gap in the system's many barriers and safeguards. Once an error has occurred, the countermeasures will include (a) detection, (b) diagnosis, and (c) mitigation of error consequences. Once an incident or an accident has occurred, it carries a lot of valuable information for both, the organization and the individual. Organizations can learn most from an

incident or accident if they focus on the organizational and contextual factors: Whereas individual unsafe acts are hard to predict and control, the factors that promote "human error" are present before the occurrence of an incident or accident. As such, they can be analyzed and converted into valuable knowledge for an organization. With the powerful tool of an IRS this form of error management focuses on organizational learning.

If unsafe acts or incidents are reflected upon immediately after the event, individual coping as well as individual and team learning are emphasized. Debriefing is an example of this kind of learning.

15.4.1 Incident-Reporting Systems

15.4.1.1 Learning from Incidents

An incident is an unintended event which reduces, or could reduce, the safety margin for a patient. At any time and any given place within a healthcare organization incidents happen. They are like the base of an iceberg – hidden below the surface (◘ Fig. 3.3). In contrast to accidents where a patient suffers from an adverse outcome, an incident has the potential to cause harm but does not unfold because safety barriers are effective; mindful healthcare professionals detect, diagnose, and correct them before they can threaten patient safety (and sometimes pure luck plays a role, too). The improper connection of the PCEA pump is an example for such an incident. Incidents can be triggered by individual errors, the patient's pathophysiology as well as organizational-process deficits. Normally, incidents and the corrective efforts remain below the "surface," where they would become visible to everyone. As a result, organizations appear, from an outsiders' perspective, to be error free and safe, and to produce the desired outcomes. Because healthcare providers constantly intervene and take corrective actions, the paradoxical situation arises that incidents do not "surface," although they constantly occur in organizations.

Despite their potential hazard to patient safety, incidents are nevertheless to some extent useful. "The vitality of erroneous actions lies in the extension of the behavioral repertoire" (Wehner 1992). Every time people commit an error they are given the opportunity to learn something new. Because the incident of the improper connection has no serious consequences, the hospital receives a "lesson for free" on patient safety: The incident indicates that the resources available (e.g., trained staff, equipment, process organization) are insufficient to ensure adequate quality of patient care. If an organization wants to get the most out of these lessons, it has to collect the information from the incident in an appropriate way, analyze it, and take measures to respond (❑ Fig. 15.4). In the past decade many hospitals and healthcare organizations have introduced IRS as part of their quality improvement efforts. The collection of data, however, is not an end in itself: The most important step for the acceptance and spread of IRS is to close the gap and acknowledge the consequences from the reported data. Members of an organization have to accept that their reports are read, analyzed, and have consequences (Hofinger and Waleczek 2003).

15.4.1.2 Development of Incident Reporting in Healthcare

The technique of critical incident analysis was first introduced by Flanagan in 1954 as an outgrowth of his studies in aviation psychology (Flanagan 1954). Incident analysis was further developed by the aviation domain into a voluntary reporting system which collected, analyzed, and responded to aviation safety incidents. The incident reporting technique was first applied in the medical community to address the issue of anesthetic equipment malfunction (Blum 1971) and was adapted a few years later to uncover patterns of frequently occurring incidents in an anesthesia department (Cooper et al. 1978; Williamson et al. 1985). The first organization in healthcare that started using the critical incident technique on a national scale plan was the Australian Patient Safety Foundation. As early as 1987 the Foundation launched the Australian Incident Monitoring Study (AIMS; Webb et al. 1993) to collect information on mishaps during and after anesthesia. The AIMS has been the cutting-edge project in incident reporting in high-stakes medical care and has inspired many societies and organizations to follow suit.

15.4.1.3 Characteristics of an Incident-Reporting System

Incident-Reporting Systems can only be helpful if the surrounding organizational culture supports a safety culture with a systemic approach. The basis for the collection of information about incidents

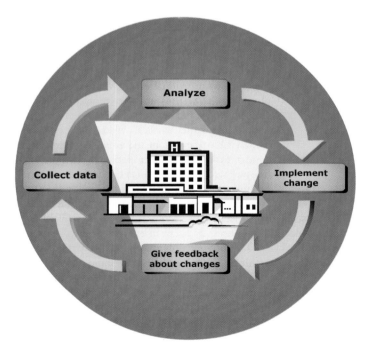

❑ **Fig. 15.4** Incident-reporting system: steps involved

and minimal events is a formalized reporting system. If it is to be successful, it has to be (Hofinger and Waleczek 2003):

- Voluntary: In contrast to the obligation to report accidents and mandatory legal aspects of an incident, the IRS depends on the voluntary report of members. Organizations can facilitate voluntary reporting if they communicate clearly to their members that any information submitted will not be used against them.
- Anonymous: Incidents can be reported without any link to the sender.
- Confidential: Any information concerning people involved, events, and actions taken will be handled confidentially in the further course of the evaluation.
- Nonpunitive: No report will have disciplinary consequences. Whoever reports an error or an incident must not fear punishment by the employer.
- No cases pending in court: In many countries the question remains unsettled as to whether or not legal authorities can access and use data which has been entered into an IRS (e.g., in many European countries). In these countries any accident pending court examination should not be reported.
- Support by the management: Whenever an IRS is introduced, the management has to support it strongly. The implementation is a top-down process. Leaders have to demonstrate the advantage of working through errors and make the necessity and implications of an IRS clear.

> The characteristics of an IRS are as follows:
> - Voluntary
> - Anonymous
> - Confidential
> - Free of legal consequences
> - No cases pending in court
> - Support by the management

If a voluntary reporting system is to be successful, the organization has to take heed of the following practical steps (Billings et al. 1998; Runciman et al. 1993; Staender 2000; Hofinger and Waleczek 2003):

- A hospital/healthcare institution should communicate relentlessly and convincingly to their staff that a policy of "no blame" be pursued. Staff members must be confident that no disciplinary action will be taken in reaction to a report, except in cases of gross misconduct or criminal negligence.
- All clinical and nursing staff should receive an induction training on risk management and incident reporting.
- The initial training should be followed by continuing education on the aims and importance of risk management and incident reporting.
- Every healthcare provider, regardless of profession and grade, should be aware of the fact that safety cannot be delegated to a single person (e.g., to the risk manager). A clear statement should be made that all members are responsible for reporting if patient safety is to improve.
- Incident reporting forms should be "user-friendly" and readily accessible for entry. Compliance with regular reporting will decrease if staff members are forced to take great additional efforts if they want to report an incident.
- Staff members should be encouraged to report any incident they find worth communicating irrespective of the assumed relevance or severity.
- Staff members should receive regular feedback on the consequences of their report.

15.4.1.4 Define the Content of Reports

The purpose of an IRS is a detailed documentation of *what* happened, *how* it happened, and *why* it presumably happened. From a technical perspective an IRS can consist of paper-based forms or a Web-based system. The reporting form should provide room for narratives rather than simple check-boxes for default options.

As for the content of the report, the informational value of a report depends highly on whether or not it is possible to elicit relevant contextual information in addition to the description of the event itself; therefore, the documentation should cover details about situational context, function, and experience of the healthcare professionals involved, the flow of information, and any action on behalf of the healthcare provider. Information about how decisions arose, which role teamwork played in the incident, and which information was accessible are just as important as those questions concerning equipment, drugs, and diagnostic or therapeutic steps. The previous history of an incident may further help to elucidate a situation. Great care should be placed on adequate formulation of questions and categories. This is especially true for human factors-related categories: Terms such as "situational awareness" are incomprehensible psychological jargon for the average healthcare provider. In contrast, categories such as "communication" may be much too general, because communication will always contribute to a critical situation in one way or another.

In addition to providing insight into factors contributing to unsafe conditions, an IRS also presents an opportunity to look for recoveries from dangerous situations. A category "recovery" may be helpful in documenting the strategy by which the incident was managed without patient harm. In addition, reporting systems should allow for suggestions as to how similar incidents can be prevented in the future. Questions concerning a perceived need for change might be helpful, too, because healthcare providers on the "sharp end" may have a profound insight into the system's weaknesses and strengths.

15.4.1.5 Promote Change

The documentation of incidents is only the first step in the process of organizational learning. In order to be able to draw consequences from an incident, the next steps have to be clarified: which group within the organization will evaluate the reports, in which way this will be done, and how will the results of the evaluation return to the organization. It is recommendable to establish a group of members who have a position of trust within the organization. The main tasks of this group consist of the work-up, classification, and presentation of reports, and in suggesting consequences. As the IRS group should not consist of managers, its task is ended with suggestions. Then it is up to the managers to implement change and provide information about changes to the whole staff. It is vital for any IRS that reports show consequences visible to those who reported. Because change generally takes time to take effect, it is just as important to make the current state of considerations visible, as it is to change the system.

The IRS uncover singular errors or problem constellations and indicate which resources were not sufficiently available. Every case is an indicator for a general structural problem. If a similar problem is encountered again and again, the assumption of a systematic error is probable.

On the other hand, good solutions can show where and how resources can be activated. This potential should intentionally be strengthened.

The study of recovery strategies and successful management of critical situations is the second equally important aspect of IRS. "What saved the day?" is the appropriate question to ask when an organization wants to learn how a potentially dangerous situation was prevented from progressing to a bad outcome (Staender 2000). Not only the weak aspects of systems, but also the innovative activities that empower humans at the "sharp end" to perform effectively provide a wealth of information which will help to improve patient safety.

15.4.2 Debriefing

15.4.2.1 Purpose of Debriefings

While many authors write about the debriefing process not all use the term "debriefing" to denote the same thing. Debriefing as a post-experience analytic process is variously defined as (Lederman 1992):

- Appraisal and generation of knowledge from experiences in work-related tasks
- Learning through reflection on a simulation experience
- Emotional recovery from a critical incident

In the context of work-related tasks debriefing provides healthcare providers with the basis for understanding why and how the new knowledge they acquired relates to what they already know. Team performance can greatly be enhanced by implementing regular debriefings at the end of every shift.

In the context of a simulated educational experience debriefing helps to facilitate learning for those who have been through the experience and those who have watched it (Dismukes et al. 2006). The process involves getting the participants to tell the story the way they experienced it, to describe the feelings elicited by the experience, and to reflect on one's own taken-for-granted assumptions, mental models, and professional work practice. In an environment that feels both psychologically safe and clinically challenging professionals improve their nontechnical skills by "reflective practice" (Rudolf et al. 2006).

Because accidents can pose an enormous emotional strain with serious long-term consequences (e.g., posttraumatic stress disorder), many organizations now offer a multistep coping concept following a critical event (e.g., critical incident stress debriefing; Hammond and Brooks 2001). Debriefings help individuals to come to terms with a situation by letting them describe what happened and allowing for emotional ventilation. In addition, early signs of a stress response syndrome can be identified (Hoff and Adamowski 1998; James and Gilliland 2001).

15.4.2.2 Competence for Debriefing

The purpose of debriefing is not to lecture or expound but instead to facilitate self-awareness, maximize group interaction, and foster idea development (Steinwachs 1992). Leaders who debrief staff members cannot do this by keeping to conventional hierarchical patterns. In contrast, it is necessary to learn specific competencies: Debriefings demand a high role flexibility as one is obliged to be teacher, critic, moderator, and enquirer all at the same time (McDonell et al. 1997). If possible, every team member should participate in the debriefing process. Positive feedback on successful performance as well as analysis of things gone wrong should be formulated by the team members themselves. The most important method to achieve this are good questions. Questions foster self-reflection. The debriefer should acknowledge and encourage every team member for what they have done well. Often the issue of "personal failure" and inadequacy will arise; therefore, it is especially important to amplify positive performance in order to enable the competence for future critical situations.

☐ Figure 15.5 summarizes possible measures to avoid the occurrence of, and manage the consequences of, errors.

15.5 Imagine the Future: Safe Acute Medical Care

15.5.1 Change Organizations Actively

The two fundamental components of risk management are changing individual and team behavior toward safer care and changing organizations toward higher reliability. These changes do not occur spontaneously; they have to be intended, and they have to be triggered by learning, which takes place at the level of the individual health professional, at the organizational system's level, and at points in between.

Organizations in acute medical healthcare influence the performance of their members, the incidence of errors, and the management of errors. If patient safety is to be an unquestioned part of the organizational culture, a change in the way processes and structures are handled is necessary. The same is true for the self-concept and the interaction of all members. Organizations continuously

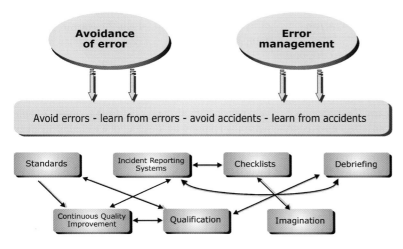

☐ **Fig. 15.5** Error avoidance and error management

change because they adapt to the changing environmental requirements. If these changes occur in a goal-directed and systematic way, they need a conceptual framework. Concepts of organizational development offer such a framework which has been validated in other organizations (Argyris and Schön 1996; Nonaka and Takeuchi 1995; Probst and Büchel 1998; Schreyögg 1999; Senge 1990).

Organizational development implies that organizations are strategically planned and systematically changed with the aim of increasing an organization's effectiveness in solving their problems. Organizational development is a long-term undertaking and requires the participation of all members.

The direction of change can only be developed within the healthcare organization. Organizations are not developed from the outside; instead, they themselves move towards their envisaged goal. Major issues in organizational development are "knowledge," "learning," "quality," "leadership," and "flexibility." In the context of a high-stakes medical environment patient safety, patient well-being, a transparent treatment chain, participation of members, and competition among healthcare institutions are superordinate goals (Bellabarba and Schnappauf 1996). Organizations try to change structures and processes with which the core process, patient treatment, is carried out. The most important resource for an organization which wants to achieve change are the people who work in the organization; or more precisely: the knowledge, experience, motivation, and cooperation of all staff members.

15.5.2 Toward a Learning Organization

A successful organization must be able to respond to changing environmental demands. To maintain a tight fit to the environmental changes, relevant structural and behavioral attitudes must change as well: The organization has to learn. This statement may sound strange at first because learning is an activity generally attributed to living beings and not to an abstract entity such as an organization; however, it is the interaction between individuals and organizations that is the basis for *organizational learning* (Argyris and Schön 1996). Although organizational learning begins with individual learning, it is more than the sum of its individual participants' learning: Members come and go and leadership changes, but certain behaviors, mental models, norms, and values are preserved in an organization over time. They define a stock of acceptable behaviors, which apply throughout an organization (i.e., "the way we do it") and which are frequently inherited by new generations of employees: In this respect organizational knowledge will remain long after original learners have departed and contribute to the organization's collective memory. In similar ways change will spread throughout an organization. Every time a problem arises (e.g., because a regional pain therapy does not relieve pain but instead threatens patient safety) several people within the organization will reflect upon causes and consequences of the incident. This way changes in procedures, flow of information, rules, and resources will result. Because many members of the organization will experience this kind of change, it is appropriate to say that "the organization" has learned its lesson from an incident.

The concept of the Learning Organization (Senge 1990) is that a successful organization intentionally applies learning strategies to adapt and respond to changes in environment. A Learning Organization constantly challenges its processes, instructions, assumptions, and even its basic structure, thereby redesigning itself constantly. In its totality organizational learning can be experiential learning: Organizations adjust their activities and mental frameworks based on experiences, both successes and failures. The structure of experiential learning is simple: Actions are taken, the environment responds, and implications for future actions are drawn on the basis of the feedback and the current mental framework. Experiential learning differs in the degree to which the learning cycle is completed.

15.5.2.1 Single-Loop Learning

Whenever something goes wrong, most people naturally respond by looking for a different strategy that will address the problem. This new strategy is based on (like the one that failed) well-known theories and works within established patterns of thought and familiar behavioral patterns. Processes and actions directed at the problem are optimized with regard to existing goals, values, plans, and rules which all remain unchallenged. Because the characteristic feature of this kind of learning is the single loop, which exists between problem recognition and action, this learning cycle has been called single-loop learning by organizational theorists (◘ Fig. 15.6; Argyris and Schön 1996). Single-loop learning is like a thermostat that learns when it is too hot or too cold and turns the heat on or off. The thermostat can perform this task because it can receive information (the temperature of the room) and take corrective action. Single-loop learning is present each time goals, values, frameworks, and, to a significant extent, strategies, are taken for granted. As a result, thinking is directed toward making a familiar strategy more effective. Single-loop learning in response to the misconnection of the PCEA line is primarily directed at the technique and making it more efficient: New labels are attached to the lines and staff members are retrained in patient-controlled pain therapy.

15.5.2.2 Double-Loop Learning

An alternative response to an error would be to question the mental models which underlie the actual perception; thus, in contrast to single-loop learning, double-loop learning corrects errors *and* changes basic assumptions within an organization. Such learning may lead to a shift in the way in which strategies and consequences are framed, and it will lead to new goals or priorities. If an organization is able to view and modify those basic frameworks, it will be able to go in new directions and think previously unthought-of thoughts. Because double-loop learning implies a process of relearning basic assumptions, members of an organization may find

it difficult at times to embrace this kind of learning. In view of the PCEA misconnection, double-loop learning could imply that basic assumptions about continuous education and retraining staff members would have to be questioned. The consequence could be a proactive training which addresses existing gaps in knowledge before insufficient experience can threaten patient safety.

15.5.2.3 Deutero-learning

In a final step organizations can go beyond revising strategies (single-loop) or analyzing underlying mental frameworks (double-loop) and focus on the learning process itself. By developing a competence for analyzing the efficacy of different approaches to learning, organizations can learn how their members learn. The identification of successful patterns within the learning cycle can facilitate learning under similar conditions and initiate a profound restructuring of behavioral patterns and norms. This concept of learning is referred to as *deutero-learning* (Bateson 1972; Schön 1975). Evidence of deutero-learning within a healthcare organization includes (Bedeian 1984):

- An explicit commitment to educational ideals in organizational policies, procedures, and programs. The organization allocates sufficient resources for such purposes.
- Daily work routines are designed in a way that healthcare providers can realistically expect to improve their knowledge and skills.
- A culture with an emphasis on curiosity and a capacity for learning as well as on teamwork skills (e.g., communication, collaboration).

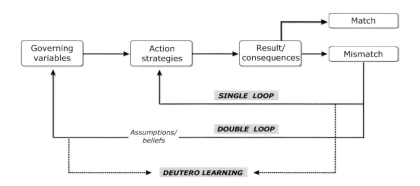

◘ **Fig. 15.6** Different ways by which an organization can learn from incidents

— A genuine participative philosophy and practice, such that members can share their learning experiences and enter into collaborative processes of decision-making and problem-solving.

— Design and management of learning environments in which members are willing and able to view one another as learning resources.

15.5.2.4 The Importance of Teamwork in Organizational Learning

Learning can take place at the level of the individual health professional, at the organizational systems level, and at points in between. One of the points in-between that is important for improvement in the management of risk and quality is the level of teamwork. Organizations have been shifting their focus from the individual to teams and their leaders as a means of improving organizational outcomes such as productivity and safety. This emphasis is most evident in teams operating in High Reliability Organizations (HROs): They have learned to balance effectiveness and safety despite the complexities of the environment (► Chap. 14). Encouraged by the results of other high-stakes industries, the healthcare community has begun to examine High Reliability Teams (HRTs) as a model for the complex domain of acute medical care (Wilson et al. 2005): Teamwork seems to be *the* essential component in the pursuit of achieving high reliability in healthcare organizations.

Because improvements in patient safety and better quality of medical care are inseparably related to the process of organizational and individual learning, a recent interest has emerged in teams as the place where organizational learning takes place and where cultural changes can most effectively be addressed. Learning occurs as an interaction between the organization's members and their environment. This learning cycle can be triggered by:

— Problems: Organizational learning is typically problem oriented (i.e., experiential). Problems may raise doubts about prevailing strategies and call for alternative responses.

— Opportunities: Unforeseen events may provide opportunities to learn and thereby may stimulate innovation.

— People: The interaction with other members serves as a strong stimulus for learning. Actions of team members as well as differing opinions and mental models can challenge organizational participants to reconsider their understanding of the issue.

15.5.3 Approaches to Knowledge Management

If healthcare organizations try to change into a "learning organization," they will have to face the question of how to restructure so as to facilitate learning and the sharing of knowledge among members or employees. Industry has addressed these issues by drawing heavily on theories of process and knowledge management. There is no generally agreed definition of "Knowledge Management" (KM). Most often, the term refers to a range of systematic practices that support and achieve "the creation, sharing, retention, refinement, and use of knowledge; generally in an organizational context" (Edwards et al. 2005). One of the unifying elements across most KM theories is a shared understanding of knowledge as *the* intellectual capital and as a central factor in achieving improved performance and competitive advantage (Bali and Dwivedi 2006). Knowledge in this context includes both the experience and understanding of the people in the organization and the information artifacts, such as documents, guidelines, protocols, and reports, available within the organization (Stefanelli 2004). Modern information technologies (IT) have provided organizations with the necessary tools to create and distribute knowledge within their sphere of influence, thus promoting the learning process of their members. These IT solutions include expert systems, e-learning, knowledge bases, corporate intranets and extranets, and other health IT infrastructures (e.g., computerized physician order entry, decision support systems; Handler et al. 2004); however, it is not enough to simply collect data and then distribute it unaltered, because knowledge is not tantamount to information: Only after information has been selected and processed to meet defined criteria is it knowledge in terms of KM. From this perspective, KM can be regarded as the art and science of transforming data into useful knowledge.

Which knowledge exactly, though, is of interest for KM systems? Despite the diversity of their theoretical frameworks, most KM practitioners share the distinction between tacit and explicit knowledge (Nonaka and Takeuchi 1995): *Tacit knowledge* is subconscious and internalized knowledge and involves physical as well as perceptual skills (e.g., complex surgical interventions, situation assessment, diagnosing an X-ray). Individuals are unaware of what they know and how they obtain particular results. *Explicit knowledge*, in contrast, is conscious and can be codified: A person is fully aware of what he or she knows and is able to communicate this information to others (e.g., calculating the i.v. dose of a drug, generating differential diagnoses).

The task of KM is, on the one hand, to convert internalized tacit knowledge into explicit codified knowledge in order to share it with other members of an organization. In a second step the knowledge offered by a KM system has to be retrieved, understood, and internalized by individuals. This way, explicit knowledge is absorbed and results in new personal tacit knowledge. On the other hand, KM theories try to solve the problem of how an organization needs to be designed to facilitate knowledge processes. In other words, how the "right" information can be brought to the "right" people at the "right" time to enable the "right" actions.

During the past decade healthcare organizations have adopted KM theories and have recognized knowledge as their main intellectual capital and the strategic management of both medical knowledge and care processes as the key to success. In their attempt to adopt KM strategies from industry to healthcare and initiate KM solutions, these organizations had to face and answer several big questions:

- How can knowledge be synthesized from medical information?
- Given the many independent "silos" within a healthcare organization, how can the sharing of knowledge be facilitated?
- What methodology works best for sharing various types of knowledge?
- What is the optimal role of information technology in facilitating this sharing?
- What are the cultural, structural, or other barriers which healthcare organizations have to face in their effort?

With regards to *medical* knowledge many initiatives focusing on increased sharing of knowledge have emerged across the health sector. This knowledge is processed for both, the patient (who can better understand his or her disease and the diagnostic and therapeutic steps involved in the treatment) and the healthcare professional (who has unrestrained access to critical information). Especially intensive care physicians often find themselves in clinical situations where a patient's clinical condition rapidly deteriorates and they have to make decisions based on the patient's medical history, a myriad of diagnostic test results, concurrent medications, and past treatment responses. The implementation of KM applications is a way of providing healthcare professionals with an immediate access to fresh information in order to support their effective problem-solving (Bali and Twivedi 2006). In addition, IT-based knowledge management systems can support patient care by "pushing" information to doctors, rather than having them search for it. Such "just-in-time" systems have helped clinicians to reduce serious medication errors by 55% by checking drug prescriptions for any interaction with the patients medical history, known allergies, or interaction with comedication (Davenport and Glaser 2002; Melymuka 2002).

As far as the care process is concerned, KM strategies aim at improving the interaction and collaboration among healthcare professionals. By focusing on the complete chain of patient care, global patient information systems can support the different organizations and professions who provide care for a patient. Emergency medical care would be an example for a high-stakes environment where different groups of staff across several organizations (e.g., ambulance crews, emergency department staff, and intensive care staff) interact and continuously create new information which adds to the already existing data and "snowballs" with the patient. As important data can easily be lost at the many interfaces between the parties involved, an obvious need to communicate exists. This systemic approach in which emergency care is seen as *one complete process* in which many organizations play a part will help healthcare professionals to focus their attention on the information and knowledge which needs to flow through this process (Edwards et al. 2005). Knowledge management will become one of the most important strategic assets that will improve patient safety in healthcare organizations.

Knowledge management is part of an informed and safety-oriented organizational culture. This brings us full circle with regard to our first topic: Safety is no faint dream of the future. The tools for making acute medical care a safe undertaking are already available.

15.6 "Reliable Acute Care Medicine": in a Nutshell

— The concept of a safety culture implies that all organizational structures and processes, all working places and equipment, the qualification standards of all staff members, and the relationship among the staff are shaped in a way which enables safe behavior at any time at any given working place.
— Reliability and safety are not static, once-and-for-all features; instead, they have to be seen as "dynamic nonevents."
— Safety and reliability cannot be delegated to single officials: They are in every single member's area of responsibility.
— "Organizational culture" defines the shared values, norms, and expectations that govern the way people approach their work and interact with each other. It is an amalgamation of the values and beliefs of the people in an organization.
— The culture of an organization is positioned at the heart of the system-vulnerability problem because of its role in framing organizational blindness to risk.
— "Safety culture" can be equated with "informed culture." An informed culture deals with the potential accidents and errors in an organization.
— High Reliability Organizations (HROs) operate in a high-stakes environment and still manage to cause very few accidents. The HROs achieve their high safety standard through mindful attention to ongoing operations.
— Skills and knowledge of healthcare professionals are decisive human resources for an efficient and safe delivery of patient care and the avoidance of errors. The systematic enhancement of staff qualifications by providing knowledge and training opportunities can be a major investment in patient safety.
— Simulator trainings are a valuable tool for staff qualification.
— Quality assurance and continuous quality improvement efforts focus on the structure, process, and outcome of medical care.

— A clinical audit is a systematic and objective evaluation of an organization by internal or external auditors that aims to improve patient care and outcomes.
— A quality circle is a small volunteer group of healthcare professionals who meet at regular intervals to identify, analyze, and resolve workplace and patient-care-related issues.
— Standardization, the deliberate strategy to maintain a high similarity in task performance, is aimed at guaranteeing the highest possible quality patient care in routine tasks.
— Instruments of error management are Incident-Reporting Systems and debriefing.
— An incident is an unintended event which reduces, or could reduce, the safety margin for a patient. Incident-Reporting Systems serve the purpose of collecting, analyzing, and responding to safety incidents.
— Debriefings are defined as the generation of knowledge from work-related experience, the learning through reflection on simulated experience, and the emotional recovery from a critical incident.
— The concept of the Learning Organization states that a successful organization applies, adapts, and responds to changes in environment by learning processes. This is done by constantly challenging its processes, instructions, assumptions, and even its basic structure.
— "Knowledge Management" refers to a range of systematic practices that support and achieve the creation, sharing, retention, refinement, and use of knowledge in an organizational context.

References

Arbous MS, Meursing AE, van Kleef JFW, de Lange JJ, Spoormans HH, Touw P, Werner FM, Grobbee DE (2005) Impact of anesthesia management characteristics on severe morbidity and mortality. Anesthesiology 102:257–268

Argyris C, Schön DA (1996) Organizational learning II: theory, method and practice. Addison–Wesley; Reading, Massachusetts

Bali R, Dwivedi A (2006) Healthcare knowledge management. Issues, advances and successes. Springer, Berlin Heidelberg New York

Barrett J, Gifford C et al. (2001) Enhancing patient safety through teamwork training. J Healthc Risk Manag 21:57–65

Bateson G (1972) Steps towards an ecology of mind. Chandler, New York

Bedeian AG (1984) Organizations. Theories and analysis. Saunders College Publishing, New York

Bellabarba J, Schnappauf D (1996) (eds) Organisationsentwicklung im Krankenhaus [Organizational development in hospitals]. Verlag für Angewandte Psychologie, Göttingen, Germany

Billings C, Cook RI, Woods DD, Miller C (1998) Incident Reporting Systems in medicine and experience with the Aviation Safety Reporting System. National Patient Safety Foundation at the AMA, Chicago, Illinois, pp 52–61

Blum LL (1971) Equipment design and "human" limitations. Anesthesiology 35:101–102

Buerschaper C, St. Pierre M (2003) Teamarbeit in der Anästhesie – Entwicklung einer Checkliste [Teamwork in anaesthesia – development of a checklist]. In: Strohschneider S (ed) Entscheiden in kritischen Situationen [Decision-making in critical situations]. Verlag für Polizeiwissenschaft, Frankfurt/M., pp 25–38

Conell L (1996) Pilot and controller issues. In: Kanki B, Prinzo VO (eds) Methods and metrics of voice communication. DOT/FAA/AM-96/10. FAA Civil Aeromedical Institute, Oklahoma City

Cooper JB, Taqueti VR (2004) A brief history of the development of mannequin simulators for clinical education and training. Qual Saf Health Care 13 (Suppl 1): i11–i18

Cooper JB, Newbower RS, Long CD, McPeek B (1978) Preventable anesthesia mishaps: a study of human factors. Anesthesiology 49:399–406

Cooper JB, Cullen DJ, Eichhorn JH, Philip JH, Holzman RS (1993) Administrative guidelines for response to an adverse anesthesia event. J Clin Anesth 5:79–84

Davenport TH, Glaser J (2002) Just-in-time-delivery comes to knowledge management. Harv Bus Rev 80:107–112

Dismukes RK, Gaba DM, Howard SK (2006) So many roads: facilitated debriefing in healthcare. Simul Healthcare 1:1–3

Edwards JS, Hall MJ, Shaw D (2005) Proposing a systems vision of knowledge management in emergency care. J Operat Res Soc 56:180–192

Eichhorn S (1995) Risk management, quality assurance, and patient safety. In: Gravenstein N, Kirbi RR (eds) Complications in anesthesiology. Lippincott-Raven, Philadelphia, pp 1–15

Firth-Cozens J (2001) Teams, culture and managing risk. In: Vincent C (ed) Clinical risk management. Enhancing patient safety. Br Med J Books, London

Flanagan JC (1954) The critical incident technique. Psychol Bull 51:327–358

Fletcher GC, McGeorge P, Flin R, Glavin R, Maran N (2002) The role of non-technical skills in anaesthesia: a review of current literature. Br J Anaesth 88:418–429

Flin R, Maran N (2004) Identifying and training non-technical skills for teams in acute medicine. Qual Saf Health Care 13 (Suppl):i80–i84

Frankel AS, Leonard MW, Denham CR (2006) Fair and just culture, team behavior, and leadership engagement: the tools to achieve high reliability. Health Serv Res 41:1690–1709

Gaba DM (1996) Simulators in anaesthesiology. In: Lake CL, Rice LJ, Sperry RJ (eds) Advances in anaesthesia, vol 14. Mosby, St. Louis

Glavin R, Maran N (2003) An introduction to simulation in anaesthesia. In: Greaves JD, Dodds C, Kumar V, Mets B (eds) Clinical teaching. A guide to teaching practical anaesthesia. Swets and Zeitlinger, Lisse, The Netherlands, pp 197–207

Halamek LP, Kaegi DM, Gaba DM, Sowby YA, Smith BC, Smith BE (2000) Time for a new paradigm in pediatric medical education: teaching neonatal resuscitation in a simulated delivery room environment. Pediatrics 106:E45

Hammond J, Brooks J (2001) Helping the helpers: the role of critical incident stress management, Crit Care 5:315–317

Handler JA, Feied CF, Coonan K, Vozenilek J, Gillam M, Peacock PR Jr, Sinert R, Smith MS (2004) Computerized physician order enty and online decision support. Acad Emerg Med 11:1135–1141

Harrison KT, Manser T, Howard SK, Gaba DM (2006) Use of cognitive aids in a simulated anesthetic crisis. Anesth Analg 103:551–556

Hart EM, Owen H (2005) Errors and omissions in anesthesia: a pilot study using a pilot's checklist. Anesth Analg 101:246–250

Helmreich RL, Merritt AC, Wilhelm JA (1999). The evolution of Crew Resource Management training in commercial aviation. Int J Aviat Psychol 9:19–32

Hoff LA, Adamowski K (1998) Creating excellence in crisis care: a guide to effective training and program designs. Jossey–Bass, San Francisco

Hofinger G, Waleczek H (2003) Behandlungsfehler. Das Bewusstsein schärfen [Reporting treatment errors]. Dt. Ärzteblatt, 44/2003:2848–2849

Howard SK, Gaba DM, Fish KJ, Yang G, Sarnquist FH (1992) Anesthesia crisis resource management: teaching anesthesiologists to handle critical incidents. Aviat Space Environ Med 63:763–770

Jha A, Duncan B, Bates D (2001) Simulator-based training and patient safety. Making health care safer: a critical analysis of patient safety practices. In: Shojania K, Duncan B, McDonald K, Wachter R (eds) Making health care safer: a critical analysis of patient safety practices. AHRQ-Publication 01-E058, Rockville, Maryland, pp 511–518

James RK, Gilliland BE (2001) Crisis intervention strategies, 4th edn. Wadsworth/Thomson Learning, Belmont

Kim J, Neilipovitz D, Cardinal P, Chiu M, Clinch J (2006) A pilot study using high-fidelity simulation to formally evaluate performance in the resuscitation of critically ill patients: The University of Ottawa Critical Care Medicine, High-Fidelity Simulation, and Crisis Resource Management I Study. Crit Care Med 34:2167–2174

Klopfenstein CE, Van Gessel E, Forster A (1998) Checking the anaesthetic machine: self-reported assessment in a university hospital. Eur J Anaesthesiol 15:314–319

Kumar C, Dodds C (2003) Educational supervision and mentoring. In: Greaves JD, Dodds C, Kumar C, Mets B (eds) Clinical teaching. A guide to teaching practical anaesthesia. Swets and Zeitlinger, Lisse, The Netherlands, pp 197–207

Kumar V, Barcellos W, Mehta MP, Carter JG (1988) An analysis of critical incidents in a teaching department for quality assurance: a survey of mishaps during anaesthesia. Anaesthesia 43:879–883

Laboutique X, Benhamou D (1997) Evaluation of a checklist for anesthetic equipment before use. Ann Fr Anesth Reanim 16:19–24

Langford R, Gale TC, Mayor AH (2007) Anesthesia machine checking guidelines: Have we improved our practice? Eur J Anaesthesiol 30:1–5 Epub ahead of print

Lederman LC (1992) Debriefing: toward a systematic assessment of theory and practice. Simul Gaming 23:145–160

Mantovani F, Castelnuovo G, Gaggioli A, Riva G (2003) Virtual reality training for health-care professionals. Cyberpsychol Behav 9:245–247

March MG, Crowley JJ (1991) An evaluation of anesthesiologists' present checkout methods and the validity of the FDA checklist. Anesthesiology 75:724–729

McDonell LK, Kimberly KJ, Dismukes RK (1997) Facilitating LOS debriefings: a training manual, NASA Technical Memorandum 112192, March 1997

Melymuka K (2002) Knowledge management helps cut errors by half. Computerworld 36:44

Miller GT, Gordon DL, Issenberg SB, LaCombe DM, Brotons AA (2001) Teamwork. University of Miami uses competition to sharpen EMS team performance. J Emerg Med Serv 26:44–51

Morey JC, Simon R, Jay GD, Wears RL, Salisbury M, Dukes KA, Berns SD (2002) Error reduction and performance improvement in the emergency department through formal teamwork training: evaluation results of the MedTeams project. Health Serv Res 37:1553–1581

NHS Executive (1996) Promoting clinical effectiveness. A framework for action in and through the NHS. NHS Executive, London

Nonaka I, Takeuchi H (1995) The knowledge creating company. Oxford University Press, New York

O'Connor RE, Slovis CM, Hunt RC, Pirrallo RG, Sayre MR (2002) Eliminating errors in emergency medical services: realities and recommendations. Prehosp Emerg Care 6:107–113

Pizzi L, Goldfarb N, Nash D (2001) Crew resource management and its applications in medicine. In: Shojania K, Duncan B, McDonald K, Wachter R (eds) Making health care safer: a critical analysis of patient safety practices. AHRQ-Publication 01-E058, Rockville, Maryland, pp 501–509

Powell SM (2006) Creating a systems approach to patient safety through better teamwork. Biomed Instrum Technol 40:205–207

Probst GJB, Büchel B (1998) Organisationales Lernen. Gabler, Wiesbaden, Germany

Reader T, Flin R, Lauche K, Cuthbertson BH (2006) Non-technical skills in the intensive care unit. Br J Anaesth 96:551–559

Reason J (1990) Human error. Cambridge University Press, Cambridge UK

Reason J (1997) Managing the risks of organizational accidents. Ashgate, Aldershot

Reznek M, Harter P, Krummel T (2002) Virtual reality and simulation: training the future emergency physician. Acad Emerg Med 9:78–87

Reznek M, Smith-Coggins R, Howard S, Kiran K, Harter P, Sowb Y, Gaba D, Krummel K (2003) Emergency medicine crisis resource management (EMCRM): pilot study of a simulation-based crisis management course for emergency medicine. Acad Emerg Med 10:386–389

Robson M (1989) Quality circles: a practical guide. Gower, Aldershot

Rosenberg M (2000) Simulation technology in anesthesiology. Anesth Prog 47:8–11

Rudolf JW, Simon R, Dufresne RL, Raemer D (2006) There's no such thing as "non-judgemental" debriefing: a theory and method for debriefing with good judgement. Simul Healthcare 1:49–55

Runciman WB (1988) Crisis management. Anaesth Intensive Care 16:86–88

Runciman WB, Merry AF (2005) Crises in clinical care: an approach to management. Qual Saf Health Care 14:156–163

Runciman WB, Sellen A, Webb RA, Williamson JA, Currie M, Morgan C, Russell WJ (1993) The Australian Incident Monitoring Study. Errors, incidents and accidents in anaesthetic practice. Anaesth Intensive Care 21:506–519

Salas E, Wilson KA, Burke CS, Wightman DC (2006) Does crew resource management training work? An update, an extension, and some critical needs. Hum Factors 48:392–412

Sawa T, Ohno-Machado L (2001) Generation of dynamically configured check lists for intra-operative problems using a set of covering algorithms. Proc AMIA Symp 2001:593–597

Schön DA (1975) Deutero-learning in organizations: learning for increased effectiveness. Organizational Dyn 4:2–16

Schreyögg G (1999) Organisation: Grundlagen moderner Organisationsgestaltung [Organization. Principles of building modern organizations]. Gabler, Wiesbaden, Germany

Senge P (1990) The fifth discipline: the art and practice of the learning organization. Doubleday, New York

Small SD, Wuerz RC, Simon R, Shapiro N, Conn A, Setnik G (1999) Demonstration of high-fidelity simulation team training for emergency medicine. Acad Emerg Med 6:312–323

Staender S (2000) Critical incident reporting. With a view on approaches in anaesthesiology. In: Vincent C, de Mol B (eds) Safety in medicine. Pergamon Elsevier Science, Amsterdam New York, pp 65–82

Stefanelli M (2004) Knowledge and process management in health care organizations. Methods Inf Med 43:525–535

Steinwachs B (1992) How to facilitate a debriefing. Simul Gaming 23:186–195

Thomas EJ, Sexton JB, Lasky RE, Helmreich RL, Crandell DS, Tyson J (2006) Teamwork and quality during neonatal care in the delivery room. J Perinatol 26:163–169

Vozenilek J, Wang E, Kharasch M, Anderson B, Kalaria A (2006) Simulation-based morbidity and mortality conference: new technologies augmenting traditional case-based presentations. Acad Emerg Med 13:48–53

Webb RK, Currie M, Morgan CA, Williamson JA, Mackay P, Russell WJ, Runciman WB (1993) The Australian Incident Monitoring Study: an analysis of 2000 incident reports. Anaesth Intensive Care 21:520–528

Wehner T (1992) Sicherheit als Fehlerfreundlichkeit [Safety as error friendliness]. Westdeutscher Verlag, Opladen

Weick KE, Sutcliffe KM (2001) Managing the unexpected: assuring high performance in an age of complexity. Jossey–Bass, San Francisco

Weinstock PH, Kappus LJ, Kleinman ME, Grenier B, Hickey P, Burns JP (2005) Toward a new paradigm in hospital-based pediatric education: the development of an onsite simulator program. Pediatr Crit Care Med 6:635–641

Williamson JA, Webb R, Pryor GL (1985) Anesthesia safety and the 'critical incident technique'. Aust Clin Rev 6:57–61

Wilson KA, Burke CS, Priest HA, Salas E (2005) Promoting health care safety through training high reliability teams. Qual Saf Health Care 14:303–309

Yule S, Flin R, Paterson-Brown S, Maran N (2006) Non-technical skills for surgeons in the operating room: a review of the literature. Surgery 139:140–149

Subject Index